Routledge Handbook of Elite Sport Performance

The *Routledge Handbook of Elite Sport Performance* is the first book to examine a broad span of performance and support issues in contemporary elite sport; including coaching, sports science and medicine, leadership and management, operating in different societies, living in the system as a performer, and future developments in the domain.

The book is written by authors with elite-level experience, expertise, success, and status across individual and team sports, including football, NFL, track and field athletics, rowing, and rugby, in professional, Olympic, and other elite domains. The book also considers the integration of systems at micro to macro levels, from working with individual athletes to developing national organisations and policy, and features in-depth case studies from real sport throughout.

This is an essential reference for any researcher or advanced student with an interest in elite sport or applied sport science, from sport injury and sport psychology to sports coaching and sport policy. It is also an invaluable resource for coaches, managers, administrators, and policy-makers working in elite sport, offering them a "breadth first" guide to how and why specialists may work together for maximum effect.

Dave Collins is Director of Grey Matters Performance Ltd and a Professorial Fellow at the University of Edinburgh. As a practitioner, he has supported over 70 world or Olympic medalists, and worked at the highest levels of professional sport and other performance domains. His current support roles include Chelsea FC, Gloucester RFC, and Snowsports New Zealand.

Andrew Cruickshank is Lead Psychologist for British Judo, Sport Psychologist for England Golf, and consultant for other elite sport organisations and governing bodies through Grey Matters Performance Ltd. Andrew is also Researcher/Lecturer within the Institute of Coaching and Performance at the University of Central Lancashire in the UK.

Geir Jordet is Professor in Sport Psychology at the Norwegian School of Sport Sciences, Norway, and regular consultant for several European football associations and professional football clubs. He is co-owner of cognitive training software company BeYourBest.

The Routledge International Handbook Series

Routledge Handbook of Elite Sport Performance

Edited by Dave Collins, Andrew Cruickshank, and Geir Jordet

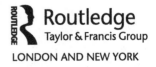

Routledge
Taylor & Francis Group

LONDON AND NEW YORK

First published 2019 by Routledge

2 Park Square, Milton Park, Abingdon, Oxon OX14 4RN
605 Third Avenue, New York, NY 10017

Routledge is an imprint of the Taylor & Francis Group, an informa business

First issued in paperback 2021

Publisher's Note

The publisher has gone to great lengths to ensure the quality of this reprint but points out that some imperfections in the original copies may be apparent.

British Library Cataloguing-in-Publication Data
A catalogue record for this book is available from the British Library

Library of Congress Cataloging-in-Publication Data
A catalog record has been requested for this book

ISBN: 978-1-138-29030-3 (hbk)
ISBN: 978-1-03-217810-3 (pbk)
DOI: 10.4324/9781315266343

Typeset in Bembo
by Swales & Willis Ltd, Exeter, Devon, UK

Contents

Contents

Contents

Illustrations

Figures

Tables

Contributors

Helen Alfano is a specialist in sport physiology and currently works as Performance Lead for England Netball, having previously worked across various sport science and support roles in professional, Olympic and Paralympic sport.

Andy Barr is the founder of Innovate Performance and a high-performance advisor for Orreco, having previously worked in high-level medicine, injury prevention, rehabilitation, and performance roles across a number of elite environments, including New York City FC, NY Knicks, and Manchester City FC.

Alex Baumann is a former double Olympic champion swimmer and, since moving into high-performance sports administration, has held numerous positions, including CEO of High Performance Sport New Zealand and Canada's "Own the Podium" programme. Alex now works in a high-performance strategic leadership role for Swimming Australia.

Clive Brewer was formerly Head Strength and Conditioning Coach for Widnes Vikings, national S&C coach for Scotland Rugby League, and a consultant to a number of high-performance organisations. Clive is now Assistant Director of High Performance for the Toronto Blue Jays in Major League Baseball.

Veronica Burke specialises in organisational development and executive coaching and consults on these and other areas internationally. Veronica is also currently Director of the Cranfield General Management and Talent Development programmes.

Christopher Carling was previously a performance analyst for Manchester United FC and Lille OSC FC, among others. Christopher continues to consult in elite sport and also works within the Institute of Coaching and Performance at the University of Central Lancashire in the UK.

Rosie Collins is a performance psychology consultant for iZone Driver Performance and England Golf, as well as a number of other elite sport organisations and clients through Grey Matters Performance Ltd. Rosie is also a lecturer and researcher in sport psychology at Oxford Brookes University in the UK.

Fergus Connolly is a performance consultant to sporting organisations, elite military units, and corporate leadership teams around the world. He has previously worked full-time in soccer (Liverpool, Bolton Wanderers), professional and college football (San Francisco 49ers, University of Michigan), and rugby (Welsh national team).

Mads Davidsen is currently technical director at Shanghai SIPG Football Club in China, having previously had different roles in Danish professional football.

Steve Fairchild is a former NFL and American College football coach with 34 years of experience. He is currently the owner of FairchildQBTraining.com and trains quarterbacks of all ages – youth to NFL. He is also a consultant to numerous football organisations.

Kieran A. File is a sports communication consultant, operating as Reactive Sports Media, as well as a researcher within the Centre for Applied Linguistics at the University of Warwick in the UK.

Tore Andre Flo is currently a technical coach at Chelsea FC, having previously played at the highest levels in Norway, England, Scotland, and Italy, as well as representing the Norwegian national team at the World Cup and European Championships.

Ian Graham has worked for Liverpool FC as Director of Research since 2012. He was previously head of football research at Decision Technology. Before working in football, Ian completed a PhD in Physics at the University of Cambridge.

Bruce Hamilton has previously worked as Chief Medical Officer for Athletics Australia and UK Athletics, as well as Chief of Sports Medicine at the Qatar Orthopaedic and Sports Medicine Hospital. More recently, Bruce was appointed Medical Lead and now Director of Performance Health for High Performance Sport NZ and the NZ Olympic Committee.

Mike Hay is a former international curler and was the first full-time national coach to be appointed in Great Britain for the sport. Most recently, he served as Chef de Mission at the 2018 Winter Olympics for the British Olympic Association.

Guus Hiddink is a former professional footballer and current head coach for China's U21 football team, having previously coached a number of successful national and club teams at the highest levels of the sport.

Sinéad Jennings is an Irish, multi-World medallist rower who finished sixth in the lightweight double sculls at the Rio 2016 Olympics, having also almost qualified for the London 2012 Olympic Games in the team pursuit in cycling.

Andy Jones is Professor of Applied Physiology and an Associate Dean at Exeter University in the UK. With more than 250 original research and review articles, Andy has also consulted with a number of governing bodies of sport or commercial companies, including UK Athletics, the English Institute of Sport, Gatorade Sports Science Institute, and Nike Inc. He was most recently involved in the attempt to break the two-hour barrier in the marathon.

Tim Jones is currently Head of Elite Development for British Swimming and was, most recently beforehand, Performance Director for the UK's Olympic gymnastics and Paralympic athletics programmes.

Ruben Jongkind is a consultant on talent development, working with clients worldwide, and was responsible, as Head of Talent Development of AFC Ajax, for implementing Plan Cruyff.

Stuart Lancaster has led, managed, and coached at the highest levels of club and international rugby union, including leading the English national side, and is currently Senior Coach at Leinster Rugby.

Áine MacNamara is a specialist in talent development and applied sport psychology, and has worked with a variety of elite and development-level organisations and clients across a range of domains. Áine is also a Reader in elite performance, working within the Institute of Coaching and Performance at the University of Central Lancashire in the UK.

Barrie-Jon Mather played at international level for England's rugby league and union teams before working as Assistant Academy Manager for London Irish and then Head of Player Development at the Rugby Football League. Barrie-Jon is currently General Manager at New South Wales Rugby League.

Graeme Maw has over 20 years of experience leading elite sport programmes and is currently a performance management consultant and Para Swimming Programme Leader for Paralympics New Zealand. Previously, Graeme's roles have included performance director for British Triathlon, the Welsh Rugby Union, and Triathlon New Zealand.

Neil McCarthy is a former England international rugby player and academy manager/head for Leicester Tigers and Gloucester Rugby. Neil is currently Performance Pathway and Talent Manager for British Skeleton.

Toni Minichiello is a highly experienced athletics coach based in the UK and former UK Coach of the Year. Toni specialises in coaching decathlon and heptathlon in particular, and has worked most notably with Jessica Ennis-Hill.

Phil Moore is currently Director of Performance Support at the Irish Institute of Sport, having previously fulfilled sport science, sports medicine, and sport psychology roles in a number of elite sport environments.

Egil Olsen is a former international footballer and manager of numerous club and international teams, most notably the Norwegian national side, who he led to two World Cups and number two in the FIFA rankings.

Anne Pankhurst is a consultant to a number of elite sport organisations, specialising in coach education and player development. Among numerous other roles, Anne previously held the positions of LTA Coach Education Director and USTA Coach Education Manager.

Frédéric Paquet is currently CEO of AS Saint-Étienne FC in France's Ligue 1, having previously fulfilled this role for Lille Olympique Sporting Club.

Nico Porteous is a freestyle skier from New Zealand who won bronze at the 2018 Winter Olympics in the men's halfpipe, subsequently becoming New Zealand's youngest medallist at an Olympic Games and first male New Zealander to medal at a Winter Olympics. His brother **Miguel Porteous** is also an international halfpipe skier, having medalled at the highly prestigious X Games.

Dave Rotheram has a background in playing and coaching at the elite levels of rugby league. Previously Head of Talent and Player Development at the Rugby Football League, Dave is now Head of Coach Development in the same organisation.

Dean Smith is a former professional footballer and, after coaching and managing Walsall FC and Brentford FC, is now Head Coach for Aston Villa FC in England.

Tynke Toering is a sport scientist and sport psychology consultant who has worked across a number of elite performance environments. Tynke also currently works within the Institute of Coaching and Performance at the University of Central Lancashire.

Olaf Tufte has competed in multiple rowing events across the last six Olympic Games, winning four medals to add to six World Championships medals in single and double sculls.

Peter Vint served the United States Olympic Committee as Senior Director of Competitive Analysis, Research and Innovation, High Performance Director, and Senior Sport Technologist. Following this, he held a senior role for a Premier League football club in England, and now he is a consultant to leading professional and Olympic sporting organisations.

Tom Willmott is a former international snowboard athlete. After transitioning into coaching, Tom is now Head Coach of the "Park & Pipe" programme for Snowsports New Zealand.

Foreword

As an elite performer you rely directly on a small but crucial band of supporters. First in line, and often directing other matters, is your coach. This relationship then sets the tone for work with other "A Team" members, which will always have a physio and medical doctor, supplemented by other specialists such as strength and conditioning coaches, analysts, physiologists, and psychologists.

Importantly, however, there are at least two other teams behind this group. For a start, the people who run the setups that provide you with the A Team supporters. In many cases, this includes national sport organisation and institute managers, plus Performance Directors. As another tier, there are media specialists, coach developers, and the people who direct the support systems to even better service. Of course, you may well have experienced different types, styles, and methods as a developing athlete, especially if you came up through the academy systems traditional in team sports. Finally, all this must operate in a way that suits the culture, both of the sport and your home country. How things operate in the UK is likely to be very different to what goes on in, say, China or even the USA. And, of course, Scotland!

My point is that, behind any successful athlete or team, there are a lot of specialists. Some are fairly obvious whilst others might never be mentioned by, or even known to, the performer or the public. Yet, optimum performance from all can underpin your results. One link in the chain failing or performing sub-optimally and the knock-on effects, whether more (e.g. coach) or less (e.g. National Sports Leadership) direct, can be catastrophic.

So, reflecting this complexity, I am happy to contribute to a book that covers all the members of the performance orchestra, wherever they are positioned, and take the opportunity to thank all those who supported my journey.

Shaun Maloney
Scotland, English and Scottish Premiership player
Assistant Coach Belgium

Introduction

Defining, delineating, and driving elite performance

Dave Collins, Andrew Cruickshank, and Geir Jordet

Before we get into the job of addressing the content suggested by our title above, we should possibly explain what this book is trying to accomplish. Furthermore, it is probably a good idea to explain what you shouldn't expect. This text is one of many Routledge Handbooks; all of which use an edited format with invited chapters to provide an excellent, in-depth, and state of the art viewpoint of the topic identified in the title. As such, at least as far as we can see, the content is written by experts, for experts or, perhaps more correctly, those wishing to gain expertise in that particular subject.

Now it so happens that all three of us are performance psychologists. Indeed, all of us have contributed to other handbooks, commenting on our "day job" work in talent, expertise development, adventure sport, or whatever. Clearly, this is also reflected in our research interests as publishing academics. In the present text, however, we take a very different stance. Rather than produce a book on psychology for psychologists, performance analysis for analysts or even institute management for managers, we have deliberately avoided such specificity. In fact, our aim is breadth rather than depth! A text in which psychologists may learn about analysis and management, managers about psychology and analysis. . . you get the picture.

So, the text reflects our experiences, most of which are positive, of work in the complex, always exhilarating and sometimes paranoid jungle that is elite performance. Our aim is to provide a broad view of how the various disciplines interconnect and how different aspects of the elite milieu might co-act to influence optimum behaviour.

In doing so, we have sought a diverse range of expertise and experience. These include practical scientists, executives, managers, coaches, and, most particularly, the performers themselves. Reflecting our aim, we intend for the book to be read by specialists and generalists alike. Perhaps those seeking "enlightenment" on how this complex world might operate!

Defining elitism

As explored by several of our authors, elitism must not be confused with level of performance. It should be clear that a world champion in, say, underwater polo (we hope this doesn't exist!), is going to be at a somewhat different level than a gold medallist in the 100m event at the Olympics. In short, level of performance is clearly a relative or perhaps comparative term.

In using the elite tag, however, what we are driving at is a status achieved by being world class at your job. Accordingly, as you read the brief pen portraits of our authors, we hope that our claim to their status is clear. We have spread the net widely and, although the geographic spread of authors does reflect our personal networks of contacts, we are confident that the presentations they make, in tandem with their achievements, will justify the elite status.

Delineating elitism

For many of the professions presented in this text, professional associations offering accreditation provide another means of identifying elitism. Once again, there is an interesting and informative spread across our authors. Some hold high-status certification in their chosen area of expertise, in addition of course to a plethora of academic appellations. Some others have ignored the pursuit of such, and rather, rely on their achievements to speak for themselves. Others operate in spheres where there are, as of yet anyway, no such schemes. For example, joining the CEO or Performance Director clubs requires neither a vote by members nor a professional accreditation, just an appetite for perpetual professional challenge and a bullet proof vest! Once again, triangulation of methods, with accreditation a "necessary but not sufficient condition" for high status, will provide the reader with the best method for delineating expertise.

For performers, in contrast, things are arguably comparatively simpler. Achievement at high level is clearly apparent from one's competitive CV. Even here, however, we have gone for breadth rather than depth. Our performers' section includes athletes of all shapes and sizes, ages, and status. Hopefully, this breadth will offer you, the reader, some useful opportunities for a "compare and contrast" reading of their experiences.

Driving elite performance

These caveats or qualifications notwithstanding, everyone in this book possesses two significant commonalities. These are a passion for and commitment to the pursuit of excellence; notably, in their chosen sphere but also, most crucially, how this impacts on their own or, in most cases, others' performance outcomes. As such, and once again, we suggest that looking for commonalities across the subsections, and between disciplines on a section by section basis, will provide some strong indicators on how performance may best be driven. We have offered a breadth without comment on the qualities of one system over another. Those interested may seek out the data which indicate the "performance epidemiology" of the various systems and make their own decision. If we may suggest, however, even this is not without its difficulty. Recent history shows how the relative successes of national systems or sports have waxed and waned in association with a complex set of precursors. Frankly, this is far more than just a case of revenue expenditure! As but one of many variables elite status must surely include some consideration of population size and involvement.

Finally, as recent media attention has shown, elitism is a challenging topic. In presenting our overviews we have avoided philosophical debate on the desirability of winning over participation; of fair governance over "no stone left unturned", put simply of medals over morals. We leave these more complex arguments to another text.

In conclusion

In concluding this introduction, we must acknowledge the selfless contributions made by our authors who have, in friendship and in the absence of inebriation, agreed to contribute. Indeed, many have come through secondary contacts and we must confess to our excitement at the quality of people who consented to take part. Each author has presented his or her personal viewpoint, working against a minimal structure and broad guidelines. Chapters vary in length but completely because that is what each author or authors felt was needed to address their issue. Given the quality and, therefore, heavy workload of our authors, we have in several cases interviewed them, and then used their words to construct the chapter. Their approval for the end product reassures us (and hopefully you) of the veracity of the content. In all cases, we have presented their views without comment or editorial modification. As such, there are some contradictions between authors as might be expected, albeit that these are surprisingly both rare and small-scale. You will also find some ideas or messages repeated in several contexts: once again, this should just add to the "rich picture" provided.

So, as you read over the contents list, we hope you are impressed by the coverage provided. Of course, this is in no way comprehensive – those involved in elite performance will immediately recognise the gaps as much as they acknowledge our attempt to provide an adequate coverage. Importantly, however, there is enough here to provide you, the reader, with a sufficiently full picture into the marvellous, hyper-dynamic jungle of elite sport.

Enjoy

DC, GJ, and AC

Part I
Coaching elites
Art and science

Given that the performers or teams who take to the competitive arena are the most important in any elite sport system, it follows that those who work most closely with them are (or at least should be) essential ingredients for success. Indeed, coaches are fundamental to the way in which performers and teams prepare, perform, and learn. In this sense, the main role of the elite sports coach is to develop and optimise the performance of individuals and/or teams in pursuit of personal and/or collective success. Of course, this success is relative to the performers and team in question; however, in essence, the nature of the job requires the coach to help them 'succeed more', 'succeed better', and often 'succeed again'.

Consequently, for coaches across elite sport, the focus of their work is invariably tipped more towards performance outcomes than a broadly 'positive sporting experience' for their performers and teams (although both will sensibly be targeted as valuable extras). For clarity, coaches will still look to foster wider outcomes (e.g., positive well-being; broader personal development), but these are usually viewed as a complimentary pillar to achieving the main goal of performance success (i.e., not the main goal itself). In this way, successful coaching in elite sport is often gauged by the performance of their performers/teams (especially in meaningful competitions, events, games or moments), the progression and/or consistency of this performance, and, of course, hard results. Intensifying the challenge, these outcomes often need to be delivered as fast as possible! That said, while the broad outcomes of coaching are similar across different elite sport environments, the *ways* in which coaches work to deliver them can and does, of course, vary a lot. As such, this section has been designed to provide a broad overview of coaching across the elite sport landscape, as perceived by our group of high-achieving and high-profile coaches. Tying in with our approach throughout this book, these perspectives focus less on *what* the coaches do and more on *how* they work and *why* they work that way with specific sports, performers, and teams.

More specifically, the first chapter from our practising coaches comes from Toni Minichiello and is focused on being the personal coach; particularly his experiences of working with Jess Ennis-Hill. In this chapter, Toni reflects on the history and evolution of his role with Jess, the nature of his work, others involved in the journey, the challenges of 'managing upwards' in the system, the skills required to be an effective personal coach, and differences between the personal coach and other top-level coaches.

Moving from the level of personal coach to national coach in Olympic sport, Mike Hay presents an overview of his approach and experiences while the first, full-time national coach of the British curling team. In this account, Mike provides a perspective on the challenges faced in this new role, the steps taken to build this system, the introduction and integration of greater science, the subsequent progression of the sport, reflections on leading, and reflections on some key innovations brought to the sport, and advice for others taking on similar roles. Continuing with the national coach theme, but moving from an Olympic sport to a professional sport context, Egil Olsen then reflects on his time with the Norwegian men's national football team with Geir. In this chapter, Egil describes how he took this national side, a small country with just about five million people, to punch way above its weight in the 1990s to at one point being ranked number two in the world. In this account, Egil's messages centre on his philosophy on playing style, with a robust basis in empirical knowledge about what wins games, as well as being in front with analytics, adopting a match-by-match way to play to the style of the opponent, and his principles of leadership and communication.

Having considered some important factors in coaching on a national level, Chapter 5 then moves to present Dean Smith's perceptions of coaching week-to-week in professional football, as based on his roles with Walsall FC, Brentford FC, and currently Aston Villa FC in England's Championship. Beginning with an overview of the roles and responsibilities of head coaching in professional club football in the UK, Dean then provides a summary of the outcomes that he tries to deliver as a coach, followed by the general processes and skills which help him to achieve this. To conclude, Dean then considers two particularly important requirements of the head coach in professional football: 'building your base' when appointed and the importance of consistency for longer-term survival and success.

Providing another – and perhaps more significant – contrast, Chapter 6 then sees Tom Willmott describe his role as Head Coach of the "Park & Pipe" programme for Snowsports New Zealand. To contextualise his contribution, Tom summarises the transition of action/adventure/extreme sports into the 'mainstream' and the particular challenges of coaching in this environment. From here, evolutions within the Park & Pipe performance pathway are considered alongside other routes into elite-level competition, plus recent innovations in the domain – including the application of emotional periodisation, development models, and 'team coaching'.

Having considered the nature and scope of work undertaken by head coaches in Chapters 3 to 6, we then return to the 'personal coach' level, but this time with a focus on the 'specialist coach'. More specifically, Steve Fairchild provides a perspective on his work coaching quarterbacks in NFL, college, and high school, covering the role of the specialist coach, evaluating quarterback performance, developing quarterbacks, training approaches (including cognitive training) and, finally, some reflections on the broader demands on players. To offer a final contrast, this section then concludes by moving from the coaching of senior elite performers and teams to the development of the 'elites of tomorrow'. To achieve this, Ruben Jongkind presents an overview of Johan Cruyff's player development philosophy, which guided Ruben and Wim Jonk as management of the AFC Ajax Amsterdam Youth Academy between 2011 and 2016. In this account, Ruben introduces Cruyff's ideas, how they were conceptualised and implemented in the academy, the role of supporting theory and data, and the politics, relationships, and personal challenges involved in the delivery process.

As will be shown, coaching in elite sport can be a highly rewarding but challenging endeavour. In this sense, it involves much, much more than the 'staple diet' of organising training schedules and sessions to aid the development and refinement of physical, technical, and tactical skills for competition. We therefore encourage the reader to keep a number of points in mind when reflecting on the messages offered by our contributors: namely, the type of performance or performer that the coach is trying to support, the outcomes that deliver this performance, the processes required to deliver these outcomes; the challenges and roadblocks that have to be accounted for; and how these areas vary in relation to each specific sport and environment. In addition to these, the next chapter sees Dave highlighting a few other important themes that run throughout this opening section. More specifically, Dave introduces some important characteristics and processes of coaches who work with elite performers and teams, as well as coaches who are 'elite at coaching' itself. These include the role of knowledge, experience, and openness (as some important *characteristics*), as well as that of professional judgement and decision-making, equal expertise, intuition, and innovation (as some important *processes*). So, without further ado, onto this 'scene setter'!

The principles of elite coaching
Blending knowledge, experience, and novelty

Dave Collins

Coaches and coaching at the elite level: some initial thoughts

Although I have never coached at the genuinely elite level, my work as a psychologist has provided the opportunity to observe and interact with some superb coaches. In addition, work as a coach to national level, as a coach educator nationally and internationally, and as a researcher into coaching and teaching have offered the chance for critical refection and, perhaps most importantly, input from others. All this has helped to shape the perspectives offered in this chapter; perspectives which, wherever possible, are supported by published research evidence.

Please don't get too concerned, however. My aim here is neither a reference-rich literature review nor a diatribe. Rather, I would like to raise some issues and questions which might prove useful as a backdrop to reading through the other chapters in this section. These are chapters which are, importantly, written by coaches who have worked and/or continue to work at the elite level: those who both have the T-shirt and deserve the accolades!

So, any general thoughts before I present some underpinnings? Well, I think it is important to define what we are talking about in using the 'elite coach' term. As highlighted by Nash and colleagues in 2012, elite coaching and coaching expertise have proved to be somewhat overused in the literature, most notably in people confusing the elite coach term with coaching elites! The confusion is, perhaps, understandable. After all, if the athlete/team is performing well, then the coach associated with the outcome must also be quite good. This confusion has led to the (until recently) socially accepted idea that, as you improve as a coach, you move up the ladder. Gratifyingly, recent coach accreditation proposals have started to recognise that a coach can be absolutely superb, a genuine elite, but be focused on different levels of performer. Personally, I would highlight Pete Sturgess from the English FA as one such individual, a passionate and extremely effective coach (and coach educator) who has consciously focused his energies on young players of 12 years old and under.

The other issue is that the quality of performance does not necessarily relate directly to the quality of the coach. There are a number of factors involved in the outcome, including scouting and recruitment, or playing on a team or squad to further your career as an athlete. So this is another common misnomer . . . because X is a great athlete then Y must be a great coach.

Often true but not always. So, to summarise my points, elite athletes don't necessarily equal elite coaches, and coaches can be elite without working with high-level performers.

So, having made that distinction, what are the implications for the chapter, especially as it is in a book on elite performance? Well, as with so much else in the human sciences, it means that we are best focusing on characteristics and process rather than outcome. Accordingly, the chapter explores the characteristics and processes of coaches who are both elite (i.e. good at their job) and coaching elites, athletes who are good at theirs! For clarity, I have split these two as separate parts, with the underlying concepts presented as sub-headings.

As you read through, however, please note the message which is reiterated in the conclusion. The effective elite coach is elite because of an optimum blend of all the ideas presented; a blend which she or he is constantly drawing on but also refining both retrospectively and proactively. Like the sports they work in, if elite coaches stand still they go backwards; if they work hard they stand still and it is only by careful and creative thought that they get ahead!

Part 1. Characteristics

Knowledge

Clearly, one of the things that distinguishes elites is their level of knowledge. In simple terms, this is probably best considered using the coach decision-making structure presented in Figure 1.1 below.

I talk more about the process in Part 2 of the chapter, and will refer back to this figure then, most particularly the DK (Declarative Knowledge) aspect. For the moment, however, it is worth noting that the coach's actions will be determined through drawing on three broad bodies of knowledge, sport specific (the WHAT to coach), pedagogy (the science of learning – so HOW to coach it), and knowledge of the performer (sometimes referred to as the 'ologies'), which helps *fine tune* the actions to the individual context. These three bodies of knowledge help the coach to generate a response, which can be an immediate action or a longer-term plan. However, for many, the final action will also be influenced by the norms or mores of the setting – in short, what is expected by the athletes in that particular context.

Based on this model, the elite coach will almost always have high levels of knowledge in all three areas, albeit that this knowledge might not be 'formally academic' (e.g. "Marks and Spencer" wrote about that!). This is a clear marker in that lower ability coaches will usually have one or more 'weak suits'; for example, many coaches have surprisingly low levels of knowledge (and even interest) in pedagogy. The elite coach will also be relatively unbiased by the expectations influence unless there is a clear benefit to doing so – for example, working to the accepted and well-respected cultural norms of the team. Finally, it is worth mentioning that most elite coaches will be well aware of any weaknesses that they may have in these knowledge structures, and will take steps to ensure that these weaknesses are covered – perhaps by the use of an assistant coach with specialist knowledge in that area.

Experience

A common-sense approach would suggest that elite coaches will have a wider experience than their less able counterparts. Importantly, however, a quick review of those often identified as better, or even elite, coaches will challenge this assumption. The reason for this contrast is down to the exact meaning of experience, which goes beyond mere length or breadth of

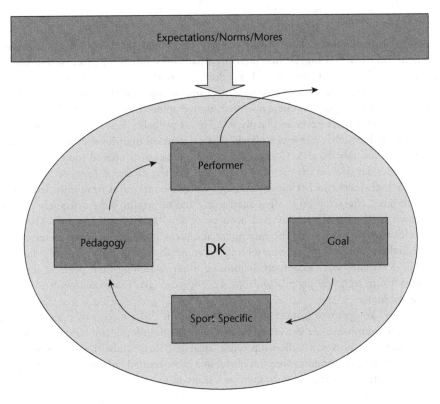

Figure 1.1   A simplified coach knowledge base for decision-making

service. "Experience is not what happens to you, it is what you do with what happens to you". This well-known quote from English author Aldous Huxley underpins the role which the individual must play in critically synthesising learning from what they experience. This idea is also reflected in the almost apocryphal saying "20 years of action without reflection is 20 years of the same substandard stuff".

My point here is that truly elite coaches will, as a trait characteristic, be constantly reviewing and refining what they are doing, hence making each episode a learning experience. I can recall fellow university lecturers who were still using slides marked 1975 in the 1990s! Or coaches who would be so consistent in their approach that you could set your watch by them. . . "OK, its March so XXX will be using that practice and that session plan". I even had the pleasure of playing high-level rugby under a coach who used the same drill every Tuesday for the whole season. Worse still, we still couldn't do it, even after that! Needless to say, none of these would fall into the elite category, even though they were undoubtedly working with high-level performers (notwithstanding our poor performance on a certain Tuesday drill!).

So, in addition to a wide knowledge base (or assistants to address the weakness), elite coaches will be aficionados of the critical reflection process. There is one caveat to the type of reflection, as I will explain later. For the moment, however, true elites will demonstrate their experience by (usually) openly describing their mistakes and describing how they progressed from them.

Openness

Openness to change is also a characteristic of elites. Some may see this as just another feature of experience but I would suggest that there are small and subtle differences which can make a big difference. To illustrate my point, I will draw on another Huxley quote: "There is only one corner of the universe you can be certain of improving, and that's your own self". My main point under the openness element is that, in my opinion, true elites will display a very particular style with their peers and 'acolytes'. This is probably best demonstrated by some work we did with coaches a few years back, that categorised high-level coaches as vampires or wolves (Collins, Abraham & Collins, 2012). The paper also offered some good insights on how coaches develop on the pathway to the top. For the moment, however, the relevant point is how high-level coaches sought out, and were open to, ideas from outside their own sphere. Vampires, characterised as often charismatic and successful, were extremely confident in their own methods, which they had been using for "a number of years". They rarely shared (at least openly) and were also infrequent attendees at conferences and in-service educational activities, unless they were presenting! In contrast, wolves almost literally 'hunted in packs'. These coaches were extremely acquisitive, often watching their peers in sessions or competitive warm ups, and happily and openly 'copying' (BUT see comments in the next section) good ideas.

So, it seems like openness (some may prefer humility) is also a marker of elites. Please note that both the vampires and the wolves were operating at a high level, and most were very successful. Importantly, however, follow-up work suggested that, whilst the wolves went from strength to strength, the vampires were successful in a more limited fashion; notably, often with specific sorts of athletes/team and even then on a short-term basis.

Part 2. Processes/systems

So, if elites have a level of knowledge, experience, and openness, how is this applied? In more depth, exactly how do they work and what can others learn from this? Well, once again there is an expanding research literature which offers some useful pointers. In this case, four systemic features which seem to characterise or even, perhaps, help to make coaches achieve elite status.

PJDM

This is, for me at least, a crucial construct which lies at the heart of expert practice. In fact, to be more accurate, employing this approach is both a marker and a causative factor in expertise. The letters stand for Professional Judgement and Decision-Making, and they represent the way in which almost all elites will operate.

The basic idea is that all professions involve some form of judgement and decision-making in planning then executing what is required. In the coaching context, this means that choices must be made between a number of options, so that the eventual provision to the athlete generates the optimum changes and outcomes. This judgement will happen across a wide variety of circumstances and time courses. At the macro or longer duration level, planning across a year, quadrennial or even longer will often work backwards from the desired outcome, phasing or periodising activities to work steadily but effectively towards the goal. This process is matched at the medium-term or meso level, with sub-phases addressing the longer-term agenda but also catering for specific issues or challenges (e.g. change of venue, weather, injury) which may occur. Finally, at the short-term or micro level, activities are planned to take

Level	Exemplar Objectives	Timeline & Activity			
Macro Quadrennial: Socio - Politico- Strategic	• Medals at OG (1), Worlds (1), Euros (4) & Junior Worlds (2) • Establish group as major player	1 Year Years	2 Years		3 Years	4 Years

Consistency in Competition

Level	Exemplar Objectives	Weeks 1 – 6	Weeks 7 – 12	Weeks 13 – 18	Weeks 19 – 24
Meso Seasonal: Socio- Tactical - Motivational	As above plus: • Consistent placing in semi final level at World Cups • Ability to rationalise and learn from results • Confirmation of racing style • Confidence in preparation, systems and coaching • Maintaining training/practice load • Individual goals and plans established	Focus on Practice Behaviour	Lower level events, training through	Two targeted events, with reviewed and revised schedules	One World Cup Performance, with mini-peak

Building confidence through understanding

Level	Exemplar Objectives				
Micor Sessional: Idio - Tactical	As above plus for example: • Talk through planning and debrief				

Figure 1.2 An example of nested thinking in short track speed skating

Source: Adapted from Abraham & Collins, 2011

account of the macro and meso agendas, whilst also adjusting for short-term influences like athlete health, variation in training readiness, etc. This approach necessitates the coach keeping all three agendas in mind as she or he designs, deploys, fine tunes, and reviews the daily coaching episodes. This 'nested thinking' approach is presented in Figure 1.2.

The figure illustrates the way in which the coach, making decisions on a day-to-day basis, must keep the different level goals in mind. So, at the micro level my sessions are planned to get the athletes on board with, and confident in, the tactical and technical agendas and practices associated with these. Importantly, however, the coach's PJDM will also be influenced by the meso (we have got to achieve consistent results) and macro (we want a medal!) goals. This balancing act is a feature common to many professions but coaching is certainly a good example.

Given the centrality of the DM process, this is worth specific focus. So, I return to Figure 1.1 and the DK or Declarative Knowledge base which underpins the knowledge and PJDM of the coach. If Procedural Knowledge is the how to do something, which is clearly fairly important, then DK is the *why this* is to be done. As such DK, knowing why or why not particular approaches might be optimum for this particular athlete in this particular situation at this particular time, is the absolute keystone of PJDM. So, the knowledge of any coach, and particularly the elite ones, must be built on an 'it depends' structure which enables decisions on which action will best fit the context.

This emphasis of fitting the what and how based on the why is a key feature of truly reflective coaches. Furthermore, as highlighted by Schön (1983; 1987), the truly effective critical practitioner will set up mini experiments to test ideas. In coaching, this is often seen with coaches wanting a bigger squad so that ideas can be genuinely tested.

If you follow this 'experimenting' approach to its logical conclusion, and reflecting my comments earlier about the need to work hard to even stay still, it becomes obvious that elites will be acquisitive and perhaps even collaborative in developing new ideas. There is a lot of talk about 'communities of practice' at all levels of coaching, and the elite level is no different. Indeed, in my experience elite coaches will also be characterised by a 'little black book' of contacts, both in coaching and in other relevant disciplines, with whom they will regularly connect. Holding an annual 'brains trust' is a common feature for many top sports teams; a similar if more interdisciplinary approach.

Finally, especially against the 'let's try it' approach described, it is important to note that elites' critical reflection usually takes place against very clear and well operationalised criteria. As a consequence, their PJDM is evidence-based, or at least as evidence-based as cutting edge stuff can be. On this topic, it might be more accurate to describe elite developments as evidence grounded rather than based directly on peer review published material. The brains trusts will often work this way. "You know, it might work if we. . ." is a common start to an entirely original thought experiment that may provide the next edge. Just for interest, it is worth pointing out how important this strong basis is for coach reflection at *all* levels. Without the grounded/evidence basis, plus a genuinely scientific approach, all sorts of strange ideas get promoted and enter the public consciousness as 'obvious because they work'!

Equal expertise

Reflecting the characteristics listed above, elite coaches usually preside over an 'equal expertise' environment. Across nations, cultures, and sports, coaching can be a very hierarchical structure. The overt difference and (hopefully) embedded respect for the head coach's word is a good example of this. Indeed, as shown in Figure 1.1, this expectation/more that 'the coach knows best' is often a factor in how information needs to be presented. In short, athletes in some contexts get worried when they are asked for their input or opinion! Of course, the truly aware coach (and elites almost always are, even if they don't show it) will adjust delivery to fit the optimum blend of the three knowledge elements (sport, pedagogy, and ology) *together with* expectations.

This condition notwithstanding, however, elite coaches will almost always work towards a model of equal expertise: one where each member of the team, whether performing, coaching or supporting, is assured that their contribution is both welcomed and valued. This structure may often be hidden, the culture/expectation being but one factor in why, but at the heart of the matter, the elite coach will look to consult widely and acknowledge what members can bring to the party.

Equal expertise environments are often associated with another characteristic of effective groups; namely, role clarity. In simple terms, everyone will know why everyone else is there, what she/he can offer and how/when/why the individual should be involved. Note that this model is certainly not the antithesis of a hierarchical structure. Indeed, the acknowledgement of expertise in others does not lead to a debating society. In fact, the leader and his/her opinion is even more valued as the one who takes the ultimate decision. It's just that, on the way to that decision, there is a more overt solicitation of opinion; a process that usually also adds substantially to group buy-in.

Intuition

Seen by some as the complete opposite to the 'it depends', critical reasoning approach, many wax lyrical about the degree to which elite coaches and leaders just act from intuition. This may follow from our fascination with people who just 'seem to know' what to do and the general praise and respect which is associated with decisiveness (cf. Tetlock, 2005). Of course, there is no doubt that coaches at several levels employ the quicker style DM described by Klein and colleagues as Naturalistic Decision Making or NDM (e.g. Klein, 1998). In fact, some of this decisiveness may be down to a quicker and more effective recognition of exactly what is needed (cf. Klein & Hoffman, 1993). Despite the seductive attractiveness, however, mainstream psychology has shown us that almost all effective decision-makers employ a combination of quick (NDM) and slower more deliberative approaches (cf. Kahneman & Klein, 2009) which are often referred to as Classical Decision Making or CDM.

Interestingly, this seems to be the approach which coaches adopt. A combination of NDM and CDM is adopted, with one or the other employed in different contexts. The style selected and applied is often for pragmatic reasons such as time pressure but also, sometimes, for reasons of preference. Notably, however, our research with elite (or at least, reflecting the arguments presented in the Introduction, high-level) coaches suggests that a 'combination' approach also takes place with short-term challenges, where 'snap decision-making' is the style required.

Given our interests, Loel Collins and I, assisted by Howie Carson, took a look at the quick-fire decision-making reported by high-level adventure sport and rugby coaches (Collins, Collins & Carson, 2016). In keeping with other views, the coaches in our sample all reported making snap decisions 'intuitively', using an NDM style. Notably, however, and an important distinction to the ideas suggested by some other authors, the sample reported the importance of using a 'check review' in slower time, using a more deliberative CDM type approach. For example, one adventure sports coach said:

> [T]rying to convince the students [articulating the dilemma] that that was a really serious day and the decision making, they all thought it was fantastic and it was a really exciting adventure, but you know, it's trying then to tell the students, actually . . . there was some wrong decision making going on there. There was some gut decision making that was . . . that basically was fine up to a certain stage [limitations of a given approach], but then it's the conditions and the environment changed [situational awareness, change, and impact] and so I was stuck, having to make gut decisions [other processes may have been better suited], and realizing that I was now in a situation that wasn't good [audit].

The point was that, rather than just stick with their decision, the high-level sample took every opportunity (or at least said that they should!) to internally review their decisions whenever time permitted. Depending on the time and challenge constraints, this might take place immediately or, where circumstances dictated, a while later. Importantly, however, and reflecting the ideas presented in the PJDM section above, all were able to articulate (albeit sometimes post hoc) the whys and wherefores of their decisions. Indeed, several used mentors, peers or assistants as 'sounding boards', checking their reasoning chain and making adjustments as appropriate. For example, a premiership rugby coach reported:

> In the heat of battle, I say and do all sorts of things. My coaching team and analysts often look at me strangely to think "why the f*** has he done that?" But I can always run the

replay in my head afterwards, with total recall, and explain the logic of why, when, and how even though I wasn't aware of it at the time.

Finally, it is worth considering specific research on adventure sport and how, given the hyper-dynamic, fast changing environment and high levels of consequence (i.e. risk of injury) they work in, coaches work to 'give themselves time' for reflection "on action-in context" (Collins & Collins, 2016). In other words, and despite the natural inclination for coaches to make snap decisions, coupled with the clients' liking for such 'decisiveness', elite coaches seem to either avoid the necessity for this and/or give themselves time for the essential post-decision reflection.

Novelty

As stated earlier, the ability to innovate and introduce novel ideas seems to be another marker of elite status. As just one example of this, I would highlight the elite coach's capacity to effectively deal with, and indeed help to flourish, the challenging but mercurial athletes often described as mavericks. It is interesting that, whilst almost all involved in sport identify creativity as a valued characteristic, many coaches find it 'challenging' (to say the least) to fully support, exploit, and develop those who stand out for their creativity and originality. As such, I would suggest that the elite coach will demonstrate an ability to fit, and form effective relationships with maverick players. For the moment, consider how many elite teams often fail to pick such innovative thinkers, often because they 'just don't fit'!

In conclusion

I hope that this brief overview has offered some evidence and ideas to stimulate perspectives on who genuinely deserves the elite label. Reflecting the role of thought on the craft and process of coaching, I would come back to some of our own work and the role that metacognition (literally, thinking about thinking) may play in helping the pathway to elite-dom (Collins, Carson & Collins, 2016). For the present purpose, my point is that a tendency to regularly review your process is an essential feature of the committed-to-upwards-mobility coach. IF coaching is a cognitive art/decision-making game, and there is a growing body of research that says it is, then metacognition is a key element in the development process.

Importantly, there are features of both characteristic and skill in metacognition: a characteristic in that the individual will have a tendency to engage in critical reflection which, because of the rigour and criteria applied, will be a lot more than mere navel-gazing; a skill in that the process will get easier and more impactful with practice, especially when facilitated by an external agency. Good quality colleagues, mentoring and/or communities of practice can all play a role in this, yet another aspect which stresses the importance of the social milieu in coach development (Stoszkowski & Collins, 2014).

In addressing the 'who is really expert/elite' conundrum, you might consider the criteria suggested by Nash et al. (2012) shown in Table 1.1 below. It is worthwhile considering the criteria they suggested against some of the content in this chapter.

As a final point, I should stress that my research colleagues and I see much of this chapter as applying to elites across the sports spectrum. However, many of the ideas in this chapter can be extended and applied to other professional disciplines. Indeed, readers might like to apply some of the ideas in this chapter, and/or the table above, to what the scientists, managers, administrators, and senior leaders have to say. In summary, elite status is perhaps most obviously a way of

Table 1.1 Proposed criteria for identifying and operationalising expertise in coaches (adapted from Nash et al., 2012)

Criteria	Essential/Possible	How exhibited in coach
Focuses on PJDM, using a broad declarative knowledge base and in line with the structure recommended by Abraham et al. (2006)	Essential	**Knowledge** could be checked by formal qualification or exam **Application** PJDM could be assessed through a combination of observation and interview/oral exam
Application of perceptual skills, and mental models as the basis for critical reflection and review	Essential	Use of ACTA techniques to provide a knowledge audit (what they know) and how it is used (what they do)
Ability to work independently and generate considered solutions. Innovative where appropriate	Essential	Observation showing consideration in PJDM Record of innovations Peer recommendation
Effective reflection and experimentation as per Schön (1987) PJDM which allows for own strengths and limitations	Essential	Peer recommendation. Record of development (including video of coaching at different stages of development) Personal drive for development of professional expertise.
Manages complex planning process	Essential	Runs mental simulations in advance, checking for potential issues and countering them proactively where possible
Track record of developing athletes (e.g. from development to world class standards)	Possible (although expertise may become focused on one particular stage)	Coaching portfolios

working or approach, rather than just the position held or CV content. See what you think as you read through the various sections and chapters in this book.

References

Abraham, A. & Collins, D. (2011). Taking the Next Step: Ways Forward for Coaching Science. *Quest*, **63**, 366–384

Collins, D., Abraham, A. & Collins, R. (2012). On Vampires and Wolves – Exploring and Countering Reasons for the Differential Impact of Coach Education. *International Journal of Sport Psychology*, **43**, 255–271

Collins, D., Collins, L. & Carson, H. J. (2016). "If It Feels Right, Do It": Intuitive Decision Making in a Sample of High-Level Sport Coaches. *Frontiers in Psychology*, **7**, 504. doi: 10.3389/fpsyg.2016.00504

Collins, L., Carson, H. J. & Collins, D. (2016). Metacognition and Professional Judgment and Decision Making in Coaching: Importance, Application and Evaluation, *International Sports Coaching Journal*, **3**(3), 355–361. doi:10.1123/iscj.2016-0037

Collins, L. & Collins, D. (2016). Professional Judgement and Decision-Making in Adventure Sports Coaching: The Role of Interaction. *Journal of Sports Sciences*, **34**(13), 1231–1239. doi:10.1080/026404 14.2015.1105379

Kahneman, D., & Klein, G. A. (2009). Conditions for Intuitive Expertise: A Failure to Disagree. *American Psychologist*, **64**(6), 515–526

Klein, G. A. (1998). *Sources of Power: How People Make Decisions*. Cambridge, MA: MIT Press

Klein, G. A., & Hoffman, R. R. (1993). Seeing the Invisible: Perceptual-Cognitive Aspects of Expertise. In M. Rabinowitz (Ed.), *Cognitive Science Foundations of Instruction* (pp. 203–215). Hillsdale, NJ: Lawrence Erlbaum Associates

Nash, C., Martindale, R., Collins, D., & Martindale, A. (2012). Parameterising Expertise in Coaching: Past, Present and Future. *Journal of Sports Sciences*, **30**(10), 985–994. doi:10.1080/02640414.2012.682079

Schön, D. A. (1983). *The Reflective Practitioner: How Professionals Think in Action*. New York, NY: Ashgate

Schön, D. (1987). *Educating the Reflective Practitioner*. San Francisco, CA: Jossey-Bass

Stoszkowski, J. & Collins, D. (2014). Communities of Practice, Social Learning and Networks: Exploiting the Social Side of Coach Development. *Sport, Education and Society*, **19**(6), 773–788

Tetlock, P. (2005). *Expert Political Judgment: How Good Is It? How Can We Know?* Princeton, NJ: Princeton University Press

2

Being the personal coach

Toni Minichiello

Editors' introduction

Following a career in the Civil Service, Toni followed his love of coaching to secure a full-time post with UK Athletics (UKA). He has enjoyed considerable successes with his athletes, most notably with triple World Champion and Double Olympic medallist, Jess Ennis-Hill. Still practising as an athletics coach, Toni has diversified his activities through a broad range of presentations, whilst joining the UKA Board as a coach representative.

My role – how it started and how it evolved

As requested, my chapter will focus on my role as personal coach to a single athlete; in my case Dame Jessica Ennis-Hill. I first met Jess when she was nine years of age and she got involved with athletics through coming down to the athletics track and taking part in a summer camp. Jess had received some coaching at school and at an after-school club. However, after a change in circumstances, she came to me at 13 pretty much full time and stayed through to her retirement: 18 years in total! I think because of the length of time coaching one person you end up coaching Jessica Ennis the person as opposed to or greater than coaching the performance. In short, it was about Jess being better at being Jess.

Of course, the balance between these two elements changed through the years. For example, the way you deal with and work with a nine-year-old compared to a 16-year-old who's questioning whether they even want to stay in the sport and what the future holds for them. It *has* to be different. In the early stages it's very direct and instructional because you're telling them what to do because they've no experience of factors or processes of how to throw a shot put, they've not got experience. After a while you move to "well what do you think? How do you think that could be better?" At that stage it becomes more coaching and then eventually more mentoring and it steadily becomes more of a partnership. The reality is that, as the relationship matures, I had to recognise that the balance changes across teaching, coaching and mentoring. It also depends on where their confidence is: either their confidence associated with the particular event, or with the particular situation. And that can change day to day and it varies so much that you step in in different ways.

The relationship is not fixed and you have to be so much more fluid I think as a coach to deal with the person, because you also find yourself dealing with stuff away from the track. I might spend time even within the middle of a session having discussions about her relationship with parents. School exams were another classic: "I'm struggling with my lessons". OK fine, I've got to chop the training sessions up or I've got to give you time off so you can manage your school work. So we adjust the pressure of coming to training. When it got close to exam time, I just said we'll train once this week.

So, as things developed, I would flex back and forth between teaching, coaching, mentoring, and life supporting. However, I would also always have an eye on the core goals which, especially in something as complicated as multi-events, is always going to drive a careful planning process.

In parallel to the modifications for personal circumstances, you've also got an eye on the next four years of well. The next benchmark is 5,800 points for an Olympic Games so what do I need to do today that lays a foundation for me to capitalise on in 8 to 12 years' time? So, you must consider where the athlete is and where she or he can go. With Jess for example, we already had an event, high jump, at 1.80 metres, which is world-class Heptathlon high jumping. She was weaker as a thrower so we needed to lay a foundation and grow a technique that would throw 14 metres in the shot put because that's world class Heptathlon shot-putting, as well as spinning the plate of 1.80 metres in the high jump. What do I do today? What are the skills that she will need? The auxiliary skills, not just the skills associated with an athletic technique, and how do I plan the skills associated with strength and conditioning? She is going to have to do cleans, probably one and a half times body weight, so you're going to need a good technique. In short, it's complicated!

The personal focus

In the early stages, before the fame and the resources, you are on your own as *the* coach, fulfilling a multitude of roles. As the personal coach, you are also much more heavily invested in the personality development of that athlete. We used to have lots of conversations about what matters and what doesn't matter. We would talk about if you won then how do you earn money out of a sport. If you win medals money takes care of itself. I think a lot of athletes are just trying to become famous for being famous as opposed to dealing with the performance, so you start to have conversations about what it would be like, what expectations should be or about controlling the controllables.

I think a turning point for Jess was when she was nine or ten. They had an international fixture at her home stadium, one of these televised events, and the javelin thrower Mick Hill signed an autograph for her. It made a big difference to her and led to a conversation. "You see how that affected you. . . now remember if you succeed how you will affect kids". I'd like to think it had some influence on Jess and how she is so personable, so approachable to kids, because she understood the effect that something like that had had on her.

Personal development *from* the sport is also important. Your time within sport will always be really, really short. Your window of great opportunity is probably about eight years. If you're lucky it's eight years that go Olympics, Olympics in the middle and Olympics at the end. If you're unlucky it covers two Olympics so roughly you've got eight years probably at your peak, ten if you're exceptional. If you're lucky you're not going to die until you're 80. Make sure you get everything you can out of it; enjoy every experience but realise there's a lifetime after that. Education in the broadest sense is critically important, adding to the rich tapestry that makes you who you are. As a personal coach, you try and give people the best experience and add as much value as you can. That value is not only the winning and the medals but who they are and how they approach life.

You also have to recognise how the athlete's other relationships are impacting their development – both as an athlete and as a person: the effect that everybody around them in their circle will have. You're a fool as a coach if you're not having a conversation with Mum and Dad. For example, in the early part of the athlete's career they are the nutritionist, the lifestyle consultant, kit supplier. . . they are their everything! I wouldn't have a conversation with the nutritionist or the psychologist or the funder. I'll have a conversation Mum and Dad as they cover all those things in the early stages. That also sets you up for keeping them involved and 'on side' later.

Keeping parents and family in the picture is crucial. For example, I recently had a conversation with a father of a heptathlete. I'm judging numbers on a sheet of paper but what I'm hearing from the father is that he feels isolated from the coaches in that he doesn't know what's going on anymore and therefore he's asking me questions. This is a bit disappointing for me as a personal coach because I would usually have sat down and gone "this is our plan for this year. . . this is our plan for four years and in year two this is our plan for year two, it's shifted a little bit now this is our plan for four years, or actually we were over ambitious we're stepping back a bit that injury has affected this". You take people with you on the journey!

Of course, there will always be difficult conversations; stuff where you're going to agree and you're going to disagree. I like the viewpoint that there are opinions. . . no such thing as positives and negatives. There are opinions; some of which you will like and some you will dislike. Those you dislike, you might say people are being negative. . . no, they just have a different opinion. The question is whether the opinion is valid, what it's based on, and who's the opinion coming from – have they got validity? If the answer to any of those is actually "that's interesting" then it's a stone you should turn and should examine.

Who else comes on the journey?

What I'm looking for is somebody who can add value to my training plan. Because it's my training plan, ultimately I'm looking for somebody who can work with me. I'm going to present this person to the athlete as an expert and somebody to be trusted so I've got to get on with them first.

So, having established that we can work together, what can you offer and can you present it in an athlete-friendly fashion? Tell me what you can do and what you are doing and can you explain it to me simply? Explain it to me like I'm an eight-year-old! I know you know wonderful technological words but if I don't understand it, trust me I'm not going to sell it to the athlete. This was also a big thing for Jess: did she get on with the person; were they pushy? I often talk about a sport scientist who was a brilliant guy. Jess got on with him, I got on with him. I've known him for years but he was the kind of guy who'd come with 15 new things. He's like a travelling salesman, open up his suitcase and he's got tens of things and Jess was woah. . . she's very risk averse and doesn't like huge amounts of change.

So, we kept the flow of input to careful and manageable levels. We would pick one thing and work down that one, get it sorted then embed it. Now the following year we would pick another one and so on. There was an important message here for support staff. We can't change ten things in one go so we need to get people to work in a way that I think adds value *and* works to the athlete's agenda; working to the athlete's rhythm.

And that's how I approach a lot of the sport sciences; namely, so what's new? What could we do this year that could give me an extra couple of percentage points? As crucially, however, is the athlete open to that and then how does that fit within the whole group? My main aim is to fit things into an overall master plan. . . this idea of gestalt that it's organic and that it grows. I've always seen the support team as cogs within a machine, like an old-fashioned clock that varies at some points in time based on what the problem or situation is. In certain circumstances or in a particular phase you're going to be a big cog – you're going to be a big mover in it because it's more in your field. At other times, you're a small cog but you're still turning and you're still adding value to the overall outcome. It's understanding that team ethos – park your ego at the door, today I'm big cog, tomorrow I'm small cog, but I need to be there supporting and investing in that.

Extending the cog idea, you can often have people who are not only driving their own area but who act as a catalyst for others. For example, when Jess was injured in 2008 we were looking to make a number of changes. One sport scientist member of the team was covering nutrition, which many would think of as a small cog in relation to an injury. She was in a room with all these other people, some of whom were not even sure why she was there. You could see people thinking "what's nutrition got to do with how we change right foot to left foot take off in in terms of long jump?" But then she said a couple of things in response to what somebody else said and it sparks somebody else and it sparks somebody else and all of a sudden "Woah this works!" It was a small cog turning a big cog and I suddenly realised "that's how I want the team dynamic to be".

So in summary, what I look for is whether somebody can work! Firstly, can they explain it to me simply like an eight-year-old? Can they add value to the agenda that I set as a coach and then can they be part of a bigger dynamic? Finally, and crucially with regard to the team dynamic, do they understand that and that they are not going to be the primary deliverer every time? Are they happy to be exerting little nudges and encouraging movements which makes the whole machine work?

Managing upwards and downwards – issues with 'the management'

Increasingly around the world and certainly in the UK at present, personal coaches need to work within a system. Inevitably perhaps, that system will evolve and leadership will change. . . in terms of individuals, personality, direction, the lot. So you might have loyalty to the person who's supported you in employing you and then you have loyalty to the person that you're probably more committed to because you've spent ten years working with them. However, the whole thing becomes very results-focused. The really bizarre thing is that the outcome of the athlete defines you whether you like it or not; as a coach, you're a good coach if they win, you're a crap coach if they lose. So, often irrespective of other issues, you become very utilitarian. My own personal ego says that I need my athlete to win so I'm going to do this, and support that above all else. But, as a consequence, you get torn in at least three different directions in terms of loyalty, and so managing upwards becomes a key part of the challenge. In my own situation, you're trying to act as a buffer between the governing body and the athlete, in addition to playing a game with the overall funding agency and support provider – in my case UK Sport and the English Institute of Sport respectively. You have to be aware of the agendas, both overt and covert, and how they might subtly or not so subtly change with changes in personnel.

Personally, I felt that the governing bodies changed to a certain extent with a new Performance Director (PD). They wanted to have a one to one relationship with the athlete and they were trying to cut the personal coach out. With the PD up to 2008 it looked like a three-way conversation. . . PD – Athlete – Me. However, from 2009 onwards it suddenly became two separate conversations. The governing body, personified as the PD, would have a meeting with the athlete. It often felt like this was to convince them of a desired change or new direction. Notably, I was not allowed in the room. I was really concerned about this as, almost inevitably, it tears the athlete in two because of the obvious tensions. After all, she also has an ego investment, together with a desire to maintain or enhance the levels of support whilst retaining selection. In most systems today, the PD holds all the cards.

How the relationship works between athlete, coach and PD is an important factor. A 'divide and try to rule' style is not a smart way of working. You piss me off, the athlete sees me pissed off and they inevitably feel conflicted. This person's helping me be as good as I can be but this person over here is my paymaster. All you do is create angst – it's non-leadership leadership. In our situation, things became awkward. I think that the PD underestimated the strength of relationship between me and the athlete and my understanding of the externals around that. He had a particular role and geographical location in mind for me and, to meet his agenda, both the athlete and I would have to move. From a personal perspective that worked. . . that's fine for me because at that time I had no attachment in that particular location. Crucially, however, that wasn't good for the athlete because I knew what a home girl she was, plus a whole raft of other private stuff. Possibly through not doing his homework, possibly for other reasons, the PD went ahead with the 'private conversation' with the athlete. After that happened, he was on totally stony ground he wasn't going to win. Even worse, he then came back to me and tried to 'encourage' me to take the decision. I know that in my position, in that situation, many would crumble or fold like a deck chair because they're not in a position of any level of strength or they don't have the strength of character to say "get stuffed".

What I did was delay the decision until after the World Championships. I thought the successful performance would 'buy us some space'. Unfortunately, however, even that didn't work as the pressure just came back. Personally, I felt very little loyalty from and, unsurprisingly, to an organisation that treated me and the athlete as such a 'commodity'. Frankly, if Jess had not been world champion it would have been a much tougher route and we would have had to conform. I would have to say that, if that had happened, she probably wouldn't have won the medals which she won, because we'd have had to try to beg, borrow and steal to make things happen.

Thankfully, external factors took a hand. Having been world champion, Lord Coe (at that time, head of the successful London Olympic bid) described Jess as the face of the games and that swung it in our favour. Unfortunately though, the relationship with the PD was spoiled and never recovered. I think there are a few lessons in this tale. From my perspective, the need to stand up for what you think is right; from a management perspective, the need to carefully consider all the angles before trying to impose change. Certainly, given the strength of relationship between Jess and myself, the approach of the first PD I mentioned was far more sensible. . . dealing with us together and collaboratively. In fact, he had also asked me to relocate my coaching as an employee of the national organisation. In that case, however, we had reached a compromise whereby my personal coach role did not suffer.

Being the personal coach – skills required

Reflecting the complexities listed above there is quite a lot to the role. However, I'll try to offer an informed overview. From a general perspective, I think you need to understand human nature; what motivates people. With the specific athlete (or athletes) in mind, you need to understand the athlete on a good day and on a bad day. Even more importantly in that respect, you need to understand yourself; to recognise what you're like under pressure, how you behave and then how those behaviours are interpreted by the athlete. Jess and I once completed a personality psychometric which was quite useful because it gave us a platform for discussion.

Obviously we knew each other very well already and the details didn't offer any big insights. Importantly, however, the platform offered us a chance to explore all sorts of things to move the relationship and her performance forward, things like how to best present information, how to coach to fit her learning preferences, her moods. . . that sort of operational stuff.

In this regard, it's clearly about how you sell the message. What I often found with Jess, perhaps because of the number of years we worked together, is that it often wasn't the message you were trying to get across, it was the messenger; i.e., it was me! I would never be able to sell physiology ideas because I'm not a physiology expert and she recognised that. OK. . . so let me bring in the new messenger, the physiologist; now let him explain: ooh oh well this is new and shiny. Now she is hooked! "Oh, I like science; wow it's really sciencey, oh OK ooh I trust the idea". Now I'm happy you telling me about it and we'll work towards a plan.

So, in the personal coach role, you're always having that kind of bobbing and weaving: understanding how they want the information delivered, understanding what they can cope with; but it isn't only them. . . it's also going back to understanding yourself. What are you like under pressure, how are your behaviours and how *should* you behave when the 'S' has hit the fan! It's kind of, what am I going to be like under pressure? One of the best stories that characterises this is the London Olympics in 2012. She's leading after the first day. The gold medal hangs on the result of this next event, but we'd had a problem with the long jump. It was perennially something we were trying to fix but it was the critical thing that, at that particular moment and that event, would mean whether she won or lost a gold medal. Up to that point we'd got too much speed on the runway. We had tweaked it and we'd worked biomechanics, so we went from a 19-stride to a 17-stride run-up. There had been several 'in parallel' changes of course. In a course of a couple of years, we'd tweaked the run-up and we'd having changed the take-off foot. There were all sorts of anxieties and stuff but we'd got to a point where she had a standing start approach. She ran down the runway in warm up and looked fantastic. We moved back a couple of shoes and "yeah you've made your adjustments that's it. . . two runways away there you go". The first runway, she came down, jumped, and jumped reasonably well, and I thought "thank goodness" because all season to that point she'd been fouling jumps; overreaching and fouling.

I looked at it visually and thought "easy. . . just move it back a bit". But then she's at the bottom of the runway waving at me, having only jumped 5.90 and it was like "we've got points on the board we're happy here. Not great but it'll do". OK, let me just look at the video footage A big reality check, however!! The biomechanist is going "she's taking 19 steps on the runway". I said "don't be stupid. . . for two years we've been running 17 steps, let me have a look at it". Meanwhile, she's waving at me because she wants immediate feedback. I play delaying tactics – "put your t-shirt on, I'll come and talk to you". So I look at the film and I go 16, 17, ooh 18, 19 and the biomechanist (who has been with us for several years and is what I would call a 'large cog') just turned around and said, "what are you going to say to her?" I said "I haven't got a clue, but I'll work it out by the time I get to the bottom of the steps". And I walked down to the bottom of the steps and I'm thinking just don't trip, look in control because I'm sure there's a TV camera on you, but what are you going to say? And it's at that point you're like "coach what you see". In other words, exploit the relationship and trust but don't spook her with too much data! OK, she was crowding the board but she doesn't know whether she's taking 17 or 19. . . she's not that kind of athlete.

So, reflecting these considerations, my response initially was "how did that feel?" She was alright, but "it's not enough". My response was both supportive and informative. . . "exactly. . . yeah OK you're crowding the board, you're leaning back at take-off. These are problems that we worked with in training. . . no worries, just move it back a couple of feet, then make sure you're upright, in the runway and take off". That was it; I walked back upstairs, made no mention at all and that the next two jumps she jumped further and she jumped further still and that was fundamentally where I think the gold medal from a coaching point of view was won; based on that judgement which was based on years of personal knowledge and interaction.

The following day we were in hospitality at Adidas and I said "Look. . . how many strides did you take on the runway?" She said "17" so I went "you look at the film, you took 19". She looked at me in disbelief, like "oh yeah". BUT what do you think she said? "Well I won didn't I?!" And that was it.

My initial feeling was "that's it?! That's all you're going to say?" But, it's at that point when you ask what you need to know. . . it's kind of like how's she going to behave if I run down and in a panic and shout . . . "you're taking 17 steps". But if I'd done that then, at that particular point, she'd have lost the gold medal. In any case, who can guess how many feet you change to run a runway for two strides?!

My point here is that the stresses I am under are irrelevant because I don't want to give my stress to her. I must, actually, accurately and optimally, judge what does she actually want and what information will help her jump a little bit further and nail this competition? You and your athlete are on the biggest stage of your lives so the personal knowledge and trust helps you to solve the issues and move forwards.

Differences between personal coaches and other top level coaches

I think it might be useful to stress the differences between the personal coach role and other, albeit successful on average, high-level coaches. My point here is that the level of relationship, trust and everything two-way that goes with it, is different. When an athlete moves from one coach to another, something that is increasingly common and increasingly encouraged, it would be what you might call a normal coach relationship as opposed to you where you are a personal coach relationship.

As a personal coach, I coach the person first and the event second. Clearly, I use a lot of the same approaches; the careful consideration and planning, for example, in the same way that the normal coach does. It's just that I am far more focused on the individual; his or her needs, growth, foibles, etc. As a personal coach, I have a method of working that might work for you but might not work for you. Crucially, however, I'm willing to flex it. When I look at successful and highly rated coaches who attract a number of 'transfers', I think it's different. It ends up being "here is my method. . . let's see if it works for you". I see the successes as why well-established coaches recruit so incredibly well but achieve very little with many of the athletes that they work with. They are very successful with three or four but, frankly, that is enough! These coaches are often rather formulaic. . . run lift run lift run lift and that's that. But when it comes to the VERY bespoke stuff, around the design of the competition programme for example, things just don't vary. "It worked for athletes' X and Y. . . why wouldn't it work for you?!"

Thinking about it, this might just be a systematic difference between two sub-species of coach. . . one systemic and one personal. Even when athletes have joined me late, say at the ripe old age of 23, I still try to employ the personal coach approach as I feel it is the best way. This might come from my previous experiences as a basketball coach. With a team game like basketball, you would always look offensively and defensively at where your strengths and weaknesses are. If you've got a short team that's really quick, you'll probably coach in a particular way, but if it's a big team that is slow, then you'll probably coach the team differently. If you've got big players and if you've got a great shooting team you'll have the option of a great 'run and gun' game. If you've got bigger players, you'll probably play offensively more of an inside game. You shape your tactics to what you have and that's the way I've always approached athletics.

Of course there are fundamentals. There's a definitive way to throw a shot put biomechanically because that's physics and you can't beat physics! However, if the athlete is long-legged and short-bodied and they can't flex in a particular way, you'll kind of tweak it but are still focused on, fundamentally, release speed, angle of release, how you get across the circle, and so on. So, you mould it a little bit but fundamentally you have to stick to the 'basics'. In simple terms, I think the difference is down to how much and how well you can mould, as opposed to how set your standards are.

In summary

So, in an attempt to delineate the distinguishing characteristics, I think it's firstly about understanding the individual that you are trying to add value to, and that you're adding value in a number of different ways. The competition performance is not the only value you add. Their interaction with people within the group can add value; their experiences can add value; developing their ability to train adds value. The experiences of those things and more are all how you add value to them as an individual. As the coach you know the messages about ethics, morals, interpersonal standards, and social relationships; being a role model, and how they approach life. As the personal coach, you are always adding value in some way and recognise that coaching is not just about the win.

3

Being the national coach in an Olympic sport

Mike Hay

Editors' introduction

As outlined in the authors' bios section at the start of this book, Mike was the first full-time national coach to be appointed in GB for the sport of curling. Very much a Scottish sport, its arrival into the Olympics opened a number of new avenues, with a rapid professionalisation and change to attitudes. As a highly committed international player, Mike played a leading role in taking the sport forwards: work that continues in his current role with the British Olympic Association where he served as Chef de Mission at the recent Winter Olympics in South Korea.

Getting started: the background to my appointment

In the summer of 1998, the Scottish Institute of Sport (SIS) was being formed, based on the much-hyped Australian Institute of Sport model. There were to be seven core sports, six summer sports, and one winter. The winter sport was to be curling, based partly on a relatively successful medal return at Europeans and World Championships. The sport had also made its modern debut in the Olympic Winter Games (OWG), Nagano 1998, or at least a return after a lengthy absence despite it being one of the sports included at the inaugural Winter Olympics in 1924.

I had been coaching junior teams at World Championships whilst still competing at international level. The opportunity arose for a full-time national coach, GB performance director, based out of and line managed from the SIS.

In the early 1990s I took up a job offer working in the lumber industry in Vancouver, Canada, taking out Canadian residency at the time, but things didn't work out and for personal reasons I came back to Scotland. A period of short-term jobs followed and I struggled to find a career that gave me the fulfilment I was looking for.

Our team had just won the European Championships in December 1997 and were favourites to win the British Championships in early January for the right to represent GB at the OWG in February in Nagano Japan. Unfortunately, it was not to be as we came up short in the final; a crushing disappointment in what had been a very successful playing career.

The time felt right to retire, I was 35 years old, looking for a new challenge and I was excited by this opportunity to go after this first full-time coaching role. I was giving up the relative safety as a sales engineer with Air Products, but that didn't bother me, I wanted to take this chance to raise the profile of our great game and challenge myself to right the many wrongs, I believed, I had experienced as a player in the national team.

I got through the interview stage, mesmerising the panel with my vision on acetates and a borrowed overhead projector. Things have come a long way!

The appointment was a major culture change for the sport and faced some questioning, at least unofficially, in many curling circles. To give you an insight, the appointment of a coach for a team going to the Worlds was not seen as a significant appointment from the National Governing Body point of view. To that point, teams winning the national championships basically duly signed the Royal Caledonian Curling Club's (RCCC) players' contract, meaning we would be under their jurisdiction at the worlds. The president's word was final on all matters. They gave us the kit, told us to train hard and that they would see us at the airport on such and such a date to fly out to the Worlds. We usually took the cheapest route, with little time for acclimation or training in-country. We could choose our own coach and fifth player (substitute) as long as the RCCC committee (blazer brigade) approved those candidates. To be fair, some of the presidents were great guys, but few of them really understood performance sport.

Depending on the president of the RCCC they may take you out for a dinner during the championships, but the big focus was their Scotch Whisky party which was the hot ticket of the week during the World Championships for those who loved the social aspect of attending a Worlds. It was mandatory for the team to attend, irrespective of what time you played the following morning, in full formal wear, making small talk with the VIPs who, armed with hindsight and a lifetime of experience, would try to explain why we should have adopted a different strategy which would have led to a win!

In summary, just the appointment of a National Coach was a culture shock, let alone the ideas to professionalise preparation and raise performance which I was so keen to implement. Interestingly, I don't think that cultural challenges *are* so rare, occurring even for new appointments to well-established sports with a longer tradition of applying science. But let me describe my journey and the many different components of the job which also typifies any national coaching role.

Into the new role: the challenges

I had just left the ranks of the players and now I was hoping I had enough credibility and respect from the players, some older than I, to initiate a new elite programme that would demand much more of their time, both in training and competition.

It is also important to consider how curling was selected to be an Institute sport. As is so common in sport, there were elements of luck and interpersonal 'pressures' but also the drive of clear-thinking visionaries. The major reason for curling being that one winter sport to be accepted as a core sport was down to one person, Gareth McKenna, the RCCC's development officer. Batting way above his station, he made it his personal crusade to get curling into the Institute: he was thinking big way before his time. This is set against a background when the RCCC didn't bother to apply for Sportscotland's (the national council that oversaw sports) grants for the development of the sport. The RCCC had around 20,000 members at the time and didn't like any conditions that might come with government funding.

Like in every sport, the politics were never far away. Curling's decision-making process mirrored its ancient history; a large committee made up of geographically elected branch members, rather than a skills-based smaller committee, ruled the sport. High performance was not top of their agenda. Most were more interested in tours and traditions such as the Grand Match (an open-air tournament held on a frozen loch and, consequently, rather dependent on the vagaries of the Scottish climate). It didn't help that most had never delivered a competitive stone. They didn't like change and had the structure to defer and defeat the most determined upstarts. Against this backdrop, I needed to learn some diplomacy and make some allies quickly if I was even going to reach the corridors of power and persuade them to promote some change.

In addition to these interpersonal issues, there were several political and organisational issues. For example, the status of curling as a SIS core sport meant that our programme sat within the Institute; meaning I was one step removed from the National Governing Body (NGB). I was line managed by the SIS's high-performance manager who, in turn, reported to the Executive Director. We of course had a relationship with counterparts at the RCCC which we endeavoured to strengthen in order to have allies within the NGB. These relationships were usually cordial; some were even positive but, on a broader basis, there was little in the way of a vision coming from the political leadership of the sport.

Building the system: first steps

So now I was appointed, with a pretty blank page, it was crucial to make the first steps really count. As such, actions had to be logical so that they would appeal and win support. Accordingly, the challenge now was to select teams to invest in and work with to try to achieve podium success in major championships on a regular basis. There had been successes before (my own team as an example). What we needed was consistent achievement rather than relying on the inconsistency and sometime brilliance that one or two teams were capable of producing, rather than trained for.

So, as a first step, we invited existing teams (or rinks as they are known in curling) to apply for an open recruitment process. This was important as it offered the opportunity to one and all. Interviews were held with teams and their coaches, the selected teams had annual/monthly planners that sat alongside their competition and training plans. The commitment was agreed alongside the investments but the excuses were also being rehearsed; after all we are only part-time curlers, we have jobs and careers to think about! Throughout this period, however, I was insistent on a single focus: "what will it take to be a world or Olympic champion?"

The 'interview' process was very thorough and, deliberately, included some challenge. The teams came in and said "we want investment. . . this is our team". I would say to them "do you know what, I don't think your second player is good enough. . . if you're looking for investment I think you might need to change them and here's a couple of options". So even though the bidding process was from already existing teams, I was trying to influence their thinking along the lines of my single world/Olympic focus. It was very much installing a little bit of responsibility and ownership with the team. I think it went a long way, rather than me telling them what they needed to do. At the same time, however, I always said to the players, "I'm going to be really honest to with you: if you're not cutting it, I'm going to tell you my opinion because ultimately I'm taking responsibility and accountability for performance". I have always felt, then and since, that this level of personal responsibility and accountability is often missing in some sports. You have got to be comfortable as a national coach or performance director to take that responsibility. Ultimately I wasn't going to turn around and blame a young team or the experienced coach at a Worlds if they hadn't achieved. I was taking that responsibility, but I was also accountable for decisions that needed to be made. For example, dropping a player because either their shot making isn't good enough or what they are bringing to the team is adverse. I've got a team to think about, not necessarily the individual.

My decision-making was just one of several 'points of contention' that the new approach faced. As another example, and with regard to who got what, the curling fraternity were split, and not very evenly. The vast majority wanted the money to be spread across all competitive teams, not the few. They didn't understand what we were trying to achieve, despite attempts to explain that we were investing in the athletes and teams who we believed had the potential to win at the highest level.

As a consequence, these splits were quite apparent. The first few years there was a clear 'them against us' when it came to the national championships and the funded versus non-funded teams. I didn't mind the snide remarks, very few said it to my face, they became keyboard warriors hiding behind anonymous nicknames. They threw plenty of stones (not the curling kind either) but offered little in terms of ideas to build a sustainable and successful programme.

When you lead a programme that has change at the heart, you need to articulate your philosophy and win the hearts and minds of those you are trying to convince: athletes and support staff, but importantly those key coaches you will need to rely on and confide in when the road gets bumpy, which it inevitably would do. As such, clear communication, selling the vision if you will, was a big part of the early workload.

For those players in the programme, I needed to make my expectations clear. The bar had been raised by Canada who were the superpower in our sport, backed by more than a million people regularly playing the sport. The level of planning, the focus on fitness, the quantity of technical training and high-level competition, were all essential but very new for many involved.

Contributory factors: the appliance of (the right) science

A lot happened very quickly with membership of the SIS programme. As with most Institutes around the world, there were lots of sports scientists and practitioners eager to offer their services. I just needed to figure out if they were there to help themselves or to genuinely help us get better. Science in curling was almost unheard of – would these guys truly make an effort to submerse themselves in the sport; to really understand how they could adapt and apply their trade for our benefit?

It was also important to recognise what would offer the biggest performance contribution. This was not a time for the 'marginal gains' approach which has been so well publicised in British Cycling. Fundamentally I knew that most of our athletes, at that time, simply didn't have the basics right. They were not technically proficient and their technique was simply not repeatable under pressure. We would be kidding ourselves if we thought that any marginal gains from nutrition, strategy, strength and conditioning, or psychology would outweigh the huge gains to be made in technique and on-ice training. They would have their place but only when the athletes could prove they had sound technique: that was and always will be the biggest and easiest gain.

There was a great temptation to shop in a free supermarket for those sport sciences but I knew I had to engage them to understand and define the impact they might have. I was always benchmarking the same question; namely, will it help my teams win more consistently at the highest level?

The first science I embraced was performance analysis. It would take the video analysis a step further and provide the factual evidence that I wanted to demonstrate an athlete's improvement in certain areas. That initial meeting was with Kenny More from Elite Sports Analysis. He showed me a video he had taken of his mother and her seniors' rink playing in a Wednesday night league at Kirkcaldy ice rink. He jokingly apologised for the standard of their play but asked me to think beyond the video and what might be the categories I would want to capture in order to measure and benchmark the attributes of a winning team. This was the thought that sparked my imagination and we quickly got him on board as a key part of the structure.

Subsequent progress and evolutions

On the face of it, the programme was extremely successful, with the Ladies Team winning gold in the 2002 Olympics in Salt Lake City. It was a fantastic medal for the girls but we didn't dominate that competition. To be honest, and Rhona (the gold medal winning skip of the team) won't mind me saying this, but at the end of our last round robin game she thought we were out. We were five wins and four losses and our destiny was now in the hands of Switzerland who we needed to win their last game, to allow us to advance to a three-way tie breaker with Sweden and Germany for the last semi-final spot. We would go on to beat Germany and Sweden for the right to play Canada, who had dominated the round robin phase with an eight wins and one loss record. Of course, having qualified, we then had two great games. I can't take that away from the girls; they were superb in the semi and the final with Rhona delivering the 'stone of destiny' at the final end to beat Switzerland. So, we were Olympic champions, but we were not dominating the world. The team had won the most important curling competition of their careers and secured the first Olympic medal for the Institute. In short, it was significant and empowered me to knock on the doors of UK sport and make a pretty good case that we were a sport worth investing in. There were a lot of challenges at that Olympics but, at the end of the day, we had taken a big step forward.

It was also really useful to demonstrate that this achievement was supported by strength in depth. We were starting to win medals at Europeans and, just six weeks after the Olympics, Jackie Lockhart and her rink won the World Championships in USA. Furthermore, she did dominate, winning seven of her nine games in the round robin before going onto to win the semi against Canada and Sweden in the final. It was clear that we didn't only have one team. The rivalry was also useful in keeping momentum and the programme moving forwards.

After the challenges experienced in Salt Lake City, we started to take a new direction. Rather than interview and select existing intact teams then perhaps 'modify' the membership, we decided to select individuals then assemble teams from the best combination of in-form players. This was a major change but one which, at face value, seemed to offer a good way forward. I think in hindsight that this approach worked to a limited extent. Crucially, however, I just believe that the chemistry and the dynamic you build up in a team can't be done overnight. Even if individuals played three or four months together, you just were not getting into the psychology and the dynamic in the team. In curling it's too easy to cover up frailties and, despite my thinking that the most talented athletes together will still beat, let's say, a hardworking team with less talent, I'm not sure that is the case ultimately.

The outcomes from the experiment were rather mixed. Going into Turin in 2006, we had a very talented men's team and the choice wasn't massively difficult. In similar fashion, with the girls we ultimately tried to pick the good players out of individual teams but they simply didn't gel. I guess the answer lay in the fact that they weren't playing together in the first place because they hadn't chosen to be teammates. They were all good players in their own right but, when push came to shove, they just didn't work together the way we'd hoped they would. So, even though at the time the case for trying this was very strong, I think selecting a team is the right way to go and you just need to put the pressure on individuals within that team. If they're not good enough they'll go by the wayside but the responsibility then is very much on the team. The approach returned to this in 2014.

This might seem like a very curling-specific issue. However, I think there are wider messages for other sports. For example, national coaches need to be willing to innovate, to try things as they look for the next edge. They also need to be honest enough to objectively and dispassionately evaluate their actions without ego involvement. If it was a poor idea, then hands up, drop it and move on. I would also highlight the importance of the psychosocial side in teams, perhaps even in squad formation. Getting the group dynamic right is important, even in individual sports and absolutely in such a high-collaboration sport as curling.

Leadership in the role: what did I bring to the party?

As my number one: a determination to be successful, whatever it took. Winning brings with it a pressure to sustain it into the future, I embraced that challenge. Winning brought good times and now gives great memories. Add to this a curiosity for innovation, a willingness to challenge the norm and an inquisitive nature. A passion for the sport and a passion to see our programme teams win at the highest level. A work ethic that would challenge all those around me and ultimately myself too. A good judge of character that got the best out of those that worked with me. In hindsight, I brought good people to the programme. No one does this themselves, but they can demand a passion to succeed from those closest to the programme. In addition, an appreciation that athletes also have a voice: they are at the cutting edge of innovation and it was they who I regularly bounced ideas off.

With regard to the style and method of leadership, there were several questions for consideration. There are many ways to lead a group, but I don't believe in the contrived: I've never read a leadership book, I take my lead from my instinct and the ability to read those around me. The ability to inspire and articulate the vision to those you intend to take on that journey to your goal. You need to be credible; that's something you create subconsciously by your actions, you can't manufacture it. Most importantly you need to be comfortable that you will be accountable and responsible for whatever outcome.

Honesty with the athletes is another essential. I may have to cut you from a team if you have not shown me you have what it takes. I may have to drop you during a Championships if your play is affecting the team adversely. I might have to call you and tell you that you were not selected for the Olympic team. However, I will treat you all the same because I want you all to fulfil your potential whatever that might be. Another factor is the ability to find enjoyment in the journey, celebrate the success with your colleagues and put into perspective the setbacks. Being passionate about anything in life means you need to ride the super highs and super lows and come out the other side unscathed.

I don't know what others perceived that I brought to the programme but those are the beliefs that I relied upon and they helped bring about a period of sustained success from 1998–2006, the highlights being, Scotland's first ever ladies World Championship winning team, Great Britain's first ever women's Olympic gold medal, and two men's World Championships winning teams.

Process markers: key innovations brought to the programme

As stated earlier, seeking and establishing positive innovation is a major element of the national coach role. Clearly, curling had a lot of room for new developments. Even with this space for development, I was very pleased with the level and quantity of new developments which the programme initiated. As a series of exemplars, these were as follows:

- Performance analysis programme – competition and training feedback.
    - We developed bespoke analysis tools to provide an evidence base for evaluation of training quality and impact.
- Sweep-ergometer.
    - Designed by the arch doyen of curling innovation Lino Di Iorio, this tool enabled the first objective examination and evaluation of sweeping, helping us to improve tools, actions and training in this crucial skill.
- Innovative practice drills.
    - Based on a critical consideration of the biopsychosocial elements of technique, we were able to develop completely original ideas for training drills, ideas which have since been communicated worldwide on the jungle telegraph.
- Use of split timers for speed control.
    - We led on the introduction of handheld timers to check on the control of stone release.
- Use of a radar gun to measure deceleration.
- Worked with curling shoe manufacturer to get the best balance and friction resistant surface to slide on.
    - Equipment innovation is now a normal feature of world class programmes. We were ahead of the game.
- Stone matching device.
    - There are only a finite number of stones used in major tournaments. We pioneered the application of analysis tools to elaborate on our data sets on these.
- Various other innovations focused on the design and conduct of elite training, programming and preparation.

My point here is not to brag about my own work; rather, I want to pay tribute to the various people who have been involved and made such significant contributions. I would also like to highlight how important a comprehensive and far-reaching programme of innovation is for anyone in the national coach role.

Moving on

Not many head coaches survive to engineer their own exit under their own terms but I lasted eight years, before admitting to myself that I was burnt out and needed a new challenge. After the earlier concerns, my feeling fuelled more uncertainty but a new chapter lay ahead. It was important to me that I left the programme in good shape, with talent in the pipeline and the confidence of our funding partners that a successful track record of achievement had been established.

Advice to others: considerations for national coaches and PDs

In closing, I thought I should offer some perceptions on my experience and learning from the role. Specifically, what others can learn and apply in the future. I see a lot of new national coaches and Performance Directors (PDs) come and some of them don't last the distance to even get to an Olympic Games for one reason or another. I think the landscape has changed a lot as well. Individuals in these roles are now under a huge amount of scrutiny, with clear responsibility allocated to them. You know where the buck stops with them. Whether that in my language is fair or not, that's the reality of it, so they are under a lot more pressure. Does it detract from what they are actually trying to do? It probably does but I think they need to be fully aware of, and prepared to face, the challenge. They are there for one reason and that is to direct performance: to get a performance out of their athletes at a Worlds or an Olympic Games. Accordingly, they need to be very careful that the finite time they have in the four years or whatever is spent trying to orchestrate that. The more distractions you have, especially if you don't have the ability to delegate, the more you need to be very careful to focus solely on exactly what is your role. So please, be very clear about the clarity of your role: be very clear with the people that you're working closest with, whether that is your head coaches or science and medicine leads, that they know exactly what your role is. Importantly, however, the last thing you want to do is to be shut out of certain areas of the programme that you're ultimately responsible for.

Reflecting this subtle and often difficult balance, I'd be very careful about abdicating responsibility in certain areas. I believe that the National Coach or Performance Director is the person who ultimately will make or break their sport. I'm sure that there are other bits and pieces and the whole role thing about what they are responsible for is broken down for them by the 'powers that be'. As one example, the amount of time you spend on these certain things. But actually, and rather concernedly, you know National Coaches and Performance Directors now need to be 'shining lights' in a whole bunch of different areas, some of which are potentially unrealistic for one guy to do. I hope that this chapter has offered some useful insights into what is a crucial but very challenging role.

4

Coaching a national team in professional football

Egil 'Drillo' Olsen with Geir Jordet

Editors' introduction

Egil Olsen is a Norwegian football coach. He has managed a series of club teams in Norway, as well as Wimbledon in England, and the national team of Iraq. However, he is probably best known for having managed the Norway national team. He did this twice, from 1990–98, and again from 2009–13. Under his management Norway reached two World Cups, in 1994 and 1998, and at one point, Norway was ranked number two in the FIFA ranking. Leading a country to these accomplishments in one of the largest sports in the world is quite an achievement, especially given that Norway has a population of around five million people, and it is mostly known for being a winter sports nation.

My role

My role was the national team coach. I was clearly a more conventional, football-oriented coach. More coach than leader, you could say: I delegated the 'leader' tasks to others, even though on paper I was technically the national team leader. When we were travelling, Per Omdal took over more of the managerial functions than I did. I was in charge of football, first and foremost.

I started this position in late autumn 1990 when I took up the job as a substitute at first. After three matches, they actually hired me. We won the first three matches and had an amazing 6-1 opener against Cameroon. Then we won 3-1 at Tunisia and took a 3-0 away victory in Cyprus. I received a job contract after that and remained in the role until 1998 when I decided to resign. I made a comeback in 2009, starting once again as a substitute, and was granted an extension until 2014. However, with only two matches left, I was fired in 2013 for a very simplistic reason. And it is not exactly a secret that I disagree with that decision.

What we did in the 1990s was undoubtedly a success. Perhaps my second period as national coach may not have been quite as positive because there were a couple of losses at the end, but the fact is that in terms of results, that period was only slightly worse than the 1990s. So, when I'm giving lectures about this, I often start by saying that I'm the second-best national team coach that Norway has ever had. Then they ask, "Oh yeah? But who's the best?" I answer that

I am. I'm number one and two, if you look at all the national team coaches and look purely at their results and nothing else. So, the 1990s were the best period, and my second time in the role, the second best. After that, Nils Johan Semb would be number three, Åge Hareide number four, and then I'm not sure after that.

Philosophy of work

My football philosophy is based on a very tight and thorough zonal defence. Offensively, I am in favour of a forward-oriented, direct playing style. In addition, I am very conscientious about doing a thorough analysis of our own strengths and weaknesses; collectively, structurally, and individually. The same goes for our opponents. That was probably one of the areas where we were far ahead of most of our opponents, in the depth of our analysis. There they caught up with us a long time ago, but in the 1990s we were quite clearly advanced in that area. Thorough analysis of your own team isn't very difficult, you could more or less work on that continuously, but we were also good at collecting data from opponents and running analyses of them as well. And with this information we'd then set up a tactic that naturally utilised our strengths to the utmost extent, whilst also trying to target the opponents' weaknesses. But the foundation we used was always a zonal defence, which I still feel is stronger than a man-marking defence. Nowadays nobody is playing a clean marking defence anymore, but when we look at the highest level, I notice that the admission to marking in the midfield is quite large in some teams. While in the back defensive four, they tend to be zonal-oriented in the rest of the world. We were early at that too. In the 1990s there weren't many other than us who played the clean zonal defence, if there were any others at all. Other countries followed eventually; Germany, the Netherlands, and Italy came a long time after. They played with marking and sweepers long after we had switched to the pure zonal defence. We were certainly ahead of the game there, probably almost first in the world at this point. Not the national team, but George Curtis came to manage Rosenborg in 1969 and practically experimented with a clean zonal defence. Nils Arne Eggen (a highly successful Rosenborg BK manager) told me that he thought it was Curtis and a gang in the FA (The English Football Association) who in theory chiseled out the rules of the zonal defence, and when he came to Rosenborg he ended up with the most amazing goal difference ever. The Rosenborg goal difference in 1970 was 15-5. We are not talking about after five matches, but when the league had ended. 15-5. It was, nonetheless, only ten teams and 18 matches. It dropped like a bomb: "Wow, is it possible to play defence that way?" No one marks, nobody follows people, we just move around here and look at each other. Let in five goals in 18 matches. Amazing. And this was around the time that I started my coaching career. I started in 1970 and thought this was incredibly exciting. Then a lot of academics emerged, with Kjell Schou-Andreassen, Tor Røste Fossen, Nils Arne Eggen, and me. We made a lot of mistakes but learned quickly. The Swedes came along with Gunder Bengtsson and Sven-Göran Eriksson, who had great success with IFK Gothenburg. And so we were very early in Scandinavia, in terms of our zonal defence. We were inspired by the English and the FA, but we caught on before most of the others.

Through my career, I slowly became more focused on the offence. My forward-oriented, direct playing style has gained a bit of a bad reputation not least because it has been linked to long passing, but that's not completely fair. There was a reason why we used the long pass so often. I started by saying that we did a thorough analysis of our strengths and opponents' strong and weak sides and we often met teams which individually were better than us, with better skills. Furthermore, especially against good opponents, the long pass was effective because then you avoid good counter attack opportunities for the opponent. We also systematised the long pass more and more when we hit the long pass towards Jostein Flo (centre-forward/right-winger, 192 cm tall and very strong duel-player), so we always had players to support, and eventually also players running behind the duel. It's a bold move because you have to push many players high up in the field, and as soon as they learned to defend against Jostein, they often moved into his body. The ball would often then travel over the duel, into the space behind them, where we had Erik Mykland or another player who often got possession. We also often had a player between the duel and the opponent's goalkeeper. This was efficient and easy, but it cost a lot, above all a lot of running. We ran a lot and that's another principle that has been a priority for me: extreme, but imbalanced skill sets. To select players who were very strong at one thing, yet limited in many other areas. Jostein Flo was a great example of this with his dueling power in the air, and then you have creative players like Erik Mykland and Lars Bohinen. There were also players such as Øyvind Leonardsen and Roar Strand who were enduring and strong run-ners; who had everything. What I missed a little was speed up front, but at the same time I definitely had speed in the back. This meant that we could push up high for long periods where we allowed a lot of space behind our own defence, especially so with Ronny Johnsen and Rune Bratseth whom no one ran away from. But something I might have been missing were wingers that were extremely fast. I had Jahn Ivar "Mini" Jakobsen who I used a little, but he was not as fast as he seemed. Although Mini's legs went fast, and he told me (bearing in mind, he was also the team clown) that when we were warming up – and we often practised progressive speed runs – "I always make sure I stay as far away from Rune Bratseth as possible".

When it comes to offence, I'm in favour of quickly going forward. I believe that teaching players to evaluate balance/imbalance is very important. We wanted to make sure that every time we won the ball in open play, the first thought was to counterattack, but not at any price. If you receive the ball facing your own goal and your opponent is in full balance there is no point to immediately counterattack. But if we win the ball facing the opponent's goal and we can play it forward on the first touch, there is a very big chance that the opponent is imbalanced. The opponent is quite often in a state of weak imbalance; gross imbalance is the exception and is rare. Not to mention numerical imbalance, which is also rare. But weak imbalance can and does happen often. We tried to seize those opportunities every time, and this led of course to us often losing the ball and rarely having the ball more than the opponent. In those days we didn't have access to possession stats like we do now, but I'm pretty sure we rarely had the most possession. If we were going to compare to how things are today, we would have looked a lot like Leicester did when they became the English Premier League champions having been third from the bottom in terms of possession, and last place on pass completion (which is measured as the pass going to a teammate or an opponent). Of course we played very differently against San Marino than we did against Brazil; the entire time we analysed the opponent and what they were up to. Playing your own game independently of the opponent is one of the stupidest things I hear, because that's what football is all about; doing what is right based on what the opponent does. I think we were good at that. We had discussions about it too, because we had players who were skeptical. Not directly opposed to what we were doing, but skeptical. It's a bit typical of the creative players who were there, Bohinen, and especially Mykland. Mykland really understood football, and we could discuss things with him constructively, he wasn't hard to work with. We even had some matches where he was almost forbidden to play the ball backwards, and I would almost say that those are among the best matches he ever played because he would usually dribble off two to three players and end up hitting a backwards support pass, thus creating nothing. What's the point then, right? Even though the audience cheers and thinks it's great. Not the zonal defence, but the extreme forward-oriented direct playing style was foreign to many. It was also foreign to many in my second period as head coach. I struggled a bit more then, because I had some players in clubs that were quite passing-oriented. It was easier in the 1990s, but of course, with wins 6-1, 3-1, 3-0 in the first three matches, you'll get a flying start.

The players were aware that if they did not adapt they would not have been selected. I even told Bohinen that the goal he scored against Italy at Ullevål was not his style; it is he who wins the ball, goes straight on, and dribbles past two opponents. Most of the players accepted this so there were very few objections.

Certainly, there were some players who in those days were good enough for Rosenborg in the Champions League, but never really made it in my team. Ørjan Berg and Bent Skammelsrud are examples of this. And the same goes for Ståle Solbakken. These players had an even capacity profile, in that they were pretty good at everything. They were prominent on their club teams, and got to play national matches under me as well, but not very many. I didn't pick many such players, I think due to my preference for players with uneven capacity profiles; those who were more extreme in their talent when it came to one or a few specific skills. These players were very good at some things but similarly bad at others. I used Øyvind Leonardsen more like a running machine that had clear limits offensively with the ball, but proved invaluable to us in the way we played. We drilled the back four a lot in training, played 6 versus 4. Like I said, this was an exercise we had before every match, 6 versus 4. It was extraordinary how much more the four struggled when Leonardsen was one of the six. He was constantly heading towards the back of the defence, and when the player in possession had a little space, he would then be just about to pass the offside line. When you are 6 versus 4 it is very easy to simply roll the ball to the next teammate because you always have an available player, and you become less forward-oriented as a result. But we drilled it a lot and we often talked about how being skilled in the back four was a bit like learning how to ride a bike; once you can do it, you can do it. But to do it successfully, it must be repeated over and over.

Against an established and fully balanced defence, you either choose to play the long pass towards Jostein Flo or look for players in the space between their two back lines. In that moment you have created the imbalance, there is no question anymore. Then you just have to go for it. If you make it, you make it. Next you have to get a shot at goal as soon as possible. So, we worked with this. If imbalance was created then we would at least make it so that opponents would struggle to fully regain their balance. This approach causes you to lose the ball relatively often, but you create goal chances. This was especially true when we met opponents who clearly were not up to our standard individually. In these cases, we would capitalise on this a lot. Meeting San Marino at Ullevål, I remember, we just hit it long towards Flo, moved people high up in the field, and won the ball after the duel or when they tried to clear it. Just after this I watched San Marino play against Turkey, the match ended 0-0, though possession I would say was probably 90-10 or at the very least 80-20. "0-0, this is how we will not do it", I thought. We have seen many times that players can become very pass-oriented, because it's so easy. It is in these cases when you lose the forward orientation.

Key empirical studies

For me, this started with Charles Reep and his research. He is considered the father of match analysis. I got to know him after a while and you cannot talk football with him as he was an army guy. As a researcher, he started with paper and pencil and has completed now roughly 3000 matches. I also became very well acquainted with one of his disciples, Richard Pollard, who has written some books together with Charles. Reep had a hypothesis that the team who got the ball most times into the opponent's 'scorebox' would win the match. But, as I said, he wasn't very into football like that in general, and I don't think he knew the difference between zonal defence and marking defence. In fact, I don't think Reep had any knowledge at all about defence organisation.

With respect to defence, the bulk of this research comes from Curtis and the Swedes. While theories of offence are basically based on Charles Reep's research, who is well known in England, his work is controversial. He's almost seen as the origin of 'kick and run' football; just transport the ball forward and run after it. In certain contexts, and at certain levels, this may have once been a smart approach, but football has evolved, and a forward-oriented team – where the ball is quickly moved forward – is a pleasure to watch. I think the tendency is there in many teams to be forward-oriented, but I watch so much Spanish football and would argue that the Spanish league is perhaps most forward-oriented of the big leagues. Only a few teams in La Liga are to a certain extent possession-oriented, but as with any league there are some exceptions. With Atletico Madrid in the lead, and Real Madrid and Barcelona behind them, these teams have changed significantly compared to what they were during the grandeur of Guardiola. Guardiola has also changed to become more forward-oriented. By comparison, I'm disappointed with the professional league here in Norway. I think there are teams here that are more passing-oriented than in the best leagues.

It's not just about banging the ball up and in, because you should preferably have control as well. In these terms it's certainly not clear whether Charles Reep's findings mean that the overall smartest thing to do is to knock the ball up there at any cost. Particularly in the counterattack phase, we are talking about progressing the ball forward, quickly, and along the grass; keeping the ball central as long as possible so you have more opportunities compared to if you are on the sideline. These are important principles. There are no two counter attacks that are exactly the same. Football is so diverse. We maybe worked more than our opponent with the principle of movement. I do not forget my comeback match against Germany in 2009 (Norway won 1-0, away). I had this to say to Daniel Braaten, "If you intercept the ball going forward, don't you dare start running forward", "But isn't that what we're supposed to be doing?", he said. "No", I replied, "You're going to sprint. That's something completely different". I remember the game very well, Braaten played one of his best matches ever against Germany. If you have a counter attack option, then you must take it. There is nothing controversial about that. It was more difficult to do it against an established defence, when you got the good pass that created the little imbalance, and then be able to complete it. You also see internationally that there are many who do not grab that opportunity. They just play a support pass and give their opponent the opportunity to regain balance. This is especially true when you play against a team with a lot of individual skill. But we were very rarely in that position, when we had an opponent in imbalance then we had to seize the chance. You win some and you lose some, and I believe we won more than we lost. What you lose is ball possession, and I do not think that mattered so much. Many people believed that you should control the game and that it is an advantage to have the ball a lot. But this belief has been challenged a bit after Leicester's recent success, and for the first time in history, most of the matches in a European championship tournament (Euro 2016) were won by the team with the least ball possession. 19 against 15; there were 34 games that had a victor, and of these 19 games were won by the team who had the ball the least.

Match analytics

A community was developed in Norway by Jan Tunli and his people. Øyvind Larsen and I were also centrally involved. Tunli was no football man either, he was a researcher and computer expert. We came up with tips for him and then that tool (called Interplay) was developed and has received recognition far beyond Norway's borders from what I understand. In this regard, we were early leaders on the analysis front. I myself spent an insane amount of time watching videos. It was like a whole new world as after time we could use this to run player analyses as well. An example of how valuable these analyses could be was our DOMP analysis, which was a very simple form of analysis where we counted different types of actions in a match for each player. D stands for the number of defensive positives, O for offensive positives, M for the number of misses, and P for the number of passing errors. A player could see the analysis for themselves and if they saw something and thought that it couldn't be right, I could go in and show them. For us this was a whole new world. I especially remember the France World Cup in 1998 after we had played 1-1 against Scotland. At the time it was very clear that neither Vidar Riseth nor Håvard Flo understood the role of defensive winger and they broke with the plan time after time. As a result, we really struggled in the second half, and so we spent an awful lot of time going through these things with the players. It worked so well in training that I actually chose to start with both of them in the crucial match against Brazil (where Norway won 2-1, and with this score qualified to the round of 16), although both were substituted out after a while. This example is a good illustration of how video clearly helped us to beat Brazil. It was an approach which was new and I doubt that others were using analysis in the same way at the time.

Leadership and communication

I have never really been too concerned with leadership and communication. People ask me about management philosophy and I'm almost inclined to say I do not have one. I've in a way just always been myself and have been more focused on football itself, the style of play and those things than anything else, and less concerned about people for sure. I have seen that coaches can be divided into those who are human-oriented and those who are content-oriented, and I slowly, surely but surely – at least in the second period – became more human-oriented than I was in my first period as head coach. In this first period, I often had a very special player group in the sense that I had seven to eight players, all of whom could be the captain. I simply didn't have that in the second period. And maybe this becomes clearer when we see what has become of them since the 1990s; more or less all of the players in that former group have become leaders and coaches.

That said, I have always been very focused on feedback, and if in any way I have a strong point as a leader, I think that's where it lies. I was very concrete. All players received feedback after all matches, though unfortunately they did not get it until the next match because when the match ends, most players disappear back to their clubs. However, they did receive a DOMP analysis and in my second period it was mandatory that they look at and review the analysis with either me or Ola By Rise (my assistant coach). At least once a year I had a good solid conversation with each player about their strong and weak sides; about their ambition level and such things. I remember before my first match against Cameroon at Bislett, I also had a proper conversation with each player. I spent a lot of time, hours even, going through the principles and persuading players to try to play that way.

I did not have a conversation with each player at every single national team gathering, but in reality it was probably not that far off. I spent a lot of time on feedback and spent that time well, utilising every bus trip on our way to training. I always sat in the first row of the bus with a player and gave feedback. I never ever sat alone, I always used the time maximally. That was something a little special about me because my strong side was so concrete. I would tell the players, "This is what you're bad at", but that wasn't to be a jerk, it was because I wanted them to be better. I could be quite tough with many of the players without it becoming a problem, with respect to negative feedback. In lectures I give, I use this as an example that players are different. Some like a pat on the back and be told how good they are, but I experienced something after the Cameroon match. When the game ended, I told a player that "You played damn well". Then I got the answer: "What was not good enough?" That was Rune Bratseth (who moved on to play 230 matches for Werder Bremen in the Bundesliga and was for the most part my captain for Norway up until the World Cup in 1994). Some players are more concerned with the negative feedback: what's not good enough.

When it comes to feedback, I give both positive and negative feedback, plus I'm probably a bit of a people person after all. I know who would rather receive the positive feedback, then there are some others who'd love to take the negative. People are different. So, I do not know if I give more of one or the other (plus / minus), but we got both, and the DOMP analysis was very good for that as well.

Overall, my focus as coach wasn't really on leadership when it came to the support staff. In both of my terms in the role I simply took over those who were already there, which is unlike most others in a similar position who are generally very focused on creating or bringing their own staff. Per-Mathias Høgmo is a great example of someone who threw out everything that was there and brought in only new people. In the beginning I had Arne Larsen Økland and we worked perfectly together, but we were probably a bit too similar. We shared the same strong and weak sides. Bjørn Hansen, who came after, complimented me a little better than Arne. Arne was also like me, first and foremost focused on the football content, and together we would discuss tactics and playing principles; while Hansen was more people-oriented and concerned with some other things. It was an important difference. I believe in a relatively small and competent support staff, and I can see that Lars Lagerback (the current Norwegian National Team Coach) agrees. If there are too many people in a support staff to relate to, I think it is difficult for the players as well. This is more a gut feeling that I have, rather than anything based on evidence. I was also a little skeptical about having a so-called mental coach, but Høgmo really wanted one. I think that for individual players this may be useful, but if someone has to have responsibility for an entire group's mental approach, then no, I'm not quite sure about that. This is certainly also because I have never been very concerned with the mental side. That said, I have also acknowledged that I could have had some help in this regard after we beat Brazil in 1998, because I know from experience that it's very easy to drop a bit after a big and important victory. Despite me being very aware of this, we did not do better because we had a relatively bad match against Italy in the round of 16 – actually against a pretty poor Italian team. They would have been possible to beat, but we didn't manage it, probably because I lacked something right at the time.

When it came to communication with the media, that was not a strength of mine. I was poorly guided, unprepared, and my relationship with the media was up and down. I did not consistently have a good relationship with the media. I quickly found out, that if a half-truth sells better than a truth, the truth is chanceless. I experienced that quite a few times. And so I did have some bad experiences with the media, but I more or less learned to deal with it.

Competing with and beating bigger nations

I often competed against nations that had bigger football traditions than we have, and who had five, ten, 15 or 20 times as many people as we have. We are a small nation, of just over five million people. In presentations I give, I tend to ask the audience if they know how many countries have more people than Norway. Of course, nobody knows, but if we consider first that the UN has a total of 193 members, and there are 70 states, as well as one independent state in the world that is not a member of the UN, Vatican City. So, then in total there are 194 states.

When I watch National Geographic, they also include Taiwan, which is not a member of the UN. China has not recognised them, but they are considered an independent state, so the total becomes 195. Of these 195, Norway is in 112th/113rd place with respect to population size.

What makes football so fantastic is that you can compensate for a lack of individual skills by being better collectively, simply by being smarter. It is possible to hide your own weaknesses, whilst maximising strengths. I believe football is special in that way. A fourth division team in basketball doesn't beat a top team. I don't think it's possible. But it can happen in football. Probably because football is bigger. It is more diverse. Multiple players, bigger surface and, not least, fewer goals.

If a coach can and is good at incorporating a solid zonal defence, I can't see that anything will go wrong. But of course it is possible. Even at a damn high level, perhaps fortunately, there can suddenly be a full-back that slacks and thus destroys an offside. So, there are things that may go wrong, but that also applies to a marking-oriented team. I do notice that there currently are many teams that give relatively large concessions to marking in the midfield because they track the other players around a bit. But I cannot see that it is more effective than playing a clean zonal defence. Offensively, it has a lot to do with individual skills. Of course, you can play in a possession-focused manner and take it all the way, and profit on it, but then you must be better than the opponent individually, and both physically and technically you'll have to have the upper hand. I found out that when we met a good opponent, we struggled to create goal chances against an established defence. When we used the long ball, there was often a regaining of possession, and then it was no longer established.

We didn't have one style that we implemented regardless; our style was chosen in relation to the opponent. If we met a team that gave away lots of space behind their back four, we would play differently than if we met an opponent who tended to sit low with little space behind their defensive line. So, we would have to adapt all the way, and it's a smart approach to take. It is hard to argue against the idea that one should find the best way to play in relation to an opponent. You can certainly also be too rigid if you're going to play forward-oriented, always direct, regardless of the situation. It is situation-oriented all the way, but I see the biggest contradiction in the offensive game today as the relationship between possession and a forward-oriented style. And there are big differences. Not only between the countries, but also in the same league as well. You have the extremes in Spain, where you have both approaches. And in that league, you can also see that some of the most possession-oriented clubs are relegated, with Las Palmas in the lead.

5

Doing it week in, week out

Dean Smith with Andrew Cruickshank

Editors' introduction

After a long career in professional football, playing nearly 600 games for Walsall, Hereford United, Leyton Orient, Sheffield Wednesday, and Port Vale, Dean started his career in coaching after retiring in 2005. Starting out as a youth coach and then assistant manager at Leyton Orient, followed by the head of youth role at Walsall FC, Dean then moved into a managerial role with Walsall FC, who were in the third tier of the English football league. Reflecting his level of achievement with Walsall, Dean led the team to the final of the League Trophy and, at the time of his move to become head coach of Brentford FC in 2015, was the fourth longest-serving manager in the English football league. After successfully guiding Brentford to tenth then ninth placed finishes in the Championship, the tier below the Premier League, Dean then moved on to become head coach at another Championship – and recent Premier League – club, Aston Villa FC, in October 2018.

Based on his experience to date, this chapter presents Dean's views on working week in, week out in professional football. Specifically, these views firstly cover the overall roles and responsibilities for a team's head coach or manager, as well as the specific outcomes that Dean aims to deliver in his work (please note that 'head coach' and 'manager' are often used interchangeably in UK football, but that 'head coach' tends to indicate that the individual's balance of activities includes more 'hands-on coaching'). Secondly, Dean's views on how he works to deliver his intended outcomes are offered. From here, the third section then looks at one particularly important phase for a head coach: understanding and shaping expectations on starting a new job. Finally, the chapter concludes by looking at how consistency – both in terms of actions and messages – can work to drive longer-term success.

Overall role and responsibilities

As the manager of Walsall FC, my role was everything: to an extent, the Chairman said "there's the budget, now do the best you can with us". Originally it was to keep us in League 1 (the third tier of the English pyramid), then, as progress was made, it was to climb the league and then get promoted to the Championship (second tier of the English pyramid). However, rather than just coaching the players and the team, my role at Walsall also involved a range of other responsibilities, given the limited number of staff involved in running the football department. For example, it included things like doing the majority of scouting for players, negotiating with their agents, and negotiating with current players on their bonuses. Perhaps because of that, and the Chairman's involvement in day-to-day decision-making, I've always treated a club's money like my own – for the team and myself to be successful, I have to make the most out of that money.

In contrast to my role with Walsall, I became a head coach at Brentford and had two sporting directors directly above me; both of whom acted as the more formal link between the football department and the club's CEO and ownership. This structure is also reflected in the organisation at my current club, Aston Villa. In comparison to Walsall, my more recent jobs have therefore been more targeted at coaching the players, or at least coaching with fewer 'outside' responsibilities: trying to make them better, trying to win games each week. In this respect, I've had more help on the training ground as I've moved from club-to-club. You end up doing everything at smaller clubs with fewer resources and facilities – bigger clubs have more staff and specialists, which takes some pressure off and allows you to put more time into the players. Roughly speaking, I had around six staff working alongside me at Walsall, 30 at Brentford, and now 50 at Villa; so, for example, the sporting director at Villa will deal with the head of recruitment so that I can devote more of my time to the main aspects of my job (i.e., coaching players). In contrast, by the time that I had driven to training at Walsall, I could have already spoken to the Chairman, the CEO, a potential new player, and their agent before even designing the actual training session for that morning!

On reflection, that's probably been one of the biggest changes in the game recently in England: the person responsible for the team's performance has seen their role become more specific rather doing everything. We're now looking more at a European-style structure, with a 'CEO-sporting director-head coach' model, rather than the 'owner/CEO-team manager' model that has dominated the game in the UK to date. Of course, this step means that there is a certain vulnerability now, or at least a different vulnerability, as before there was a straight voice to the owner(s); now it's going through layers and there are less opportunities to get to the owner(s). But, that said, the 'new model' does allow the head coach to really set a focus on how the club is going to play in terms of style against a longer-term plan. With this remit, I've also been able to play a role in building clubs on a bigger scale – developing a vision on how we are going to play going forward, all the way from Under 23s down. In this respect, the most important thing for a head coach is the day-to-day work with the players, especially those who will play in the first team that week: you need to get them on the pitch ready to play for themselves first and then for you second. Ultimately, this will be based on how well you have coached them and how well you have dealt with them management-wise; because if they perform for themselves consistently then you've got a chance longevity-wise.

In this sense, I think that 'coaching' is mainly on the 'green stuff'. The 'management' side of my role is the conversations, the 'pats on the back', bringing players in and making them feel comfortable. Given the balance of my work, I think that players and staff perhaps see me as a coach who manages: 50% of my job is coaching, 50% is managing. The coaching sets the style of play for the first team and throughout the club, but you're always managing people. More broadly, you are perhaps coaching players more than you manage them, and managing staff more than you coach them; but it's difficult to separate. Either way, one vital requirement is that you know what you're trying to achieve with all of those you work with.

Outcomes of my work: what I try to deliver

When it comes to working with players, one of my main objectives is to support their ability to make consistently good decisions as, in every competitive game, they will make key decisions every second that they are on the pitch. Significantly, this ability also needs to be developed so that it can delivered under pressure. Tied in with these decision-making skills, I also want players to become leaders and take responsibility for all aspects of their performance. As one particular example, an area that is often overlooked in professional football is around set-pieces: I still don't understand how players struggle to go with six corner-kicks compared to the number of plays that American footballers and rugby players can remember! Perhaps this reflects a problem in the industry where we've done too much for them and, arguably, still do too much for them.

In this sense, one general challenge in professional football is most players' reliance on agents: not too long ago, if you weren't playing then you went to see the manager or the coach, but now you go to the agent and they, more often than not, tell you how good you are rather than helping you to learn or develop. In my view, agents should work for the players, not the other way around: agents should advise rather than tell, but they've become more and more powerful in dictating what players do (including, sometimes, refusing to play in order to force a transfer to another team, or not signing a new contract to hang on for a better deal). Building on this theme, my own goal is to help players to take responsibility for all aspects of their approach and lives. I'm a big believer that you take every day into match-day and I want players to be in total control of their future; including knowing what to eat, when to eat, how to recover, how to sleep. In short, all of the things that come into being a professional athlete.

In terms of the staff within the football department, my goal is to help these individuals to achieve or sustain excellence in their jobs so that they can be a constant driver to players; especially when confidence has dipped after a bad game, or run of bad games. I want the staff to be able to help others to start again and be persistent in making players better. I also want staff around me who want to get better and better because they'll push me as well.

Delivering the outcomes: key processes and skills

While a number of processes and skills are important for delivering these outcomes with players and staff, some do tend to stand out a bit more than others in my experience to date. More specifically, these are: *managing and engaging the person, longer and shorter-term planning, prioritising the fundamentals*, and *teaching, stimulating, and challenging players*. Each of these will now be described in detail.

Managing and engaging the person

In terms of *managing and engaging the person*, this relates to my work with players but also the wider group of stakeholders involved in the running and performance of a team. With a player-lens, managing the person is always the biggest thing: you're dealing with 18 to 35-year olds, effectively young human beings who are a bit vulnerable as they all want to be the best they can be. Of course, all players are different and you become part-psychologist to try and get the best out of them: recognising who needs a prod and who needs an arm round the shoulder. Fundamentally though, all players want to know the truth: if you're not playing them, tell them why not. In line with this, my door is always open to speak to players openly and honestly.

Of course, they can then agree or disagree but, crucially, they have now got a choice: they can mope around the training ground or go out and work hard to get back in the team. So, while you can't make them do anything, you can always help players to see what their choices are. Similarly, it's also important to value members of the coaching and support staff as I do think that many football clubs, in general, prioritise the recruitment and salary of the manager or head coach over helping staff members to become better (or be paid better). Indeed, one of the biggest problems that clubs have is the retention of good staff.

With regards to those beyond the player and staff group, all other individuals involved need to feel valued too – from cleaners, to chefs, to the CEO, and owners, it's amazing what that can do for a place. You're aiming to create a culture and environment where people *want* to work, as I think everyone in professional football wants to get better and be successful. If you have people coming in every day who feel like they're getting better and pushing themselves and testing themselves to be better then I think it makes it a better place to work. Of course, the easiest relationships to keep valuing are those you see day-to-day. Therefore, contact with those you see less often needs a slightly different approach: you need to be more proactive. For example, I speak to the owner after every game: it's their money and so they deserve to know why you made certain decisions at certain times, or why you picked a team for a certain game. As well as sharing the reasons behind your decisions, you've also got to continually find out what's making them tick. Most of those who own or lead entire clubs are successful business people who are football supporters. So, while there are lots more layers to get your voice to the owner at the higher levels of the modern game, you've got to find a way to make them feel part of it at a team-level because they're the ones that pay up.

Longer- and shorter-term planning

Moving on to *longer- and shorter-term planning*, I've always interviewed clubs when they've interviewed me as I need to know that there's a plan and strategy for how the club, as a whole, is moving forward. Without this in place, it is extremely difficult to achieve a level of consistency with a team in a year or so, which is about the average tenure for a head coach in the English leagues at the moment. In terms of working in the football department after your appointment, plans need to be made on a number of levels: from the plan for pre-season, to the plans for blocks of games during the season, to the plan for the immediate week.

Regarding the pre-season plan, this is perhaps the most important given that this is the time to really get your biggest ideas across. It has to be aligned to your style of play: here are the physical markers of what we need, tactically this is what we need, analytically this is what we need, and you have to bring all of these strands together to set you up for the season ahead (which, in the Championship, usually involves one but often two games per week). The importance of this plan is evidenced by the fact that work starts on it from January (around four months before the end of the current season), including a consideration of when the players will return from their break, where to travel for camps, and which teams to play in friendlies.

Beyond this major block of planning, during the season we work to six-week plans, which are shaped by principles of effective recovery and preparation to get players to their optimum on match day. As mentioned, games come thick and fast in the Championship; so much so that, at the time of my interview for this chapter, I've been at Villa for four weeks but have only had seven days on the training ground. As a result, the up-front periodisation of training is crucial; based on, among other things, physical, psychological, and logistical factors (e.g., whether you need to fly, take a bus, or have a hotel stay before away games). Importantly, players always have sight of the next two weeks at any given time to help with the organisation of their personal lives.

Prioritising the fundamentals

Despite the number of factors and people involved in the running and performance of a profes- sional football team, it is also important that all of your plans and activities help you in *prioritising the fundamentals*. For example, players are the most important group in any club and you can never lose sight of that: you need to provide them with the best information, support, and time so that they can be at their best. So, although everybody wants a bit of your time across the staff group – which is entirely appropriate – you need to find or make time to speak to players. Also, although your plans might be established for the next block of games, I've always found it important to focus on the next game as you can't look too far ahead in what is a 'week-to- week', 'game-to-game' world. Similarly, a certain amount of basics have to run throughout the training plan and coaching sessions: you've got maintain the cycle of 'learn, revisit, re-learn' so that the fundamentals of our approach are engrained and some of the pressure is alleviated on match-day: it shouldn't be forgotten that the basics of the game are still to score more in their goal than they score in your goal!

Teaching, stimulating, and challenging players

Linked to the cycle of 'learn, revisit, and re-learn', the ability to teach and educate is also crucial as I believe that we, as coaches and support staff, are teachers: we're passing on experiences and ideas on how to approach and play the game. The players are the ones who make decisions on the pitch and so you have to give them responsibility for their performance and learning. In this way, I get the players involved an awful lot and ask a lot of questions – I ask them and I want them to ask me. Coaching is also now a lot more 'in the classroom' as well as on the training pitch: for example, at Villa I've changed the name of the analysis zone to the learning zone, and all players can be coached after the training session using video and other tools. In this sense, the role of the analyst in professional football has also got bigger because players want and expect more feedback – which has perhaps come from changes in schooling where kids tend to be asked and involved in their learning more than in the past. More broadly, I also try to keep an eye on trends and set up wider learning, with education on social media and sport psychology seeming to be particularly relevant moving forwards. In this respect, one of the biggest chal- lenges in the modern game is social media: most players tend to be impressionable young men and it's so much easier now for supporters – and other people – to give their opinions that can affect the players psychologically.

I also want the players to learn to become leaders and, importantly, for leaders to create more leaders than followers. As one way to achieve this, at Brentford I asked the players to vote for the captain for each game. If you have a set captain then the manager and coaches tend to gravitate towards them to get messages to the players but, in effect, you're then overlooking a lot of players in the squad; players who could learn to become a leader, or a better leader, but never do because they don't get the opportunity. At Brentford, I also took part in reviews and appraisal processes with the sporting directors at the same time – with them providing feedback to me and me to them so that we could learn and progress together.

As well as introducing or shaping certain processes and activities, long-term learning and progress is best supported by an environment that stimulates and challenges players and staff on a daily basis. For example, one of the biggest recent changes in professional football has been in sport science. However, while data from heart rate monitors and GPS are useful and can give you evidence to support what your eyes see, they can also place limits on what players think they are capable of. In this sense, I don't think we can put limits on players as you never know what they can do. I've yet to see a player carried off a pitch exhausted: how do we know what they're able to do unless we've really pushed them? Many measures that we use from a sport science view often reflect what a player is *currently* able to deliver; not their *potential* to deliver something even better in the future. As such, I'm very reluctant to put limits on players and try to find ways to continually challenge them. For example, one of the things we've done at Villa is to put the players' data on public display (e.g., numbers of sprints, volume of high-speed running, distance covered). They're all competitive so they'll see someone in the same position as them and try to outperform them. Keeping things fresh when doing your week-to-week coaching plan is also important as if the players get bored then you're gone as a coaching team. It's vital to give them stimulation to help them keep getting better; especially those who grasp things quickly.

Building a base: understanding and shaping expectations from appointment

Of course, it is important to recognise that the processes and skills described in the previous section are all general features of my approach to the head coach role. To get to the point where these processes and skills have maximum effect, you need to have built a base to work from. In this way, handling the initial phase of your time with a new club is crucial for the head coach.

Significantly, this initial phase actually starts before you're appointed into the role. More specifically, being aware of expectations before you take on a job at a new club is one of the most important steps. In fact, if I've got one piece of advice for others working as, or aspiring to be head coaches or managers, then clarifying the expectations placed on you from the club is essential to then go and work comfortably – including whether the focus is results or performances, because there's a difference in these two that owners and top management sometimes don't see.

From this point, first impressions with players and staff are crucial and you need to shape the perceptions that people have of you as soon as you can. In your first meetings you need to get your message across straight away: "this is how I work; this is what I expect of you; this is what you can expect of me; the door is always open." While you have an idea of what the players can do before you come in, it's also important to reassure them that they have got a clean slate and you are a fresh pair of eyes. Additionally, when you move clubs you tend to inherit staff rather than bring them in from your prior club now. As such, you also need to deliver a similar message and, in particular, form a good relationship with your heads of department because they're going to feed what you want down into their areas. Finding out the politics is also essential: what they are; how you need to play them; who's close with who; and who's not close with who. In line with this, I always find out the staff structure early on: I want to know whether I'm a line manager of someone or whether they can go straight to the CEO – it's important to know where people are going. It's also important to give all staff an opportunity to perform as you need them to, especially as they may be better than what you've had at your prior club.

That said, if you do have someone that you feel you can't work with then you need to address it straight away, and by doing it in the right way through treating them with respect. Later on, you might have players who don't agree with your approach or tactics for a specific game, or people in the dressing room who just don't like you. If you feel that they've got the power to recruit then you have to get them out as, if they do recruit, the tide might turn in the dressing room all of a sudden. All it takes is one player on a Whatsapp group to say that they should be playing instead of someone else for things to turn. So a way to set expectations is by your decisiveness – especially in any early challenges; and while I try to be inclusive from the off, I'm not scared to make calls that will create the best environment moving forwards.

A key mechanism for the long run: consistency, consistency, consistency!

Having built a base to work from, much of the long-term success of a head coach or manager, in my eyes, comes down to consistency: more specifically, consistency in how you act as an individual and consistency in how the department works as a whole. In this sense, any new head coach has an impact straight away purely from being different to the old head coach – that's just the nature of it. So, whoever you are, you can have an instant impact; but then the longevity comes from the consistency of your approach and messages that you build within the club. In this respect, values mean nothing unless they are lived consistently, every minute of every hour of every day. If someone off the street walked into the club they should 'see it, hear it, feel it' – and if they don't then we still need to work on the culture.

For example, I'm not results-oriented with players: any professional team is focused on winning and I believe that it's the performance level that becomes the factor in winning regularly. Players can't control results as there are so many outside variables; all you can do is affect your performance and the performance of your teammates – then it becomes a chain whereby the performance will come good and the results will come good. In line with this, I always guarantee players that there will be mistakes before we play any game, but what they can control is what they do next and recognise that better players move on from mistakes quicker than others. Of course, a key factor in delivering a consistent approach and message comes from having a consistent staff. As such, heads of department need constant clarity on what's being done and why: if, for example, a physio agrees that a player should be playing then you're struggling. So I'll always ask staff for their opinions and encourage debate as I think that's healthy; and when we have made a decision then that's *our* decision – whether that decision originated with me or one of my assistants or someone else.

Another major factor in the consistency of your environment is the role of the media. In fact, one of the most important things that you ever do is speak to the media after a game: if you think cleverly enough about what's going to come, you can then set the dialogue rather than react to it. First of all, the message I want to get out to the media is a message I want to get to the players, then the fans, as they deserve to know what we're doing. Fans can clearly influence the game: if they're behind the team, they can make the players more confident; if they're vociferous, it can affect the players the other way. Complicating the challenge is that the post-match media are very reactive, based on the result, and your dialogue has to come 15 minutes after a highly emotive event (which is very different to media interactions before the game, when you have more time to prepare what you're going to say and anticipate the kind of questions you're going to get). Overall, however, the media can offer an important route for getting a consistent message out to lots of people.

Reflected in my approach with the media, a key expectation that I place on myself is being consistent in what I do, but also being consistent with myself. As I see it, there isn't 'one-way to be' as a head coach but there is a way to work that gets the best out of yourself and other people: I like to be relaxed and have relaxed people around me. Shouters aren't my style; there is a time and a place for that, but a relaxed environment encourages people to be comfortable, be themselves, and be innovative. In line with this, one of the reasons I don't go into the changing room for a long time after the game is because emotions are high and you need the players again for the next game. If I go in with an emotion that is delivered in the wrong way then I could lose them and you can't afford that.

Also relevant to consider is that the whole club can be up or down on a Monday after the weekend result and so you need to be consistent to keep doing what you set out to do. Players and staff sense when you're on the floor and it can spread quickly, so you learn that you can't change what's happened and only learn and get better. As a consequence, I feel that I need to have emotional control because if the players see you out of control then there's no way you can expect them to remain in control as well, or hit them with anything if they lose it on the pitch. To help with this, I commit to switching off away from football: spending time with my family, walking the dog, or golfing allows me to de-stress and clear my head. I'm also not on social media and don't read reports in the mainstream media. I know what I've done right and I know what I've done wrong: I've got 42,000 fans who let me know!

Concluding comments

In conclusion, coaching week-to-week in professional football is a highly demanding and challenging role. However, there are a number of processes and skills that can help head coaches to survive and thrive in a job. For me, some that stand out in particular are *managing and engaging the person, longer- and shorter-term planning, prioritising the fundamentals*, and *teaching, stimulating, and challenging the players*. To have the best chance of working, these processes and skills need to be delivered from a strong base; which the early phases of your tenure can, to a large extent, 'make or break'. From here, success is then often related to your ability to be consistent in everything that you do – and to ensure consistent approaches and messaging from within the football department as a whole.

6

Coaching in action/adventure sports

A novel challenge

Tom Willmott

Editors' introduction

Following a moderately successful career as a snowboard athlete, Tom transitioned into coaching in New Zealand first at a regional level, then at the Torino 2006 Winter Olympics in the new Olympic sport of Snowboard Halfpipe. He moved on to coach across the Freeski and snowboard spectrum, helping athletes to achieve success at major events including FIS World Cup, Global Open Series, X Games, and other major events. Tom now works as Head Coach for Snowsports New Zealand (SSNZ)'s Park & Pipe programme, heading up a growing and successful team which secured two medals at the 2018 Winter Olympics – New Zealand's best ever Winter Games performance. In his 'copious free time', Tom works as a heli-ski guide (on a snowboard) and relaxes by climbing mountains then snowboarding back down them!

Action/adventure/extreme sports and the move to the mainstream

As a starting point, and to save confusion and words, it is worth clarifying what sports fit into the adventure, action and/or extreme sports category. There has been some debate over the use of these terms but, throughout this chapter, I will use the action sports label as the overarching category. Action sports encompass a wide range of activities; such as freeskiing, snowboarding, skateboarding, surfing, freestyle motocross, BMX/freestyle BMX, mountain biking, wake boarding, and windsurfing. Moving into the adventure sport genre, examples include rock-climbing, white water kayaking, BASE jumping, and speed flying. Some of these are now seen as 'standard' sports, some are recreational pursuits that have evolved into competitive pursuits, some of them have just remained recreational. However, in almost all of these sports there is a competitive angle and also a recreational angle at the same time.

From a competitive perspective, many still see the X Games as the 'pinnacle event' for their sport. Starting in the 1990s, the X Games takes place across the globe, in various formats including a winter and summer split. In contrast, several of the sports have joined the Olympic roster, with the transition being more or less of a challenge for those involved. The most recent additions have been skateboarding, surfing, and climbing. Personally, I am involved with three different 'Park and Pipe' events, Halfpipe, Slopestyle, and Big Air, each of which is held for either freeski or snowboard with separate categories for men and women. So, 12 events in all. On the 'recreational' side there is a strong 'parallel universe' characterised by online postings or 'pay to view' videos which highlight the athlete's skills in very different but clearly related ways. As I will explain later, these two universes, what I will call the competitive versus recreational approaches, create a tension across the sport and for individuals at many levels.

It is important to note that the competitive angle for the events I am involved with is based on a subjective score – and this is based on overall impression. Judges reward athletes for the extent to which their run meets elements of the judging criteria which has five main categories – Progression, Amplitude, Variety, Execution, and Difficulty. This is different to a set of strict criteria or tariffs as used, for example, in artistic gymnastics or diving. Athletes are judged on performing manoeuvres and tricks in the air or on slopestyle features.

This 'move to the mainstream' has certainly been a challenge for the culture of the sports; a challenge for the participants and for national governing bodies. It has also required some adaptation from national funding bodies (in our case, High Performance Sport, New Zealand or HPSNZ); as they have supported new and different sports, new cultures, and new ways of doing things. As a simple example, fitness for Park and Pipe competition (hereafter P&P) was originally a 'just do it' thing – you rode or skied to be fit for snowboarding or skiing, with gym work almost frowned upon by some. This caused a clash when the sports became mainstream Olympic events, as they were typically designed for a more 'accountable' set of events. For example, the highly objective centimetre, grams, seconds (or CGS) sports where performance is based on an outcome measure, or team sports with a clear score in goals or points. Some in these organisations tried to push types and/or levels of training on performers, many of whom rejected the title of athlete with which they were labelled. It is worth noting that sport science support has been most effective, and take-up most apparent, when the approaches have been applied with a close watch on cultural and event specificity.

You can see some of these issues discussed in more detail in a paper I published on the transition, my experience of it, and what seemed to work or not work (Willmott & Collins, 2015). It is certainly worth consideration for other sports, including skateboarding, surfing, and climbing, as they approach their first full Olympic challenge in Tokyo 2020.

The particular challenge to coaching

Clearly, as arguably the biggest part of the 'system' in traditional sports, the place of coaching has also come in for its fair share of critical review (cf. Ojala & Thorpe, 2015 and my response to it Collins, Willmott & Collins, 2016). Clearly, and especially in P&P, the athletes came before the coaches, so coaching has evolved as a knock-on effect from the new greater emphasis on competition. The approach has borrowed ideas from coaching in other sports and domains but, notably, has also developed and evolved its own coaching methodologies suitable for the individuals involved and the nature of the sports. P&P typically involves an element of risk and is performed generally in a dynamic outdoor environment where weather factors, altitude, and snow conditions play a big part.

We have now been through six Olympic cycles in halfpipe snowboarding, which was the first P&P event to appear in Nagano 1998. There have been other action sports at the Olympics such as windsurfing, but snowboarding certainly pioneered the coaching profession in action sports, at least with the heavy competitive emphasis that is now typically accepted across the P&P environment.

With regard to the acceptance of coaching, we've got athletes that are being born and growing up in coaching structures versus the original situation, over 15 years ago, where athletes were starting the sport and learning from each other or in a self-taught setting. As a result, coaching is becoming a lot more accepted by the participants. There are still some smaller factions, generally coming from the recreational side of the sports, that would question the role of coaching and look with disdain at the impact and influence of coaching on their sport. Within the competitive side of the sport, however, coaching is becoming a lot more accepted. Of course, there is still a lot of coaching evolution to go on and action sports need to establish what really does work in this very specific context. There is a need to almost iron out the kinks of coaching methodologies that have just transferred directly from other sports that aren't necessarily all that appropriate.

Interestingly, the influence of coaching is also starting to impact on the other 'recreational' element of P&P. Clearly part and parcel of the sport, there's still an influence in the sport of progression, of getting better. This offers a good balance to the competitive side and, from the recreational side of the sport, there's funding from sponsors and brands, plus opportunities for athletes to showcase their skills outside of competition: to go on photoshoots and film big mountain free riding lines for example. To be honest, the levels of challenge from this element belies the 'recreational' label that I have been using. It might be better termed 'promotional' in that it offers excellent exposure to the sport for a much wider audience whilst also benefitting the performer.

Of course, performing in this sphere is also very positive for the competition side. It's all about timing: it can be very positive in terms of intrinsic motivation for the sport, getting into flow, and experiencing elements that are going to have a positive knock-on effect on the well-being of the athlete. There is also a significant movement vocabulary needed for the athlete to be capable of performing tricks in a non-structured environment. Competition is very structured and features are very similar each time they hit them in a session. In the big mountain back country environment, freeskiers and snowboarders have got to visualise and respond to the demands of the terrain in front of them, almost always at speed, a challenge which develops very good adaptation and adds to their skillset. From a mental skills perspective there's often a lot of pressure, over and above the personal risk. For example, when expensive helicopters are buzzing around and camera men are getting paid to film the clip, athletes are expected to land tricks first time and not waste time with repeated crashes and blowing it. So, when all is said and done, there is a very good crossover in terms of being able to perform under pressure that can transfer to competition; there are a number of positives. Negatives are that back country stuff could potentially impact and pull energy out of training time that's more specifically competition-focussed. So, as with most things in our sport it's all about the periodisation of those elements to make sure that they are enhancing performance in the targeted environment. Which, based on the current emphasis imposed by funding agencies, is increasingly down to the Olympics!

And for coaches. . .

As I have described above, there have been some clear cultural challenges in the move to the mainstream. For the personal coach in action sports, however, and particularly in my own disciplines of P&P, there are a number of extra issues. Of secondary importance is the technical challenge of the moves required. The ever-changing environment due to snow conditions, weather, and particular venue challenges means that athletes must be highly adaptable, with even well-embedded skills subject to significant change as conditions dictate. In addition to this, there are the usual challenges faced by coaches in any technical sport. Basically, there is the need for the coach to be developing moves that he or she may have never attempted, let alone mastered. Furthermore, and increasingly at the top end, you might be working with an athlete who is progressing towards an entirely original and innovative trick. So not only have you never achieved this as a coach but neither has anyone else. As a result, a whole raft of mental skills to do with imagery and mental simulation come into play; interestingly, for both coach and athlete, with the added necessity to form a bridge between the two. Pending the availability of Vulcan Mind-Fusion (cf. Star Trek), approaches to build Shared Mental Models (or SMMs) are particularly useful!

These technical challenges notwithstanding however, the primary problem is to do with personal safety – to what extent as the coach you are entitled to 'encourage' the athlete to give it a go when she or he are experiencing quite justifiable nerves at the prospect of a first attempt. Of note, many action sports involve personal risk and the coach is often the sounding board for the athlete, assisting with the decision as to whether a trick is on or should be shelved for another day. In P&P, fatalities have occurred and serious injuries are not uncommon.

Of course, recent technical innovations have helped to make things a lot more straightforward. Athletes now do an awful lot of their preparation work on giant trampolines then move the trick to snow through a number of bridging supports, such as water ramps or air bags. For my own team in NZ, the purchase of an enormous, progression air bag has made a significant difference. Adding to the more traditional and naturally occurring support cushions is, for example, trying new tricks in a spring camp environment where warmer temperatures and softer snow provide a more 'forgiving' environment.

Even with all these aids, however, the decision to 'go for it' on snow for the first time is often a challenge for both athlete and coach. As a result, there must be high levels of trust and good communication so that the athlete will listen to and be persuaded by the coach's advice in either direction. The trusting relationship between the athlete and coach is key, and the ability for the coach to read the athlete and help them with their decision-making as to whether it's worth pushing the risk today or not. As a support to everyone in this inevitably difficult process, we have developed objective decision-making tools including a progression checklist which asks the coach questions about the environment, the athlete's state physically and mentally, and about the preparation that has been done in order to achieve the goal. The bottom line is to help them decide whether it's the right time for the goal. We've got objective tools combined with subjective tools for the coach to be able to use their professional judgement in their decision-making to help an athlete ultimately make the decision whether they're going to go for this hard manoeuvre or not on any given day.

The performance pathway

As P&P has moved to the mainstream, the development of an effective 'performance pathway' has been a parallel evolution. This has necessitated us to consider several questions, in a similar fashion to other traditional sports. For example, how early do athletes need to start? What general and sport-specific characteristics do they need to have or develop. And reflecting these needs, what else do they do in parallel to the sport, so as to avoid the early specialisation challenges which are increasingly being identified?

Well, perhaps as a result of the relative youth of the sport, the first word in this instance must be 'normally'. There are plenty of examples of people that don't necessarily fit a standard mould but still achieve. So, I will describe what I'd call the standard mould and what we've seen successful in terms of the past, but with the important caveat that people will come in from different angles and directions but still be successful.

First steps

Without going into too much detail, the first key element is the development of general move-ment vocabulary as a youngster. I'm talking the five to ten-year zone where they should be experiencing all kinds of different 'general sporting' movements – throwing, catching, running, jumping, tumbling, gymnastics, team sports, individual sports; in simple terms, the wider variety the better. In parallel to the motoric side, and perhaps reflecting the wider elements of physical literacy, these young children need to develop an understanding for the mental elements of their sports; elements such as overcoming challenges, overcoming fear, learning skills, work ethic. All of those other wonderful elements that are positive for sport; working in a team, working with other people, dealing with winning, dealing with loss. From a wider psychosocial perspective, children evolve their interpersonal skills; developing relationships with their parents, learning how to utilise coaches. In short, a total package of psychomotor, psychobehavioural, and psy-chosocial skills, plus the practice at applying them to meet different challenges.

At the same time the children should be getting into snowboarding and skiing. They would be developing a love of the mountain environment: they would be spending time accessing snow in New Zealand, perhaps starting some trips away into the northern hemisphere and experiencing some different cultures, experiencing travel. They would be competing, ideally in some of the fundamental skill elements; so, racing, learning how to turn a board or skis left and right. These are key parts of our sport that are best learnt at a young age and developed early. Their performance snowboarding and skiing would start to evolve in that five to ten-year window in terms of specific learning.

Stage two

As the next key stage, let's look at the ten to 14 age group. Young performers will be starting to train and compete in the park and pipe disciplines. Coaching is likely to be provided through a regional coaching provider. Once again, and especially for us in New Zealand, the northern hemisphere trips are going to come increasingly into play. The athletes will be competing on the national series and developing more specific skills. At the same time, they will be keeping up their movement vocabulary with off-snow work including trampolining, gymnastics, parkour, and other complimentary sports, and also, developing their physiology through aerobic capacity enhancement during that phase. Finally, athletes will potentially be starting to compete at an international level from around the age of 12–14 years.

So, as the young athlete starts to compete internationally and come on our radar, we need to consider what sort of profile we are looking for; what's needed for us to say "actually this one might be worth it". We are looking at their performance, not necessarily looking at how much they're winning at this age, but rather how much they're progressing.

There's a number of skills that we are looking at but one of the most crucial is their work ethic and motivation. In addition, ability to progress is huge, plus the ability to learn from their exposure and their environment. Finally, we're pretty keen on evaluating that broad skillset and strong movement patterns, including very good neuromuscular control, that are going to limit an athlete's risk of injury.

As a specific element of that last factor, we look for athletes who can rotate in all four directions! On skis and snowboards there are four general directions. You can turn to the left, you can turn to the right, you can be going backwards and turn to the left you can be going backwards and turn to the right; so four different directions. We would like to see athletes at the ten to 14 year-old age bracket that are equi-skilled in all those four. They are bound to have a preference but we want to see the athletes that have the mental fortitude or mental strength to put time into their work on direction to bring it up to speed. If they start racing ahead in one direction, that helps their ego but it's not going to put them in good stead for the future.

This rotation goal is both an outcome and a process indicator. Process-wise, if they can spin in all four directions, they are going to be comfortable putting time and energy into their physicality and robustness at such time that that becomes a 'need to be worked on' factor. They're also going to be more willing to put time into their mental skills if that becomes an element that they need to work on.

Finally, we are working on their take-off patterns. In aerial sports, the landing is the easy part if your take-off is done correctly. So another fundamental skill that needs to be honed early on is a quality take-off.

Stage three: the 14–18 age band

As we get into the 14 to 18-year-old phase, hopefully they've got a strong fundamental package and skillset so now it's about accelerating their progression. It's now post-puberty so they're likely to have quite a rapid progression in terms of their skillset. The early parts of this phase may also be an introduction to competition: to travel for sustained periods where they need to learn how to be away from home for long periods of time, away from their parents, away from school. Usually, we're looking at correspondence schooling. Depending on where they're geographically located, some can maintain school; if they're able to train where they live at home if that's next to mountains. Whatever their circumstances, however, we are progressing the coaching volume and they are getting exposure to regular international events which are benchmarking their performance against their peers internationally.

Ideally, the athletes will have maintained a general on-snow diet! Still competing in all of the park and pipe disciplines, half pipe, slope style and big air. Halfway through that cycle, about age 16, they may start to put more time and energy into one of those disciplines but between 14 and 16 we'd like to see them make the most of their time in all of the disciplines. They are getting lots of time with a bib on in competition and developing their individual execution. Putting their own rubber stamp on performance, creating their own style, their own way of doing things which separates them from the crowd.

To clarify, we are not necessarily talking about P&P as an early specialisation sport. Rather, it might be thought of as an early progression or early challenge sport. Unlike some of the more formal talent development environments, such as academies, there are a lot of 'adult' challenges going on which athletes must master if they are to prosper on the nomadic existence of the World Cup circuit. That's quite an early hit because even if you were a gymnast you might well still be living at home and training in the same gym.

In terms of who is likely to achieve at the highest levels, I think you know as early as ten or 11 years. At the last Olympics, we had two sixteen-year-old medallists. Notably, however, we had been looking at them for six years; involved with them, aware of their presence, and aware of their abilities.

At the top and other ways in

As I said before, this 'normal' or 'usual' pathway is only a guide. There have been examples of some elite performances from much older athletes as well as from some who entered the sport at a young age and were child prodigies. Take Shaun White for example. Child prodigy at the age of 13, won his first Olympic gold medal in 2006 aged 19, went on to win another gold medal in 2010, fourth in 2014, won his third Olympic gold medal in the same discipline in 2018 aged 31. And he is still going, targeting the summer Olympics for skateboarding and then the next Winter Games in Beijing 2022 at which stage he'll be 35 years old. We also had Kelly Clark competing at the most recent Olympics, again in the snowboard halfpipe. She was 19 when she first won gold in 2002 in Salt Lake City. Aged 35 she placed fourth in Pyeongchang.

So, while there is early specialisation, there's also the potential for a long career; especially now that sport science – medical, psych, quality coaching, quality planning, quality periodisation, and quality training facilities that reduce the risk of injury have come on board. People can sustain long careers in the sport at the top.

With the additional funding and support for younger ages, later entries to the sports (informal walk-ons or formally identified through talent transfer schemes) are becoming rarer. I feel that the gate is getting drawn closed to an extent as the sports are maturing and evolving, and there's more funding and resource from national governing bodies tending to go deeper down into pathway. I feel that the door is closing on the 'anomalies' or the outliers of people that fit a different developmental path.

From a personal perspective, I would only see formal talent transfer searches as being useful if it's at a young enough age. I would want this within that ten to 14-year age group so that transfer could to occur in the 'middle window' that I described earlier. Of course, there might be the odd individual with exceptional motivation that could transfer. However, this is not sufficiently common to justify resourcing a programme, even though I know that some are running around the world.

Getting an edge – innovations for progress

Clearly, achieving and then maintaining athletes at the top level requires constant but really effective innovation. Accordingly, even though we are a small programme, we have a number of 'irons in the fire' in an attempt to gain a competitive edge. Planning is a crucial component; really high-quality planning that will optimise the challenge skill balance. So, we are developing skills at a high level, then challenging those skills regularly at the right level *and* having an opportunity to recover from that progression. Accordingly, herewith three examples of coaching approaches we have used to get ahead.

Emotional periodisation

We employ an approach known as emotional periodisation, in order for our athletes to progress optimally; pushing the injury threshold while not stepping over it and getting injured, either physically or mentally through burnout. We have published some of our ideas on this in an open access paper (Collins, Willmott & Collins, 2018) but, for the moment, let me present three examples of actions we use.

Clearly, P&P carries a high emotional load. Both training and competition involve personal risk, the frustration of trying to master complex skills plus the often challenging environments which must be handled day in, day out. So, in the same way that traditional periodisation varies physical load to ensure optimum development and recovery from physical training, we use emotional periodisation to optimise development whilst avoiding the short-term fatigue and longer-term chronic burnout which the inherent 'constant coping challenge' can generate.

Firstly, we use heuristics to guide our planning towards an appropriate balance. My fellow coach Sean Thompson has developed a 'Push-Drill-Play' structure, which we use as a daily, weekly, or longer element in designing the content, timing, and conduct of sessions. So certain days are identified as 'push' days – where the athletes stretch themselves to meet the challenges of new tricks at the nine or ten out of ten difficulty level. On 'drill' days, tricks at the up to eight out of ten level are drilled to promote both embedding (a lower stress execution) and adaptation; essential for handling the variations in competitive environment that I alluded to earlier. 'Play' days do what they say on the tin, helping the athletes to remind themselves of why they love their sport, the environment, their training group, and also provide an opportunity for getting creative – learning new ways to do things.

This idea is demonstrated in the performance analysis tools we use, an example of which is shown in Figure 6.1 below.

The figure records the location of training but also, and more importantly, the 'intensity' of the session as operationalised by perceived risk and the number of falls (or bails) experienced. Reflecting ideas presented earlier, we also record the equi-laterality of spins, to keep the athlete focused on her or his fundamentals. As you can see, and reflecting our three-part heuristic, 'push' days are spread out to ensure recovery.

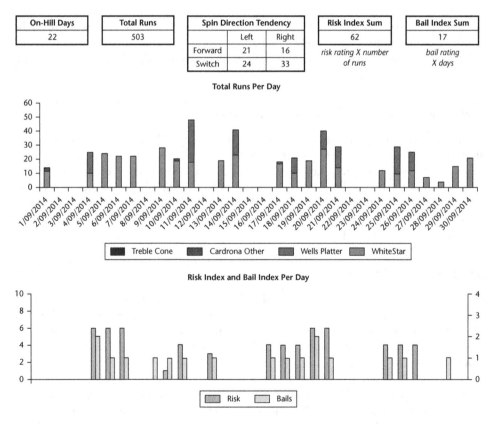

On-Hill Days	Total Runs	Spin Direction Tendency			Risk Index Sum	Bail Index Sum
22	503		Left	Right	62	17
		Forward	21	16	risk rating X number of runs	bail rating X days
		Switch	24	33		

Figure 6.1 An exemplar training workload record for two freeskiers

In fact, recovery is the third principle that helps us keep athlete development at an optimal balance. We also stress the need for acute recovery and, in the longer term, re-creation activities such as skiing or riding powder to regenerate emotions and enthusiasm. We are also very aware of the workload.

We see this approach as underpinning a very individualised programme but also a very humanitarian one. Certainly athlete health and wellbeing is front and centre of decisions on the SSNZ programme. We have a limited talent pool here in New Zealand so we certainly have more of a nurture approach rather than a natural selection. We are looking at the athletes holistically, especially with the early specialisation/challenge nature of the sport. Coaches are mentors and role models to a greater extent perhaps than in other more traditional sports. We are almost taking on a loco parentis role at times. Importantly, however, we have generally had athletes with very supportive parents that are able to buy into the team approach for the development of their child and take on board input from the specialist experts.

The 'rocket ship' approach

Reflecting the emphasis on top quality planning, we have a model of development which is basically a breakdown of different skills that we believe an athlete needs to possess at every stage. This runs from mental skills to technical skills to tactical skills to off-snow movement skills to on-snow movement skills. Within each category, we identify as different parts of a rocket ship that's going to be able to take off on a mission into space. We have identified verbally what each of those different levels are so we can explain them to an athlete. This helps us to profile where they are at, then share that with all the stakeholders to ensure a consistent focus. So, a parent can work with an athlete and profile where they're at, a coach or a support team member can profile where an athlete is at, decisions on where energy and work needs to be put into the planning of an athlete can be made and improvement can be measured against time. Figure 6.2 shows a typical profile with names and details removed to preserve confidentiality.

The team coaching approach

One feature of the New Zealand park and pipe team is the fact that we're relatively small with around ten athletes at the elite level. Of course there are both advantages and disadvantages to this. Positively, however, we have a small athlete pool that are competing in numerous different disciplines, so we have a coaching team that needs to collaborate and cross over between disciplines. We have got coaches that work across freeski and snowboard but, more importantly, we 'triangulate' our coaching input and use members of the coaching team to audit our decision-making. Utilising that team approach, which is geared towards 'what does coaching provision look like at the winter Olympics?', we backtrack from that vision and that picture of who is where or working with who, we backtrack and plot and plan throughout the quadrennial to ensure that the athletes are exposed to multiple inputs. At its simplest, the coaches who will work with athletes in high pressure situations have worked with other coaches in lower pressure situations so that the team can effectively deliver on *the* day.

However, the additional benefits of this are that any one athlete gets at least two 'perspectives' on what she or he is doing. Obviously, each coach brings something slightly different to the

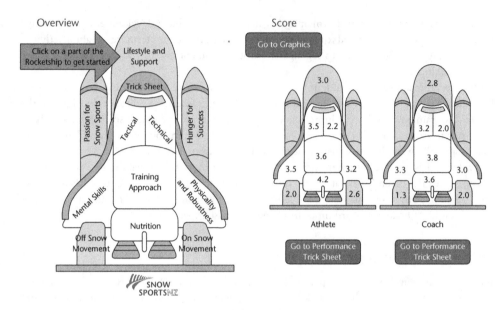

Figure 6.2 An exemplar of the SSNZ 'rocket ship' model. Note the use of athlete and coach ratings on the essential factors that make up the ship

party, and each will have a different set of criteria, a 'weighting scale', that determines what particular factors they will focus on. So, each athlete is allocated a lead coach who does the majority of the work, supplemented by a co-coach who might have a separate agenda or set of work-ons.

It has taken some time to evolve shared mental models, alignment, and a good level of challenge within the coaching team. A culture of honesty, egos in moderation but a model of 'equal expertise', means that everyone has something to bring to the party. These are all elements that have helped us to generate an effective coaching team which, I believe, performs far better than the sum of its parts

In conclusion

What I have described is a very positive holistic humanitarian type programme. But when push comes to shove we are coaching an activity which carries high risk. Trusting and autonomy-supportive relationships are key! It's knowing your athlete then encouraging your athlete to be the one making the decisions, and you're ultimately there as the 'yes man' to confirm things in the end.

In fact, I'd suggest there's more conservativism if a scenario is coach-led and you are 99.9% confident that they're going to land their trick or at least get their board down because you've been more thorough with the preparation. When the athlete takes over the leadership, you give them a little bit more leeway – depending on the individual – but you generally give them a little bit more leeway in terms of taking risks. Because, at the end of the day they're the expert; they're the ones with all of the information about them. You are providing that third eye, that external perspective, but you are not inside the athlete's head and can't evaluate every single thing that's going on in that athlete's brain. So, to put the whole chapter into one sentence, coaching action sports may be different to coaching other sports in the degree and intensity of relationship that is required.

References

Collins, D., Willmott, T. & Collins, L. (2016). Over Egging the Pudding? Comments on Ojala and Thorpe. *International Sport Coaching Journal*, **3**, 90–93. doi.org/10.1123/iscj.2015-0068

Collins, D., Willmott, T. & Collins, L. (2018). Periodisation and Self-Regulation in action sports: Coping with the emotional load. *Frontiers in Psychology*, doi.org:10.3389/fpsyg.2018.01652

Ojala, A-L., & Thorpe, H. (2015). The Role of the Coach in Action Sports: Using a Problem-Based Learning Approach. *International Sport Coaching Journal*, **2**, 64–71. doi:10.1123/iscj.2014-0096

Willmott, T. & Collins, D. (2015). Challenges in the Transition to Mainstream: Promoting Progress and Minimizing Injury in Freeskiing and Snowboarding. *Sport in Society*, **18**(10), 1245–59. doi:10.1080/1 7430437.2015.1031530

7

Specialist coaching
Coaching quarterbacks in NFL, college, and high school

Steve Fairchild with Geir Jordet

Current role

My background in the coaching profession is 34 years of college and NFL coaching. At the college level I was everything from a quarterback coach and offensive coordinator, to head coach at Colorado State University. In the NFL, I was a quarterback coach as well as an offensive coordinator. The NFL teams that I've coached for were the Buffalo Bills, St. Louis Rams (now in Los Angeles), and the San Diego Chargers (now also in Los Angeles).

As for right now, I am a quarterback trainer. I train quarterbacks from youth football all the way to the NFL. I train specifically the techniques and fundamentals, using drills that are applicable to being a good quarterback in the game of football. I do this year-round and also do some consulting based on video (looking at video tapes, grading video tapes for various organisations, from the NFL all through online organisations that do statistical analysis for the NFL and college football).

My path

I started playing youth football as early as ten years old. At that young age everybody plays every position, but eventually you become more specialised. So at a very young age I became a quarterback and played youth football through high school and then I played at college at the Division 1 level. As I looked at it, you wake up one day and you've been doing football for eight to ten years and it's a big part of your life. After I graduated from college, I made the decision to stay with football and see if that worked for me. I started coaching at a very low level. My first coaching job was at a junior college. The pay was low and I swept the stadiums after the games, and did the laundry. But I realised that I really loved the game, and it was a big part of my life, so I continued going up the coaching ladder, went through junior college to small colleges and then to bigger colleges. I became an assistant coach, then coordinator, and finally head coach. I spent 34 years climbing the ladder in the coaching profession. Having the opportunity to be a head coach at a Division 1 school in college, and an offensive coordinator where I called plays in the NFL, was a great experience.

Specialist coaching

A lot of specialist coaching now is outside the organisation. If you are Tiger Woods, a professional golfer, you are the organisation. He seeks out a swing coach, he seeks out weight training coaches and nutrition people. They are outside his organisation, but he feels the need to get this extra coaching to help him play at a high level. This is starting to happen in the game of football as well. You can't be a high school quarterback now that goes on and gets a scholarship to play college football if you just go to your high school and try to be the quarterback. Almost all players seek out specialist coaches on how to get an extra edge. Specialist coaching can help you be the quarterback of your team, and maybe go on and play in college and play in the pros. That is what I am doing right now. I am not in the organisation, but a separate entity, and people seek me out to teach them to play quarterback, to evaluate their quarterback, or to examine the pool of upcoming quarterbacks.

With young quarterback clients, I spend time with them in the classroom, teaching them the game of football, how to play quarterback. We may look at other quarterbacks on tape, and we discuss what they are doing from a tactical standpoint, as well as what they're doing from a mental standpoint. This could involve teaching them about the Red Zone, third downs, and how different parts of the game can be approached. When they come to me they are seeking more coaching, and football knowledge. Football players may want to get more training. If I work with a player one evening, we might cover the technique on the field. Then we will go into a classroom and spend an hour watching tapes and teach defensive coverages, blitz looks, and other football knowledge. This is all outside his own team and coaching.

I am also working for teams and online agencies. They send me video tapes of games and have me grade it. For example, I could grade the San Francisco 49ers quarterback at 84% and the San Diego Chargers quarterback at 92%. Those organisations digest that information to have a new set of eyes on our quarterback. Or it could be an online website that grades players. People can get online and access "who is the best quarterback in the Red Zone or the best quarterback on 3rd down".

I also grade college quarterbacks for NFL teams as they build their roster in the off-season. I write up quarterbacks in college and rank them prior to the NFL draft. They say, Steve Fairchild sees the top five quarterbacks in this order, our personnel department sees it in this order, and scouts see it in this order. When you rank college quarterbacks or NFL free agent quarterbacks and then they have to make decisions in the spring on how they build their roster, a new set of eyes or a new write-up is sometimes a good thing to have.

Evaluating quarterback performance

To perform as a quarterback, there is a certain level of arm talent and size that you have to have. If you can not throw a football a certain distance, or if you are not a certain size, you are going to really struggle. Obviously, in most sports it is like this; the bigger, stronger, faster, and more athletic people are going to have a better chance of succeeding than others. At the end of the day the quarterback has to throw the football. And this is about the arm ability, the ability to throw accurately and put the ball from their hand and to the place down the field that they want to put the ball to. That's where the real strength of a quarterback is, and that's where the technique part that I coach can make a difference. To make you able to throw more quickly and accurately.

It is very hard to see on a video tape what a true arm movement looks like. Seeing it live, in real time, is necessary. You're talking about differences of tenths of a second. For example, if you picture a quarterback from that point when he puts his two hands on the football, once that first hand comes off the football and he starts that throwing motion, it's a bang-bang type of sequence, and it's quick. Even the slow ones are pretty quick, so you're talking about the difference in tenths of a second. The smoothness and the quickness doesn't show on a video tape like you can see it in person. I do 600 hours a year of just quarterback technique training. Just standing there and watching a guy throw for that many hours, and you can see things well. I wouldn't be able to correct a golf swing in real time, but I know there are people that can do that with their eyes. I feel like I'm in that category. So it's a big advantage for me to see a quarterback in person.

When I was on the NFL coaching staff and I was going to look at a quarterback, I certainly wanted to see his delivery in real time. But also I wanted to see how he interacted with his receivers, and what type of 'it-factor' and presence he had during the workout. That is so important for a quarterback. You are so reliant of the ten other people in the huddle. You have to make those ten people better players by believing in you and the way you handle yourself. There is a lot to learn about people by their body language and communication skills when they are working with other players. You cannot see that on a tape of the workout, but you can see it in person.

Moreover, when I see players, I will look at how they present themselves, not only to coaches, but to the person running the drill. How they take coaching, and how they interact with the receivers and the people around them. Body language and voice inflection. It is like when you go in to a room with a teacher, the first five minutes you may really enjoy and be confident in this person's message or the body language and the delivery. And its just the way they're doing it, you may just say; I'm following this guy. There's a lot to that.

I think like good teachers, good coaches, good quarterbacks, they come in different shapes and sizes. Some people are a little bit more fiery, and some people are more scholarly. I want to watch the guy, and see, is he effective? Is he effective when communicating? Does he have a loud voice, or a calm voice? Is he effective in his work ethic? Is he moving and getting things done? You know a good one and a bad one when you get there.

You can have all the skills in the world – a perfect quarterback in height, arm, and ability, but he still might not be successful, because at the end of the day, that position is judged by the group's success or the group's lack of success. If you're not scoring points and as a group on offence you're not winning games and moving the football, you're going to get fired. Football is a result business, driven by the results of the group, and not the individual.

Football people in the US often question: can a guy process? Is he football smart? Can he learn the offence? What I've found through my years, is that the people who love the game are willing to study more and spend more time in the film room. They will truly master their offence as oppose to some people that like football, but they like other things as well. They are not as studious. I've been around quarterbacks that are very smart, that could learn anything, that could give you the information back if you tested them on the content of the offence. But their ability to process was ultimately what made them what they were. You may have the answer to the test and you may know what to do. But can you get to that answer in a matter of seconds, when people around you try to hit you and tackle you? It's like some people can take a test and ace the test, but if you give them the same test but with very limited time on the response and you hit them with cardboard while they take the test it's a whole different outcome. It's playing with people around you and making decisions in two to three seconds, as opposed to learning in a classroom.

I get frustrated when I talk with people in general, and people in personnel, about quarter-backs, because they keep using the word 'process'. I am thinking that people 'process' when in a relaxed environment, but can you process in a very time constrained and hostile environment? There are two things that can really help a quarterback to do this. The first is experience. The more snaps you have playing with people around you and having to see things on the run very quickly is a big advantage. Second, when you break the huddle there is probably about eight to ten seconds where you're coming up to the line of scrimmage and you're looking at the defensive line and structure. That coverage gives you some clues that you only get for about eight to ten seconds. When the ball snaps, you either confirm what you expected or it changes very differently and that play lasts for two to four seconds and in that time you digest what you're seeing. So, film study, recognition of your opponent, and knowing good looks versus bad looks, as much as you can digest before the ball hits your hands, is very important. You only have a few seconds. That's where the whole game is played. It's a few seconds and you've got to make some critical decisions and throw and perform technically well.

There is no question that really good quarterbacks are faster in their heads than other people. You've heard about point guards in the NBA making decisions on where to pass. They say that the game slows down for them. And that's what good quarterbacks say as well. The game slows for them. What would appear to be three seconds doesn't feel like three seconds to them. Everything is moving very slow and they're very comfortable with it. Is that a product of preparation, study, and experience – the number of plays you've played? I think so, but also, some guys just have the ability.

Developing quarterbacks

Any teacher-student or coach-player relationship starts with trust. Knowing that as a player, you believe in what the coach is telling you and why he's telling you to do it. If a player and coach don't trust each other they're starting down the wrong road. I think there is a personal level to this, that you have got to get to know somebody and I think it's done in a lot of different ways. There's a lot of different personalities at play here. I know even just doing the specialist coaching, if they don't trust me, then I'm not going to be successful coaching them. And then secondly, I think your ability to communicate is crucial. You may know what you want to get across, but do you have the ability to break it down and communicate it to the player? I think some people that are very smart in their industries lack that skill, and therefore lack the success they could have had.

Let's say you go to a football practice and it's two hours long. That's where you develop a lesson plan. How much do we want to take the individual, fundamental component and work on that? Because that is important. And how much of it is putting them in a team setting, where they not only have to do the individual technique, but they have to communicate with the person next to them and play the game and consider how it's going to be on game day. In football, both are important, but every team is different. You may have a veteran team and they are pretty good technique-wise, and you may have a very young team that is not very technically good so you want to spend more time doing that. Here's the part I've learned, and I have learned this late in my career. What you really need is applicable training. In football, two thirds of the game is not played in what one might call normal rhythm. In other words, a quarterback about one out of three times he throws, he's going to take his drop with three or five steps, set, and throw it to a receiver. That's what people normally train – taking the steps, dropping back, and throwing it to a receiver. But in reality, two out of three times, he's going to have to drop back, duck, shuffle up, and make a throw with his feet in an odd situation. Essentially, something happens in the situation that calls for something out of the ordinary, and this is actually the norm. To fully consider this as a coach starts with an analysis of what's going to go on in a game. If you do not practice it – you're never going to get it done in a game.

Let me elaborate a bit on this. As a coach for quarterbacks I started writing in a little notebook 30 years ago whenever a quarterback had to do an odd thing. In other words, I would look for those instances where instead of a right-handed quarterback's stepping with his left foot first and throwing, something different happens. For example, suddenly in a game somebody fell right in front of his front foot and he actually stepped with his back foot to make the throw. So, I wrote those different instances down over the years, and based on this, I probably have a thousand drills that I just made up because I saw it and it occurred in a game. And I thought, if it occurred in a game, it may occur again. We're going to practise all this odd stuff. And I found it actually make players better, because they're not in the routine where they are practising the perfect environment. They're out there practising the hard things. I still think that when I go to watch college or NFL practices, they're not doing this, and consequently, they are not training as well as they should.

Even more specifically, let's say the design of the play is for a quarterback to take five steps and to throw it to a receiver that's 12 yards down the field. What typically happens at practice in high school, colleges, and the pros, is that the quarterback takes five steps, the receiver runs 12 yards, then turns around, upon which the quarterback throws it perfectly on time and hits the receiver right in the numbers. And you feel good about it after that practice. In a game that is not going to happen though. What I do is have them take five steps and I will take a bag and I'll push it right into the front part of their body and make them slide to the left and then make that throw. And on the next attempt, I will punch the other half of the body and make them slide to the right and make that throw. Then, I may put the bag on the ground and have you step up while I'm slapping at the ball. You better have two hands on the ball or I am going to slap the ball out of your hands, but you're going to step over the bag while I slap the ball and then you're going to make that throw. I may have a thousand of those drills that when you really break it down, with respect to the biomechanics of it, are about what the quarterback actually does in a game. For whatever I see, I make up a drill, and then we drill it.

About doing this within a team setting, you still have to create this type of environment. To give you an example, if we were at practice and somebody misses a block, we don't tackle the quarterback to the ground, because we don't want to get the quarterback hurt, we bump into him and say that would have been a sack. But here's one thing that I've found: we never end the play for the quarterback, so even if the guy missed that block and the defender bumped into the quarterback, we still have the quarterback finish the play and make the throw down the field. And that became a repetition-under-duress type of throw. And it really helps the quarterbacks keep their eyes down-field and finish the play. So, you can take some of that technical stuff and put it into a team setting and still get repetitions in that regard. The other thing I will say is you go down there and say, well, we're going to take five steps and throw a 12 yard route. But are you doing that on third down against the blitzes? Are you doing that in the red zone on the 18-yard line where the field is not very big? Basically, are you playing situational football? It is important that you make sure all the situations are practised, not just against a base defence, but against different defences, different field perimeters, different times on the clock and in a variety of game situations.

A training day

In the NFL, every day for over six months there is a detailed plan and schedule. There is a time for meals, there is a time for treatment, a time for individual meetings and group meetings.

You also go out on the field and walk through what you are going to practise so that when you practise at full speed you are not making mistakes and having to do it over. That will place wear and tear on the guys' legs, especially late in the year. So actually, when you have a 45-play practice, you walk through all 45 plays so that everybody is on the same page. It's very detailed, because at the end of the day, it is about how efficiently you used your time. Then there's different topics on different days. One day there's base offence, next day is a red zone, and third down day. So, on that first day, with respect to video, you watch all first and second down defences, and the next day you watch all the red zone, and their third down defences. It is much more complex and organised than the average fan thinks. Those guys are working extremely hard, very detailed, to get as much done as they can in the time they have. Even though at college you have student athletes and they're going to class, it is very similar. At the college level if we practised in the afternoon, nobody could take a class after 11am, so you had to take a 8, 9, or 10am class so you're done at noon and at the facility at 1pm. From 1pm until 6pm, there are five hours mapped out in detail.

Each day the game plan is different with a different focus. And as you are getting later in the week, the time on the field will be reduced, so you are getting more rest for the game on the weekend. With that said, to give a specific example, let us take a normal Tuesday or Wednesday in the NFL. The team meeting may be at 7.30am or 8am in the morning. And they're going to remind you at that team meeting of some things about the opponent, the schedule for the day, what in the coaches' minds needs to be emphasised and what we did well and what we really need to improve on. And then you're going to go to position meetings after that. At 8am then you have an hour-long position meeting where we study what the quarterback needs to know as opposed to what the centre, wide receiver, or the guard needs to know. So you're spending some time on the board talking about things, you watch some film for that day – if it's a third down day, you watch all the third down play of the defence that you're playing. Then you may go out on the field and walk through it all and make sure what you're doing at that afternoon practice has been walked through and seen visually, because some guys can pick things up in a classroom, and some guys need things visual. So, you may walk through from 10am to 11am, and at 11am there may be some treatment and taping and getting whatever you need to do physically to get ready. There may be a lunch involved, and you may come back for another quick meeting about the practice and this one would be at 1pm, where maybe we will talk about the specific reps that we're going to call and how we're going to call them. And then maybe go to the field from 2pm to 4pm and get back to the classroom and watch the practice on tape from 4pm to 5pm, and then maybe dinner. It's very well thought-out.

Cognitive training

When I started coaching, you used to put the pads on when you practised. Now, in the collective bargaining agreement between the players and the NFL, the players asked for limited padded practice. So in the NFL right now, you can only have 14 padded practices once the season has started. And it's a 16-game schedule, so you have less than one padded practice per week. A lot of it is going through the motions and more the mental thing. In many ways, in the NFL, it is way more cognitive to get ready to play than it is physical.

I would give tests every night to our quarterbacks. Let's say our passing game for third down was going to have 34 plays. These are shown in diagrams, with maybe five on a sheet of paper, giving six, seven sheets of paper with five diagrams on each. We would load them into their iPads. Then I would draw it on the board and talk about it and go out and perform it. But I would take those pages, and leave the play-call on there, so it might be "red right 22 Z hook".

But the diagram disappeared and they had to go in and fill in the diagram with their own pencil. You can say they had their iPads so they could just look at their iPads. I am a little old school, but I still think that if they were writing it, there would be some learning going on. So every night after that 5pm dinner they would take their test, go home, and give it to me at the team meeting at 7.30am the next morning. I would grade it and make sure they wrote it down.

Also, lately, there has been a lot of work done with virtual reality simulations, particularly with quarterbacks where they put the goggles on and see the game in front of and around them. The applications that I have seen have been okay, a little bit like a video game. I don't think they hurt, and they probably are another way of studying. I don't know if they are any better than a written test, but you could certainly argue that it is, because it is more visual. With some of the cutting-edge virtual reality, the quarterback is actually going to move with these goggles on. I don't know if there now is anything that really simulates the game, but eventually I think modern technology will come up with something that is really good.

The demands on players

The NFL season is probably four to five weeks of training camp, then there are four pre-season games, that will take it to eight weeks. Then there are 16 games, so that is a 17-week season (because of the bye week), so now you are at 25 weeks. Then there are the play-offs that you can add to that, so it is a long time and you have to be aware of not only the physical drain, but the mental drain. And that is the hardest thing I saw with young players coming from college. They are done playing around Thanksgiving, and NFL still has ten more games to play. People have to get used to that grind and how to approach it.

Even though the season may be shorter than some of the other team sports, it feels very long for those involved. Your whole focus in life is to be up at six, go to the training facility and not get home until six at night, then have a test or some film to look at. Doing this over a continuous span of time, in a high-pressure environment that is very competitive where winning or losing could mean your job, there is high scrutiny from fans and media. There is a stress level for players and coaches, so when you are done you need some time away.

In the off-season, the NFL now will not let the players get back into the training facility until April. So when the season is over in January (Super Bowl might go to February), you literally can't go into the building until April. You cannot sit in the coach's office to watch film. You can not use the weight room, and you can not train on the field. Only if you are injured can you go in and get your treatment. So that is where I now come in, as an external quarterback coach. Let me give you an example. Chad Kelly is the number two quarterback for the Denver Broncos (he was number three last year). He could not go to the Broncos' training facility, but he could meet me. So we trained, and obviously he gets some time off in January, but in the middle of February he is back doing some things with me on the field that did help him become the number three quarterback. It is certainly not anywhere near the full regular day schedule, but the guy might lift an hour a day and throw an hour a day, and he may do some stretching, and nutrition consulting. But you are talking two to three hours a day that he puts into developing his craft, as opposed to the entire day.

8

Developing the players of tomorrow

Ruben Jongkind

Editors' introduction

Ruben is the former Head of Talent Development of the Academy at AFC Ajax Amsterdam and co-writer of the "Plan Cruyff". As the son of a Spanish mother and a Dutch father, Ruben unites the best of both worlds with his passion and strong analytical skills. Ruben holds a degree in Environmental Science from Wageningen University and a Master in Business Administration (MScBA) from Nijmegen Business School. During his academic and professional career, where he specialised in analysis, design, and change of organisations, Ruben spent many weekly hours training as a triathlete, leading him to a career as a trainer/coach. In 2006, he decided to become a full-time coach and said goodbye to his consultancy career. After a successful period in track and field and amateur football, he attained the position of individual trainer at the Ajax youth academy, first as a volunteering intern and then as a coach. Working together with Wim Jonk through various individual programmes, he helped improve players such as Christian Eriksen, Toby Alderweireld, and Daley Blind (all of whom later made the step to the top level of European football). In 2009, Ruben coached elite 800 metres athlete Bram Som back to world elite level. This process taught him so much about individual elite sports, that he decided to combine his knowledge on elite individual sports and organisational design and apply it to his work with Ajax's top football talents. Consequently, he teamed up with Johan Cruyff and Wim Jonk in 2010 and took up the writing of the "Plan Cruyff". The first thing that he did was create an explicit model on paper of Cruyff's football vision which was implicitly in Cruyff's head. The second thing was to connect the work that he and Wim Jonk had done to individualise the player development process, in this model. This mix of Cruyff's inspiration and Jongkind and Jonk's models and methods to individualise and upgrade the youth academy constituted "Plan Cruyff".

One of the main pillars of this visionary plan was the necessary upgrade and reform of the Ajax youth academy, based on an individual approach in talent development. After a period of great turbulence, often referred to as 'the velvet revolution', the club finally adopted the Plan Cruyff as its new policy in 2011. Ruben was appointed Head of Talent Development and became responsible for the implementation of the plan in the academy. Between 2012 and December 2015, he implemented the Plan Cruyff and by doing so revolutionised the academy and the club as a whole. In concert with Head of Academy Wim Jonk, Ruben fundamentally reformed the Ajax academy structure as well as its culture, introducing a new philosophy that marked the player and his development as the indisputable focal point of the academy, in all aspects of its organisation and processes. In December 2015, after a period of ongoing disagreement with the Ajax board of directors about the lack of implementation of the Plan Cruyff in other parts of the club, the involvement of Wim Jonk and Johan Cruyff with Ajax came to an end. As a result, Ruben decided to leave Ajax, lacking the belief that the Plan Cruyff would be fully implemented without Johan Cruyff and Wim Jonk.

Introduction

Developing future athletes typically requires a fundamentally different approach than facilitating or supporting athletes' current performance. In this chapter, I will address one specific perspective on the development of the players of tomorrow. Specifically, this is the player development philosophy of the legendary Dutch football player and coach, Johan Cruyff.[1] His ideas fundamentally guided Wim Jonk and I as management of the AFC Ajax Amsterdam Youth Academy in the practice during the years 2011–16. The outcomes of this period were generally very good:

- Ajax B (U23) won the championship in the second division for the first time in history in 2018.
- The players developed under Plan Cruyff are the new internationals of the Dutch Team despite their young age: Matthijs de Ligt (debut at 18), Donny van de Beek (debut at 20), Kenny Tete (debut at 20), and Justin Kluivert (debut at 18).
- The estimated transfer values of some of the youth players are: de Ligt – 50 million Euro, van de Beek – 30 million Euro. Kluivert jr. made his way to AS Roma in 2018/19 for 17 million euro (interview with Sky, 15 february 2018).
- Ajax reached the 2017 Europa League final against Manchester United (2-0 defeat) with the youngest starting line-up in the history of European finals.
- Financial results: Ajax's equity rose from 44,700,000 Euro in 2011 before Plan Cruyff to 158,900,000 Euro in 2017 after Plan Cruyff.

Johan Cruyff: the inspirator

As is evident from some of the central people in modern FC Barcelona history, the philosophy introduced by Cruyff made a big impact on this club:

> For me, he was the most relevant person in the history of Barca and the ones that are here always maintain his legacy. His philosophy is the best in the history of football.
>
> *(Xavi Hernandez, the legendary FC Barcelona player,*
> *about Johan Cruyff, in Garcia, 2016)*

> I knew nothing about football before knowing Cruyff.
>
> *(Pep Guardiola in Cruyff, 2017, cover)*

Johan Cruyff started playing football on the streets of Amsterdam. Ascending from a humble neighbourhood, to the greatest stadiums around the globe, Johan delighted the world with a brand of football that would grow to enthrall generations of football fans and profoundly influence the modern game. Johan Cruyff was the personification and mastermind of *total football*. When he played, Cruyff glided across the pitch with a grace and fluidity that made his play mesmerising. He demonstrated both technical mastery and tactical intelligence while leading both AFC Ajax Amsterdam and the Dutch national squad to world prominence in the 1970's. The introduction of *total football* in this era marks the most influential change in the history of the game and etched Johan Cruyff into the minds and memories of those who appreciate spectacular, creative, and attacking football.

After winning three consecutive European Cups with Ajax, Johan transferred to FC Barcelona in 1973. As perhaps the world's best player at that time, he immediately led the club to its first national title in 14 years, sparking a rebirth not just of the club, but of Catalonia as a whole. In 1999, Johan was elected European Player of the Century[2] and finished second in the World Player of the Century election,[3] marking just two accolades on an endless list of trophies and personal honors.

Johan Cruyff was equally influential as a coach, further developing and implementing his football philosophy at AFC Ajax and FC Barcelona. He began his coaching career at AFC Ajax Amsterdam, winning the European Cup Winners Cup in 1987 and rocketing a number of great Dutch talents to world prominence. In 1988, Johan moved back to Barcelona, where he would hold the head coach job for eight years and fundamentally reform the club to the stature it holds today: an icon of world class football and an exemplary model of the beautiful game. Gradually building his legendary 'Dream Team', Johan led FC Barcelona to an unprecedented four consecutive national titles (1991–94) as well as the European Cup Winners Cup (1989) and, ultimately, to the European Cup at Wembley stadium in 1992.

Beyond his trophies, Johan has been heralded for his innovative style of play and his unique coaching principles. He paved the way for generations of top players and entertained audiences worldwide, inspiring many great coaches to follow in his footsteps. In addition to his career as a player and as a coach, Johan Cruyff was an innovator and a football visionary. His style of *total football* invoked a revolution of the game, introducing new and more dynamic strategies for attacking and defending in which all players participated, optimising the use of space across the pitch. In addition, Johan was the strongest advocate of beautiful football, relentlessly aiming to produce both quality and results. He argued that football, in its very essence, is a game intended to entertain and bring joy to the fans.

A strong believer in playing and nurturing home-grown talents, Cruyff stood at the cradle of two of the most famous and successful academies in football history: De Toekomst at AFC Ajax Amsterdam and FC Barcelona's La Masia.

Johan's distinctive philosophy on talent development, where individual development is the cornerstone of an academy, gave birth to generations of great players and coaches. They continue to dominate the game of football today and are the living proof of an unrivalled personal football legacy.

The philosophy

The Vision laid down in "Plan Cruyff" rests on four main pillars:

1   Playing attractive football through an attacking playing style. Football is played for the fans and for the players to enjoy themselves.
2   Half of the squad should be homegrown players, developed based on a player centred approach. The academy is the backbone of the club, connecting the fans, the city/region, and other stakeholders with the players.

3   Sustainable transfer policy: direct reinforcements only, minimise blocking upcoming academy talents.
4   Create a performance organisation through a culture of continuous improvement on operational, tactical, and strategic aspects.

Only by building and integrating these four pillars you create quality and results.

The trick to mastering attacking football is to start teaching its principles to your players as early as possible. Working at Ajax between 2011 and 2016 with Cruyff, I collected and wrote down all available football knowledge with Johan, thereby creating the Cruyffian football model. This model consists of several 'principles of play', specific match tactics as well as a clear set of standards for the required player skills. I integrated the knowledge about individual elite sports, organisational design, and Wim Jonk's ideas about individual football training and translated the model into a framework and Cruyffian methodology, creating a universal language for players and coaches in the academy.

Everything starts with a playing style that you have to believe in, that is rooted in your identity. This will help create a structure and culture for all people within the club, and set standards for the academy. The next and most important step is to know what kind of players you need, how you want them to play and what this means for your youth football curriculum from six to 19 years. It's essential to create a clear methodology and coherent structure that enables a continuous feedback cycle. And match relevance can only be achieved if: (a) players have the right skills set, (b) the right players are recruited, with the potential to acquire this skillset and (c) if the game model is trained on a daily basis, at the highest level adapted to every age group and individual player.

The player paradigm

> I have never seen a team make its debut. Only individual players do.
>
> *(Johan Cruyff, personal conversation)*

Plan Cruyff's primary topic of reform was to change the academy philosophy: I clearly saw this required a paradigm shift and translated this schism in terms of a paradigm contradistinction: the team paradigm to the player paradigm. The team paradigm typically manifests itself in an academy culture that focuses on team results, on the current level of players (who is the best player today) and the importance of the coach as an instructor of the players. The absolute prevalence of the team paradigm in youth football today is underlined by the undeniable existence of the relative age effect (RAE), a clear indication that clubs and coaches are predominantly recruiting and playing the (relatively) older players, at the expense of potentially more talented, but physically weaker and younger players with less training hours and development opportunities. Typical elite academy compositions show an overwhelming majority of players born in the first half of the year, often in a 70–30 or more ratio.

Extra fuel for the more short-term team paradigm is provided by the economic system in football, with coach salaries in adult football far exceeding those in youth football, and older age groups' coaches earning more than their colleagues working with younger age groups. Such incentives create a forward feedback loop that further strengthens the team paradigm (see Figure 8.1).

In order to make the next step in youth football development, a shift to the player paradigm will be crucial. The basic premise of the player paradigm is: potentiality over actuality. The primary

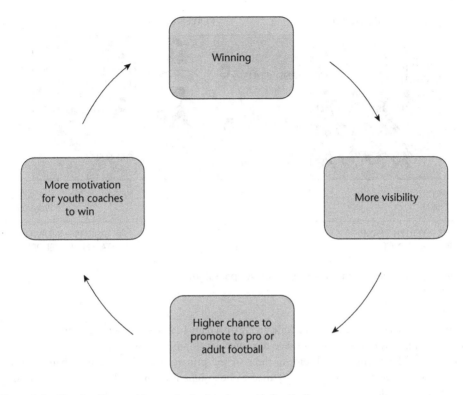

Figure 8.1   The feedforward loop of winning in youth football

objective in the academy should be to optimally develop individual players and fulfil their maximum potential, instead of focusing on current performance levels. Making the most out of a player's potential should in fact be the primary process of every youth academy.

The environment must be prepared in such a way that the environment becomes the coach. The coach takes on more of a mentoring role and has the responsibility to create that environment. Only then can true individualised learning take off. On the player level, every individual is unique. He or she will have a different learning preference, different strengths and a unique learning curve.

Furthermore, although modern football tends to demand more multi-functional players, specialists for different positions still need to be developed and they will often make the difference on the highest level. Nurturing and growing talents into specialist players requires different training methods. Unfortunately, 95% of professional clubs are still under the spell of the team paradigm and not tapping into this vast opportunity of optimal player development.

The traditional organisational structure within an academy is built around a number of teams for specific ages. At Ajax, the organisational focus was shifted from teams to three (multi) age groups, or development phases, covering the full academy which stretches from ages six to 19. Of course, a team structure was inevitably kept in place within the Ajax academy (which for example was necessary to play games against other teams), but it was no longer the main focal point. The coaches were assigned collective responsibility for the total quality of their respective (multi) age group, as well as throughput to the next development phase. Based on the premise

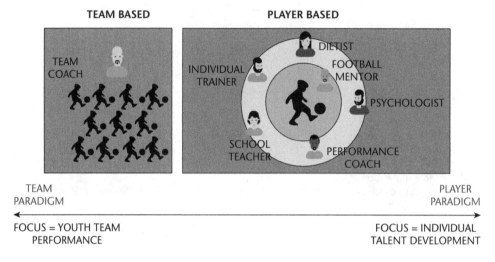

TEAM BASED   PLAYER BASED

TEAM
PARADIGM

PLAYER
PARADIGM

FOCUS = YOUTH TEAM
PERFORMANCE

FOCUS = INDIVIDUAL
TALENT DEVELOPMENT

Figure 8.2   The team paradigm and the player paradigm

that 'more eyes see more', they met collectively on a daily basis to discuss the players and playing style: a continuous interaction in service to player development (see Figure 8.2).

Parallel to the organisational reform, the coaches' primary responsibility was changed: from winning with their team, the unit they used to be assigned to for a full season, to maximising individual player development.

Although the coach 'has' a certain team in the weekend, he would switch teams over the season (rotational coaching system) and would no longer be held accountable for the team result, yet much more for the extent in which he adhered to the playing style and followed up on decisions made with the coaches in his age group to enhance player development. As a result, the typical 'island culture' within the academy was gradually broken down and replaced by more cooperation, to the benefit of the player.

The process of introducing a new paradigm in a professional football club

In introducing the player paradigm at a club, a large percentage of the day to day activities for managers is spent on change management. Important is the notion that coaches have to switch their mindset from result driven (by economic and psychosocial incentives) to development driven (by content, process, empathy, self reflection and self organisation, cooperation, and analysis). Creating such a change has to be done on three levels: the player, the coach, and the organisation.

Furthermore, at Ajax, the focus of work was changed from team performance to improving the individual player through a set of collectively defined player characteristics. By doing that the focus of the coach and parents shifted from winning the match to improving the player. To get the coaches in this different mindset, a lot of supervised discussion on a daily basis between coaches had to be organised. Whilst before each coach operated as their own independent 'island', now he had to work together with others, open himself up to feedback and ideas from others, learn to debate without using fallacies, and learn to control emotions. Finally you need an organisation which supports the role of development, both financially and structurally. For example, the salaries of the coaches of the youngest age group were raised so that they wouldn't have the financial incentive to get promoted. Hence, they stayed working with the youngest age group, which was their core competence anyway.

Role of theory

In this change management process, I relied upon multiple types of theories:

- Systems theory: understanding the nature of complex systems is very important to properly design any training system.
- Biochemistry: understanding the individuality of humans gives the insight that every individual needs a different approach.
- Organisational change theory: helps to design a process of radical change in an organisation and create acceptance throughout the organisation.
- Theory of training and biomechanics: helps to design proper training schedules.
- Theories of talent development: helps to design proper methodology.
- Theories of sports and cognitive psychology: helps to design and maintain optimal environment and helps to interact with stakeholders.

Role of data

In order to help the discussion you need facts and empirical data. Staff were encouraged to debate using logical arguments based on observation and analysis at the expense of blunt opinions and prejudice. In order to have more empirical data I designed a screening method to test players in the four areas of the total footballer: technical, tactical, physical, and behavioural. I used scientific methods to do this but also pragmatic analysis and inter subjective settings. For example, the basic skills of the youngest age group like finishing and dribbling were tested with very simple settings to determine their ball control without pressure. Furthermore, a panel of coaches was asked to determine the subjective level of both skills under pressure and game intelligence, based on the requirements of the football model. Moreover, I used a scientifically designed test (adapted from and by Jordet & Toering 2014; see also Jordet, 2016) to determine the psychological variables such as coping strategies, mindset, and self regulation. Each test was tailormade for the respective age category.

In that way test data became the subject of discussion, which fuelled the content focus on players and kickstarted social interaction between coaches. The communication developed over the years, and could be roughly described following the categories in Tuckman's (1965) team development model: in the beginning, year one, it was forming; years two and three were storming; year four was norming; and finally, year five it was performing.

Politics

An important aspect of the change management process could be discussed under the label of politics. Club politics, for this purpose, could be defined as the interaction of different interests of different stakeholders, which could be driven by many incentives and often simply by a drive to maintain the status quo. Politics had a huge effect on the way I had to organise and communicate his work. The complexity of both the formal and informal structures meant that I had to deal with dozens of different people with different interests. Specifically, there were several complicating factors:

- The historical love-hate relation between the club members and Johan Cruyff.
- The culture of striving for status and power (Machiavelli, Freud and others), which is very prominent in elite football.
- A strong Ajax community consisting of 600 exclusive Ajax members, with a relatively high average age of around 65, that constitute the majority shareholder of the club with 73% of the shares, which poses a threat to people exposing behaviour outside the common norms of this community.
- Former players who have a very strong informal power; the authority argument is unfortunately a frequently used argument in elite football development environments. As someone who depends on first principles, logic, and empirical observation it poses a huge challenge to the way I personally dealt with social interactions and decisions.
- A very complicated formal governance structure influenced by informal power structures (Cruyff, former players, media).

  o You can only become an Ajax member if two other members nominate you.
  o The members elect the club board of seven members with one president who, de facto, is the formal owner of the club.
  o The club board elects a supervisory board of five persons of whom one is president of the supervisory board.
  o The supervisory board appoints and controls a board of directors of four directors.
  o The board of directors appoints and controls a technical heart, consisting of the coach, the technical director, the head of academy, and the assistant of the first team coach with a special role of guarding the culture of Ajax.
  o From the onset it was clear that this complex structure would create inclarity and eventually structural and insolvable conflicts.

- A lack of clarity regarding tasks, responsibilities and autonomy of decision-making between and within the board of directors and middle management.
- A mismatch between the responsibilities of the management of the academy and the autonomy to make decisions about and within the framework of the academy. In other words: academy management was held responsible for the results and operations of the academy but was not allowed to make decisions on hiring and firing academy staff, spending within the assigned budget, external relations and in the last stages even about playing style of the academy teams and decisions about academy players.
- Different sides within the club had different 'media partners' with which they regularly communicated. This posed an external pressure to the academy. Specifically, within the club there were different stakeholders (change-reluctant coaches, directors, board members, parents, and club members) who had contacts with different newspapers, social media channels, and national television programmes, competing with each other. So there was one pro-Cruyff side with backing from media X, Y, Z and an anti-Cruyff side with backing media A, B, C.

As the academy management (Jonk and Jongkind) was not supported by the club leadership and we were transforming the organisation whereas the decision-making roles between supervisory board, club board, board of directors, technical heart and academy management, were not clearly defined, they were constantly putting out fires on an operational, tactical, and strategic level. This impeded their work tremendously. Plan Cruyff only started after going to court to impede the entrance of Louis van Gaal as a new CEO, which was a plan arranged behind the back of Cruyff by the club board, the supervisory board, and the board of directors. Although Cruyff won the case and the whole supervisory board stepped down, the president of the club, who knew about the van Gaal plan, remained in charge of the club. So he and his fellows where always reluctant to Cruyff having success and getting control over the academy, let alone the club. Since parents, coaches, and general Ajax employees have friendships with board and union members and some union members work as coaches, or employees within Ajax, this enables almost everyone to exert informal power over formal entities. This mingling of informal and formal power structures influenced the change process enormously. Next to this, it was unclear who was responsible for what process. Who could appoint and fire a youth coach? Who could recruit a new player and under what conditions? These uncertainties and flaws in the management and control structure created many conflicts between different layers in the organisation.

Essential relationships

In my role as head of talent development I had to develop and implement a complete new methodology throughout the whole youth academy. In this, some of the essential relationships were with:

- The *head of academy*: to formulate policies, make decisions about difficult cases, strategise on future plans, and to implement change management. For example, how to relate to parents, how often and who communicates to them, how to translate the game model into a set of individual parameters for player development, how to deal with coaching development, and how to connect different departments like technical and medical?
- The *coordinators of the three age groups, performance, scouting, and methodology*: they were the ones who had to implement the changes and guard the new norms with the staff. Why, what, who, and how to test and measure? What are the responsibilities of the medical staff in relation to player and coach? When is a player ready to train or ready to play a match? What is the role of methodology in coaching development and design of training sessions? How to connect to the talent identification system and to the player development system? How to organise coach-scout sessions to assess which player should come in, which player should stay and which player should leave the club?
- *Individual coaches*: mostly on the field and during informal meetings it is imperative to keep listening to and talking to the coaches to get feedback on their experiences of the transformation and with this feedback to alter the pace or content of the change process. What are the roles and responsibilities of the individual trainers compared to the coaches? What do they have to train and how to establish whether they have done a good job or not? How should they communicate with players?
- *Parents*: informing parents about the changes and how they can help to beneficially influence their children is essential. In what setting is communication done? Who should be present, how often, what should be communicated and what not? How to deal with problem situations, which rules to set for parents and why and how to communicate to them and enforce them? How to empower the player to take responsibility and communicate his development plan to the parent?
- *Former players* (mostly with Johan Cruyff with whom I spoke at least once per week during five years), because their informal power is so strong it is important to keep them informed

and connected to the changes and give them roles in which they can use their strengths and mitigate the downside of the authority argument.

- *Specialists*: sometimes it is better that a specialist in a certain field brings the message across, rather than the management does so. Therefore sports psychologists, former top athletes, communication experts, and medical specialists were hired to break daily habits and give an impulse to the change process.
- *Press*: everybody in Holland, as well as many people abroad, have their eyes on Ajax and particularly on Johan Cruyff. Therefore countless interviews for papers, magazines, radio, and television were done and eventually a documentary on Fox was made showing everybody the philosophy and how that worked out in daily practice.
- Last but not least, with *players*: keeping in touch with players, keeping supporting them and listening to their experiences. In the end, it is about them, so they need to have the feeling that they become better players and be able to explain why, and next to this smiling was encouraged (because football is a fun game). I strongly believe that observing and interacting with players and parents are essential to understand the effectiveness of any methodology.

Personal challenges

Being a central part of such an organisation, with these types of internal and external pressures, comes with a set of personal challenges. For me these are related to:

- Impulse control: how to control first impulses in case of irrational decisions.
- How to communicate in a way that the message is effectively transmitted.
- Agreeableness: in my case, I had to become less agreeable: making decisions which are less empathetic for the individual but necessary for the organisation.
- Coping with stress: overload on the amount, difficulty, and variety of tasks.
- Balancing the 80–100 hour working weeks with a private social life.

Conclusions

Developing the players of tomorrow is a feat that involves a large set of interactive factors. In this chapter, I have set out to explain one specific approach to this, and more importantly, how exactly this can be done within the structure of an existing club. The most important message is, you need a clear vision, stick to it and implement the changes step by step allowing for the organisation to adapt gradually to a new paradigm. Furthermore, it is imperative to have the full support of the club owner and board of directors. Without this, in a world that is opportunistic, any efforts to change are in vain. As the reader surely will acknowledge, this path is not straightforward. At the same time, the importance of the aim makes even the most strenuous path, both meaningful and rewarding. I would have done the same again, if given a chance.

Notes

1 Wim Jonk and myself were the ones to make a method/practice out of his principle that the player is the centre of the development philosophy and not the coach/team result.
2 https://iffhs.de/iffhs-history-europe-the-player-of-the-century-1900-1999/.
3 https://iffhs.de/iffhs-history-te-worlds-best-player-of-the-century-1900-2000/.

References

Cruyff, J. (2017). *My Turn*. London: Macmillan

Garcia. A. (2016). Interview on ESPN Soccer. 25-03-2016

Jordet, G. (2016). Psychology and Elite Soccer Performance. In T. Strudwick (Ed.), *Soccer Science*. (s. 365–388). Champaign, IL: Human Kinetics

Jordet, G. & Toering, T. T. (2014). Measuring Performance Psychology in Football: A Manual. Unpublished document

Tuckman, B. W. (1965). Developmental Sequence in Small Groups. *Psychological Bulletin*, **63**(6), 384–399. doi:10.1037/h0022100

Part II
The appliance of science
Uni-disciplinary perspectives

While coaching has long been a cornerstone of elite sport systems and programmes, a relatively recent evolution – or revolution in some respects – has been the formal integration of scientific principles and processes in developing, preparing, and supporting performers and teams in elite sport. In many cases, including in the more distant past, these principles and processes have been sought out by performers and coaches in their pursuit of a cutting edge, or their next cutting edge. In other cases, and much more recently, these principles and processes have been more readily offered by scientists, or 'scientist-practitioners' themselves, with a number of specialist and sub-specialist professions growing in scale and credibility. In fact, developments in both the knowledge and application of science have supported major advances or changes in how a host of sports are played or approached. It is also now rare to find a top performer or team that doesn't have any formal 'scientific input', or even multiple sources of 'scientific input'. As such, the purpose of this section is to provide insights on the role that science and scientists plays in modern elite sport, covering a range of established – and becoming established – disciplines.

More specifically, this section is made up of contributions from authors who have provided services to elite sport systems, programmes, and teams across a range of roles. In this section we focus on the work of these individuals as uni-disciplinary specialists, emphasising the exact contribution they make to the performance pie. To start, Andy Jones offers a perspective from physiology, focusing on his work in endurance. In this account, Andy explains his initial steps in the field, his work as a scientist-practitioner, the nature of collaboration with coaches and performers, requirements for doing the job well and professional practice, and, finally, reflections on how physiologists might work best in elite sport settings. Building on this physiological perspective, Clive Brewer then presents his outlook on the role of the strength and conditioning coach. Starting with a description of the role, Clive then outlines some principles of training the individual within the team, sports specificity, and athletic development. From here, Clive moves to consider the importance of clarity in outcomes, how to work in the heat of competition, developing relationships with players, coaches, and fellow support staff, and, finally, essential knowledge and skills for performing in the role of strength and conditioning coach.

In Chapter 11, a view on performance analysis in football is presented from Chris Carling. In this contribution, Chris provides an overview of the modern analyst in football, their skillset, important aspects of their working practice, including working with video and data, coaches, and performers. Staying with football, but moving onto psychology, Geir then provides a perspective on his 20 years of experience as a consultant working with numerous professional European clubs and associations. In this chapter, Geir offers his thoughts on the nature of the professional football environment, his journey and philosophy, and the nature of his work with management, the team, individual players, academies, and in recruitment and scouting. From here, and with Geir's support, Andy Barr then presents his views on how to reduce the risk and incidence of injuries, based on his experiences across a range of high-profile roles and environments. As part of this, Andy provides an overview of his path and philosophy, interactions between 'science' and 'art', elements of testing, the role of psychology, the need to adapt to different sports, typical mistakes, and the importance of communication.

Finally, and progressing to medical practice, Bruce Hamilton then offers his views on this role in relation to elite sport systems, programmes, and teams. More specifically, Bruce considers the role and organisation of medicine in modern elite sport, some important considerations when building a medical team in this environment, some specifics on the role of the team doctor, and some ethical challenges for practitioners and the discipline.

Moving through this section, we hope that the contribution and typical 'ways of working' in each discipline come across as there are certainly a number of similarities but also, inevitably, a number of important differences. More generally, it should also be worthwhile to keep in mind the type of questions that these scientist-practitioners are trying to answer, as well as the type of solutions generated. Additionally, and consistent with the objectives of this book, attention should again be placed on *how* these individuals go about their work, and *why* in this way; particularly in relation to not only technical challenges, but also operational and interpersonal hurdles. Indeed, and recurrent throughout this section, the effective application of science in elite sport requires *much* more than just 'the science' itself!

9

Physiology
Working in endurance

Andy Jones

Editors' introduction

Andy is Professor of Applied Physiology and Associate Dean for Research & Impact at Exeter University in the southwest of England. A researcher with an international reputation, he has authored more than 250 original research and review articles and is co-editor of three books. Andy is also a Fellow of the American College of Sports Medicine, the British Association of Sport and Exercise Sciences, the European College of Sport Science, and the Physiological Society. As a scientist-practitioner, he has acted as a consultant to a number of governing bodies of sport or commercial companies including UK Athletics, the English Institute of Sport, Gatorade Sports Science Institute, and Nike Inc.

Getting started – aspirations and progression

Considering the topic of this chapter, I think I'm a bit of a mix between academic researcher and applied practitioner. I actually started in applied support work, and was 100% applied for a short period of time after I'd done my PhD and my post-doc. I spent about 18 months at the Welsh Institute of Sport at the Sports Council for Wales in Cardiff. Even then, however, I never really lost my aspirations to do a bit of research so I was probably 90 to 95% applied but hankering after research. To be honest, at that time, the distinction between the two wasn't perhaps as clear as it is now. The Welsh Institute of Sport was there before the English Institute of Sport (the EIS) which now provides the vast majority of support to Olympic sports and their NGBs. It was actually a bit of a trailblazer and we were doing a pretty decent job of both servicing athlete needs and pushing knowledge forward.

I was full-time at that stage, working with a whole variety of different sports which was interesting but made me realise that that wasn't the career I wanted to do 100% of the time. I missed the research too much and I wanted to specialise my applied work in endurance sports and in running specifically, rather than trying to cater for all these different sports with different needs. So, after a job search looking for the right position and the right environment, I returned back to the academic fold at Manchester Metropolitan University (MMU). This was a very positive step: MMU was then playing arguably the leading role in sports science support whilst also working hard to establish itself as an academic centre of excellence. In parallel to my academic work, I was working as consultant physiologist for UK Athletics for the majority of that period. I was entrenched in the world of elite sports physiology at that point and even now I like to retain some of that. Even with the more fundamental research that I do, however, I like to have a bit of an applied element to my portfolio. In fact, both while I was at MMU and now, I wouldn't have designed a study that I didn't feel couldn't potentially be useful to athletes or coaches.

Moving forwards to the present, I don't do very much hands-on support any more and that's partly because, as I've climbed the academic ladder as it were, the opportunities have waned. The geography of where I work doesn't help either – being tucked away in the southwest of England doesn't really help as far as that goes. That said, the most recent very applied thing I did was the work with Nike on the Breaking 2 Marathon Project.

With respect to my working status today, I would describe myself as somewhere between an applied scientist and a scientist who does applied work! What I learned a long time ago is that I want to be able to do both equally effectively, so I wouldn't like to be 'pigeon-holed' as one or the other. I always wanted to fill that 'middle niche'. I feel that there are lots of people who want to be basic scientists who toy a little bit with applied work and, equally, there are others who want to be out-and-out applied scientists and don't necessarily know too much about the science. I actually wanted to have a foot in both camps; to be able to do what I hope is good research that actually addresses some basic fundamental physiology questions but also, like I mentioned earlier, does have some application to sport. Equally, I want to be doing some of that translation myself personally rather than having to go through somebody else to make the application.

This was a personal decision. It is a good place for me but I don't think it's necessarily the case that everybody either should do it or can do it. I think there's a specific type of person who can do a bit of both, BUT we do need the people who are the scientists who just do the more fundamental things, some of which may or may not be applicable to athletes at some late stage and we need some people who are hands-on at the coal face; I think there should be a continuum. Not everybody is equipped to do both jobs; those that are have an advantage in the sense that they are a 'one stop shop' for athletes and coaches and they can expedite the translation of new science into practice. Essentially, you can 'cut out the middle man'. I see an important symbiosis in conducting studies in the lab and delivering direct physiological support; there is cross-fertilisation wherein the athletes and coaches can inspire new studies with relevance for performance and the results of new studies can be employed in the field.

The scientist-practitioner approach: an exemplar from my research

One example of this dual approach and the benefits it can offer might be my work on dietary nitrate, which connects with both theoretical and applied issues. The original paper that stirred my interest was published in *Acta Physiologica*, a Scandinavian physiology journal. Most of the work had been done by physicians at the Karolinska Institute. They were interested in nitric oxide biology and, in particular, how it helps in human health and disease. As a group they didn't seem to have a great interest in exercise, so I think it was probably by chance that they put people on sodium nitrate or placebo and got them to perform an exercise test. They were probably interested in blood pressure but, to their surprise and certainly to mine when I read the paper, they also found oxygen uptake was lower during submaximal exercise. In other words, somehow just a few days of supplementation with this particular salt made the subjects more efficient or more economical.

That's very, very surprising and very difficult to achieve so, having read that paper, I could see the performance implications which I think had not been recognised by the authors. Simply, if you can improve the efficiency of an endurance athlete, and all else remains equal, then actually performance should be improved.

So investigating the use of nitrate, from both a theoretical and an applied angle, has generated some very interesting and impactful findings. The increased interest in the use of beetroot juice (a source of nitrate) as an ergogenic aid is one outcome of this. It also offers an example of how having your finger on the pulse of fundamental research can give you the opportunity to take your work in a completely different direction.

Working with coaches and athletes

As an applied scientist, some of my work has involved taking a role in influencing an athlete's training. I don't write the training schedules nor coach athletes directly. An important distinction here would be that the coach writes the schedules and the scientist, in this case me, advises on the impact of those schedules and how those schedules might be refined. I think that maintaining and building from this distinction is very useful in establishing good working relationships with coach-athlete dyads. It also helps that I was a competitive runner myself, albeit not at the level of the athletes I work with. One reason I think I became successful as an applied physiologist with distance runners in particular was because of my background in the sport as well as my scientific training.

The 'mechanics' of the role are pretty straightforward. Anyone can run a treadmill test so long as they follow set instructions. With a little bit of training, they can learn to adopt an appropriate protocol or collect some basic data such as oxygen uptake and blood lactate. Then you've got some numbers but that is clearly much less than half of the story. We are still missing the interpretation and extrapolation, which is where the real expertise kicks in. You have to have a feel for those numbers: what's high, what's low, what's an appropriate blend of those things for that athlete, at that time, based on their aspirations, what they're training for, and everything else. But then you need to know how to translate and interpret these numbers into something that's actually going to be meaningful to the athlete and coach. Now, you can only really interpret the numbers if you know what training they're doing at the moment, so I usually like to have sight of that. Then you need to know, if this particular parameter is relatively low, what type of training might be appropriate to bring it up and where are the potential deficiencies in the existing programme. To sum it up, this is a complicated process requiring a genuine empathy and a 'feel' for the data. Furthermore, inter-personally, there is a very fine line on how critical you can be whilst still ensuring a positive impact. You have got to have very open-minded coaches who don't mind having their programme scrutinised a bit; not necessarily *criticised* but certainly critically reviewed.

This is where that relationship becomes really important, which also places a 'common sense' red line on how much advice to offer. I am fine to give critical feedback and make some suggestions. For example, I'd suggest what you introduce to remedy that deficiency is x, y, and z – but that is where I would usually leave it. I might give some example sessions but I don't feel it's ever my role to show how that all integrates into a weekly or monthly programme. This is where you have to have that interaction with the coach.

In this situation, the athlete-coach-scientist dynamic becomes really important. Many athletes don't particularly want to *understand* the programme. They want to just be told what training to do by the coach they've got, having implicit trust in that person. So everything is best sent through the coach. You have to have that relationship with the coach. The athlete has to buy into it and trust your communications with the coach. Of course, the coach may or may not take that advice. From my perspective, however, if I have delivered the right message in an effective fashion then I have done my job and they can then programme that into what the athlete does, to a lesser or greater extent. In contrast, there are other athletes who are much more involved who almost tell their coach what it is they ought to be doing, so in that case a different approach is needed.

In both cases, as I mentioned earlier, having credibility is really useful. Clearly, that can come from people I have already worked with. However, it also helps that both athlete and coach know I have been involved personally; that I have tried out the protocols and, often, the sessions I am suggesting – that I know how much it hurts! Also, I think there's a language thing as well. I do endurance physiology so arguably the things that limit cycling, for instance, are the same that limit running performance. Notably, however, the language (jargon) is very different and whilst I may have the scientific expertise to be able to advise a cyclist, I don't have the credibility in the sport or the lingo. As a result, I wouldn't be as effective.

What do you need to work effectively?

For an applied worker or a scientist practitioner, some reasonable level of experience and performance is a big, big help to working in the field. I must emphasise the parallel need for interpersonal skills, however. Almost inevitably, there is at least the potential for conflict through the critical role which you should play. Diplomacy is really important. You shouldn't see 'disagreements' as a which-of-you-is-right issue because you both might be! You just have to have a bit of respect for one another's professions. As I mentioned already, if I give advice on the basis of some physiological test data, I'll give that advice to the best of my ability. Whether or not it is then actually used is up to the coach. You know they may dismiss it but I think they'd be foolish to not at least consider it. Indeed, I think all the good coaches will at least consider it. Crucially, however, if they've got a valid reason for rejecting it, that's fine. I'm not going to press my case on them and insist; I think if you start to do that you're on really shaky ground.

What the coach knows much better than I can ever is what that athlete's reaction to that would be psychologically. They have that day-to-day interaction and should bring a much greater and more detailed insight to the 'whys' and 'why nots' for any particular action. So, while what I might say might be true on a generic level, the extent to which that can be built into the programme is the most important element. At the elite level, it is an art really (cf. ideas in other chapters on equal expertise and Professional Judgement and Decision-Making).

The interpersonal skillset also comes into play within the longer-term relationship; for example, how much knowledge is needed of the client. A big factor when working with the coach and/or athlete is their literacy in physiology. Have they had exposure to the subject or content matter before? Have they much interest? Do they have a degree in sport science? Most importantly, perhaps, how confident are they in their knowledge and understanding – anyone lacking in confidence can often get very defensive, feeling 'pressured' by the 'wall of meaningless jargon' being thrown at them. To avoid this, you have to pitch things at the right level. Therefore, and as a crucial part of the initial agenda, you have a bit of an educational role. You have to explain things very, very simply. You don't want to be bamboozling people with jargon.

In my experience, I think this is often a characteristic of younger practitioners; perhaps they themselves are feeling nervous and a bit defensive. As a consequence, they can fall back too much on references and SCIENCE, instead of remaining confident in the quality and veracity of the advice. Things are ideally done on an easy conversational level. You start at the lowest common denominator really and then, over time, you can develop that as they learn a little bit more about what these measurements are getting at and how they're changing due to the training stimulus. As the scientist, you're taking the athlete and coach on that journey. You can become a bit more sophisticated as you go along, but you absolutely don't want to lose them straight off the bat.

In contrast, you design and apply a nested, long-term agenda of increasing their physiology literacy. You are trying to increase their understanding, so you can increase your communication in both breadth and depth. Ideally, the clients are inquisitive about the process, what the tests are measuring/showing and what that means for training. Actually the people that come to you in the first place probably have that sort of mindset unless they've had their arm twisted to come along. The best clients are also acquisitive! They have already read a bit about the area and its potential to contribute. They are aware of some of this stuff already; they're interested, want to broaden their horizons a bit, and want to leave no stone unturned.

Promoting professional practice

In a similar fashion to other sport science disciplines, you can push professional practice through three distinct but often overlapping routes; as a practitioner yourself; in a 'meta-practitioner' role in which you lead a team of providers; or through the accreditation process whereby effective service is evaluated and quality assured, usually this being through a formal or semi-formal certification.

Assuming the existence of a set of very effective criteria for you as a personal practitioner (as outlined above), both the other categories have some inherent problems. First of all, you can't really accredit the person. Of course, some are going to be stronger than others (processes, knowledge, etc.) and some will have more appropriate credentials than others. But, due in no small part to the interpersonal element, some are more effective than others and that's both hard to change and 'challenging' to rule on! You can do your best to try and mentor that individual but, when working away from you, they are on their own and their own person. As a result, their fate is often cast! They are either going to be successful at what they do or not: you can't change their background nor, particularly, teach them 20 years of lingo in six months. As can be seen in the various accreditation programmes run by sports science bodies, you can rubber stamp it to a certain extent. One common method is to use a competencies approach to accredit on behalf of the association that you work for or the national organisation. Unfortunately, however, I don't think you can guarantee that each and every one of the relationships which those providers form are going to be as effective as they might be. I have tried to do that but the extent to which people are receptive to that varies; in some cases, they think they're great already! As with so many 'person-to-person' environments, someone simply has to tell the aspirant practitioner that this isn't for them!

Another issue is the breadth of knowledge and experience which the effective practitioner might need. This can definitely include nutritional and biomechanics skills and a large dollop of psychology is also often useful. It may be that such breadth is really important at the lower levels of client. For example, I think I'm certainly more of a physiologist than a sport scientist. I know enough nutrition to advise on the basics and certainly on the ergogenic aids and such like. However, I wouldn't consider myself a nutritionist. It's been interesting getting into the beetroot juice thing – a whole new world opens up and all the nutritionists and sports dieticians want you to come and speak to them. I'm always at pains to mention that I'm a physiologist not a dietician or a nutritionist even.

Finally, and especially if you are in the meta role (e.g. overseeing a group of physiologists or other disciplinary specialists providing a service), there are issues with time and mentoring skills. When you are in that meta role, which I was for some time, you just don't get the chance to mentor or 'coach' the in-depth skills that are needed. You tend to buzz in to a venue for a day and you watch them do the test and you see work that they produce remotely and give some advice. Of course, you can sit and see how they interact. You can also get feedback 'off line' from other athletes and coaches about that relationship. But in the end you need both the skills and the time to do the job properly. To be honest, there are more chances to develop individuals through the apprenticeship-like relationship that you get with your PhD students.

In any case, I think it takes a bit of nerve to get to the point where you can say to someone "well you're good at this and bad at this". So, for example, if one of my PhD students can't write very well, I know exactly the process that I'd go through to make them a better writer. I think many mentors would need some additional upskilling for them to be able to do the same thing in their applied relationships.

This brings up a very interesting question for institutes or large organisations who want to have a 'network' structure of providers. Are they better having a head of physiology, who looks at the discipline across sports; say cycling, rowing, sailing, running, etc. Or are they better having a sport science and medicine co-ordinator who 'lives in' each specific sport, and has sufficient scope to look at the overall profile of the practitioner, and how s/he fits with coaches, athletes, other providers and management? I would have to say that the second option perhaps makes more sense, albeit that a parallel system of discipline leads can serve to offer advice on innovation.

In conclusion – using a physiologist

In closing, I wanted to offer some examples of how a physiologist might work most effectively in an elite environment. Accordingly, I would like to finish with saying something about my contribution to the Nike Breaking 2 project, in which we had the audacious aim of selecting athletes and supporting them towards an attempt at running a sub-two hour marathon. This is really the current 'holy grail', the new equivalent of the sub-four minute mile. That was the culmination for me to my scientific career so far because I used everything that I've ever learnt whether it be science, soft skills, working with and through coaches/other practitioners – the lot! To come to work with the best endurance athletes in the world to take on this incredible goal of trying to break two hours for the marathon was such an incredibly exciting journey to be part of – to work with Nike and those athletes in the way that we did for as long as we did; to see it all come together and all the logistics being it; all the different parties working together for the same goal.

This was an almost perfect mission or project (Eliud Kipchoge eventually ran the fastest marathon ever, 2:00:25, in Monza in May 2017) and exemplifies lots of the things I have talked about in this chapter. So there's a lot of background science on making the measurements and designing and delivering the overall strategy but just as important is the science-coach-athlete interaction – sitting down with athletes and coaches in Kenya and Ethiopia and getting their buy-in. In short, the hard science, the interpretation of the data, the extrapolation and the application/transfer to the real life challenge. This was a challenge I was excited by and rose to. A physiologist who is capable of contributing in all these areas is probably rare but, I'd like to think, worth finding.

10

Strength and conditioning in the elite team sport environment

Clive Brewer

Editors' introduction

Clive is the Assistant Director of High Performance (Programs) for the Toronto Blue Jays Major League Baseball Team. Prior to this, he was the head strength & conditioning coach to Widnes Vikings Rugby League Club and the National Strength & Conditioning coach for Scotland RL. Clive has been a consultant to a number of high-performance organisations, including Manchester Utd, USA Football, IMG Academy, WTA and the Wimbledon tennis championships. A masters degree graduate from Loughborough University, Clive is accredited by the UKSCA and the NSCA as a Strength & Conditioning coach, and in 2015 was awarded a Fellowship of the UKSCA. He is accredited by the British Association of Sport & Exercise Sciences (BASES) as a support scientist, as well as being a chartered scientist with the UK Science Council.

Understanding the role

The Strength and Conditioning (hereafter S&C) coach plays a unique role within the dynamics of the team environment. On paper this comes down to being the professional with responsibility for ensuring that each individual within the team is adequately prepared to meet the physical demands of the sport for which they train. In practice, the reality is a role that requires a high-energy individual, able to understand complex physio-mechanical concepts, incorporate metabolic training into sports-specific situations, be accountable for injury prevention, and create an appropriate environment where team-mates can push each other to excel.

The context and title of the role is also variable, and I have seen it used differentially across the team sports that I have worked in: in soccer the role is often labelled as the fitness coach or sports scientist; sometimes a dual role, sometimes the sports scientist is separate. In rugby it's typically the S&C coach who is also the sports scientist, and in other contexts it is different again. For example, at the Blue Jays the S&C coach is just that, but is also responsible for administering components of the sports science programme, which runs across every discipline. In other sports the role is split further, so an S&C coach may be a 'strength coach' and not leave the weight room, as is more typical within American football. The key is that the individual within the role has the necessary character and competence to deliver the functionality that is expected of them within their working context.

Train the individual within the team

Much is written about the S&C coach needing to understand the demands of a sport, or a position, with a view to enabling the team to appear at the start of each competition fully physically prepared. Definitely true, but the unwritten rule within this generalisation is that every individual is different, so whilst the team may be on a schedule to enable them to prepare game to game, every individual player within that team is different. The effective S&C coach is accountable for recognising this individual need and organising individual training loads that optimise preparedness for that player, within the structure of the team plan. The S&C coach's understanding of load and recovery parameters at an individual level is fundamental to the effective planning and implementation of any training programme in a team sport environment. As I explore in this chapter, much of this relates to the competitive schedule of the team, but as an example, consider the following scenario which was my reality at Widnes RL in the Superleague from 2012–14.

Of the 32 Players in the first-grade squad, 19 would prepare to play the game on a Saturday. 13 would start, four would be substitutes (so with interchanges typically nine players would play the whole 80 mins, four might play a cumulative total of 40–50 mins, four would play less than 40 mins). Some players may have played for 20 minutes but been involved, whilst two would have prepared to play in case of an injury in the warm-up, but other than warming up these players would have no physical role in the game. Two further players may be loaned out to a different (lower grade) team for game experience or match fitness – they may play on Sunday. We may have three players at different stages of rehab at any given time, and seven players who were not involved in any games at the weekend.

So for some, Sunday was a recovery session, for some game day, and some needed to do some training but not of sufficiently strenuous nature that they were fatigued for Monday, when the team preparation began for the following game. So it's about how the coach differentiates this preparation for each individual to be able to fulfil their role that will determine success. Individualised loading (training or games) and recovery (strategies and players' response to these) are inextricably linked; knowledge of how to manipulate the former to optimum individual levels whilst being able to measure and enhance the effectiveness of the latter enables a comprehensive and effective training plan to be implemented.

Sports specificity and athletic development

The primary ambition within the S&C programme is to create a performance training process that parallels the specific needs of each sport. Central to this is understanding the performance model for the sport – essentially answering the fundamental question "what does it take to win?" Clearly defined physical parameters set forth within the overall performance programme essentially direct the distribution of sessions and resources to this quality, as well as the nature of technical expertise to better align with this philosophy.

The nature of the sport, and the role that 'physicality' plays within it, arguably determines the function that the S&C coach plays within the overall programme: I would suggest that an expert in the physical development of players is always an essential role to fulfil in any team sport. However, the direct contribution that 'physicality' plays in the outcome of performance will determine the prioritisation that the S&C work has within the overall programme. For example, rugby league is a sport where the physical intensity of play is directly related to the likelihood of game outcome: A team can 'out-athlete' the opposition to get a result every five to eight days. So, as reflected in Figure 10.1, a high percentage of total player training time in pre-season

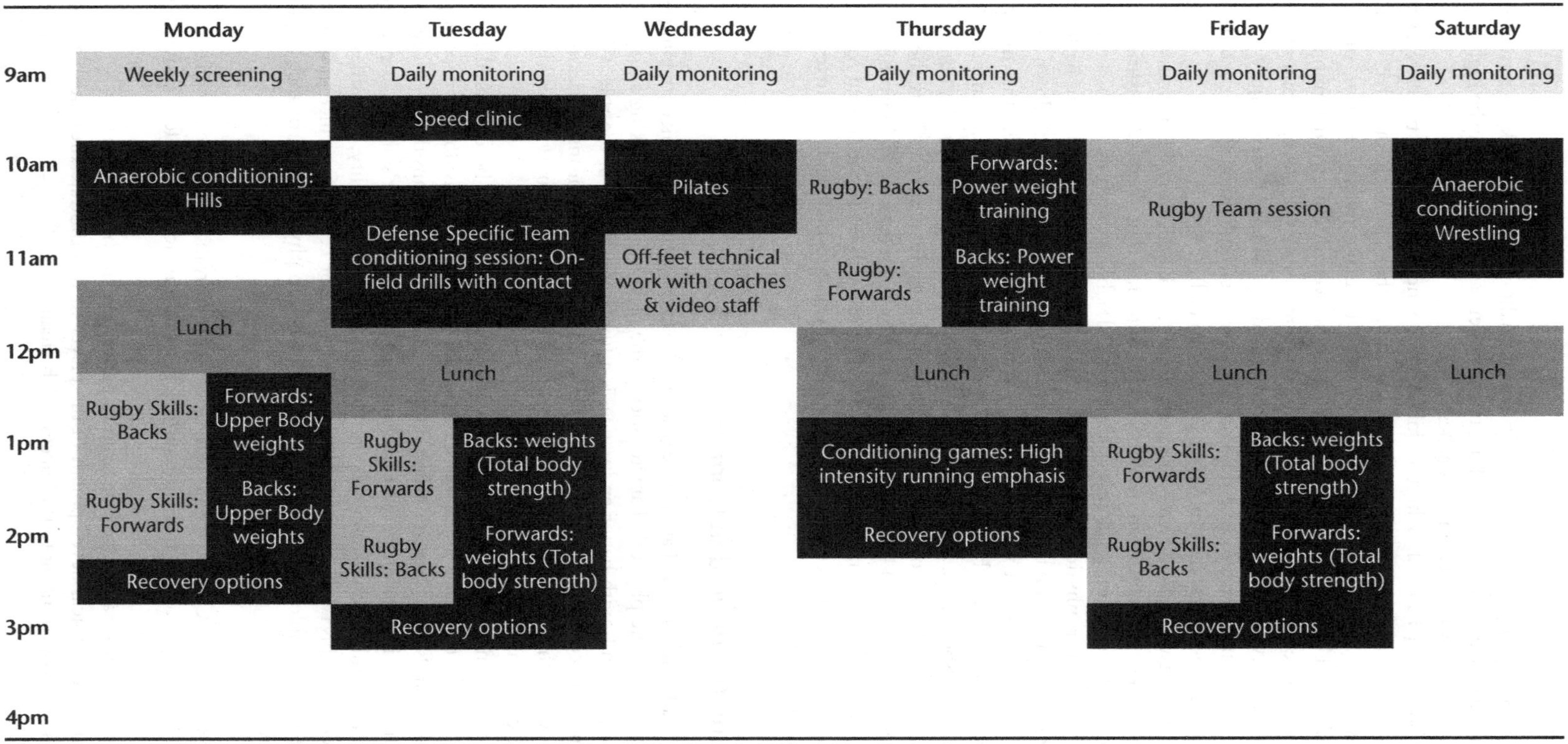

Time	Monday	Tuesday	Wednesday	Thursday	Friday	Saturday
9am	Weekly screening	Daily monitoring	Daily monitoring	Daily monitoring	Daily monitoring	Daily monitoring
10am	Anaerobic conditioning: Hills	Speed clinic	Pilates	Rugby: Backs / Rugby: Forwards; Forwards: Power weight training; Backs: Power weight training	Rugby Team session	Anaerobic conditioning: Wrestling
11am		Defense Specific Team conditioning session: On-field drills with contact	Off-feet technical work with coaches & video staff			
12pm	Lunch	Lunch		Lunch	Lunch	Lunch
1pm	Rugby Skills: Backs; Forwards: Upper Body weights; Backs: Upper Body weights	Rugby Skills: Forwards; Backs: weights (Total body strength)		Conditioning games: High intensity running emphasis; Recovery options	Rugby Skills: Forwards; Backs: weights (Total body strength)	
2pm	Rugby Skills: Forwards	Rugby Skills: Backs; Forwards: weights (Total body strength)			Rugby Skills: Backs; Forwards: weights (Total body strength)	
3pm	Recovery options	Recovery options			Recovery options	
4pm						

Figure 10.1 An example pre-season week at Widnes Rugby League

Source: Used with permission of Widnes RLFC

(60–70%) is given to the development of physical qualities (shaded black). Consequently, the S&C coach is typically part of the coaching teams' inner-sanctum, and may be higher up within the hierarchy than assistant technical coaches.

Contrast this with baseball, a highly skilled sport where players are typically expected to perform every day (with the exception of the starting pitchers, who are on a five-day rotation). Baseball players rely on athleticism to enable them to make defensive plays, or are speed-specialists who steal lots of bases, but skill is the biggest overriding factor determining win–loss. In this sport the essential role of the S&C coach is to maximise the player's ability to make the movements that they need to execute and avoid deloading (which increases injury risk) through application of minimal yet effective training doses for each individual during a heavy playing schedule (162 games in 180 days in Major League baseball).

Somewhere between these two extremes is soccer; a skilled sport where individual aspects of physicality at key moments can influence game outcome (e.g. forward outsprints defender, defender outjumps attacker, goalkeeper is powerful/flexible enough to pull of a reflex dive to save a shot). However, physicality is not something that directly impacts team performance in every game, in that a skillful team can typically retain possession and break down a fitter team. That doesn't mean to say it isn't important, I stress again it is a vital role that many athletes have neglected to maximise because they do not fully understand the performance-enhancing value of strength, speed, etc. However, the contribution that physicality plays on result is less important than the ability to execute the skills of the game at speed. Thus the qualities of fitness (speed, strength, etc.) become enabling functions to repetitive and forceful skill execution. It should also be remembered that increased fitness will lead to increased robustness and the resilience required to recover sufficiently from a game to play again in three to five days, 50–70 times per year.

Understand the desired outcomes

Many have made the mistake that the role of a S&C coach in sport is to think of training as a vehicle to improve only the physical characteristics of the player. Indeed, making a player stronger, faster, more powerful, with better endurance, is a fundamental part of the role. Conceptually, however, an S&C coach needs to think of (physical) training as a means of making the player better. This slight change in emphasis needs to encroach into the entirety of thinking relative to programme design and session planning.

So the effectiveness of the S&C programme typically needs to be evaluated by measures related to the need to 'make the player a better player'. Period. This doesn't necessarily mean that the player can 'squat / bench / insert name of lift more' – it means that we need to be able to demonstrate the impact of the S&C programme upon the player's ability to perform as an effective team member. Our outcomes are factored around availability, robustness, reliability, and preparedness. This typically comes down to three major key performance indicators showing that the player's athletic capacities are able to exceed to physical performance requirements of the sport:

1   Player availability: Consistency in team sports comes from having the best players available for the head coach to practice with and select in a formation that he feels provides the best chance for success.
2   Increased physical capacity of the team to perform at the highest level.
3   Optimise the physical development of the player to demonstrate the valuable impact that they have in contributing to the success of the team.

The role typically can therefore be broken down into two major aspects – the physical preparedness of the players during the week and in the build-up to the game, then the in-game management of the players. Typically, this chapter will focus on the former, but a brief look at the game-day process is an important context to understand.

In the heat of battle – stay calm!

This is where professionalism becomes most challenged, as stood pitch-side, with the game going on in front and the crowd screaming behind, your job is to take care of one thing – the immediate needs of the players and coaches. As support staff you cannot be a fan! You cannot be excitable and get involved in the game: being controlled and consistent is an important trait in this situation. That way you can take care of business regardless of what is going on around you. Remember that the game is for the players and the fans – your role is to support that outcome, not get involved in it!

You probably won't see the game anyway! You will typically be watching a particular player and seeing how he is moving, or trying to estimate his / her level of fatigue (especially in a game such as rugby league where players can interchange throughout the game). You may be undertaking a sideline warm-up, or running water onto the field. The role really depends upon the context of the sport: in soccer it may be more about setting up the dressing room for half-time, *then* watching the players in action (probably not the action though!) due to the

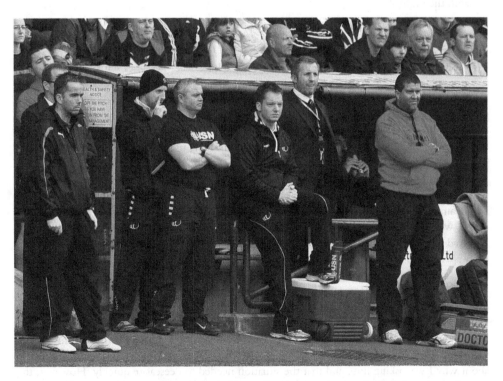

Figure 10.2   The dugout during a Widnes game: notice how the head coach (Denis Betts, suited), and medical staff are watching the action around the ball – I (in short sleeves) am looking at another player and watching how he is moving

Source: Used with permission of Widnes RLFC

level of interaction involved. In baseball the strength coaches may be helping fuel athletes in the dugout, recording key statistics such as 'time to first' or a catcher's 'pop-time', or are back in the clubhouse with a non-playing pitcher working out during the game. In rugby my role was to run the bench – get water and coaches' messages onto the field, prepare players for interchange, and keep the manager informed of any change in players' status, as well as manage the half-time routine.

Essential relationships: the player(s)

The need to be high-energy is often mistaken to mean that the S&C coach needs to be a 'motivational cheerleader'! The reality is that most coaches at the top of their professions are far from this but, as the individual who is prescribing typically the most taxing sessions for the players in the team process, you need to empower and inspire them to bring the best version of themselves to training every day. You also need to do this knowing that elite players act 'outside of normal parameters' and definitely do not exist at the average. This requires consistency, and 'knowing when to put your arm around a player, when to blow sunshine into their world, and when to let them know more is expected of him / her' in a manner in which that individual will value. More importantly, it's about creating the environment where players can hold each other accountable for their teammates to do these things. This also means that you need to be selfless – the needs of those 32 players come before anything going on in your life when you are with the players!

Trusting you with their careers!

The S&C coach in an elite team environment is a selfless role. It comes with territory where success is defined by helping others to grow, develop, and perform: everything about your role is related to making the players better! That doesn't make you a servant, but coaching is a service industry, and our role is to work with the players in order to provide them with the optimal opportunity to perform every game. Learning that you need to be friendly with the players, but not their friend, is a key lesson that typically occurs early in the life of every strength coach. They need to know that you care as a precursor to knowing what you know!

This is important, as there will be times when you are required to have difficult conversations with players, who, as superstars in the sporting world, have big egos that you need to manage. For example, I remember one session that was being overseen by a less experienced assistant coach, who wasn't having a good day at the office, and the players weren't responding with the required intensity. One of the stars of the team was getting frustrated, but rather than setting an example and showing the other players how the drill should have been done, he retreated into a shell and largely disappeared from the session.

As I wasn't a technical coach, it was my role to intervene without undermining the coach during the practice. Therefore, afterwards I went up to the player and asked him why he didn't "step up": This was after all part of their conditioning load. His response can't be printed, but "F . . . . you if you think that's my fault" was a common feature. I quickly realised that my timing was awful given his state of arousal and anger with the wasted session, his lack of understanding about why I was asking him, and that the situation needed to deescalate quickly. However, the next day, when the player came in, I asked him if I could have some of his time. We sat and I showed him his GPS data for the session, that of others around him, and what the data were like for other, similar sessions that went well. I acknowledged my mistake in the timing of my challenge, and we talked calmly about him leading by example, about responsibility leading accountability, and about how others look to him as an example to drive the intensity of the work that needs to be done – if he responds to the coach, others will.

Always be humble, not vulnerable

One important lesson to learn right off the bat is that if you are worried about making a fool of yourself, you are in the wrong job. Players will challenge any weakness that you have, and if you take yourself too seriously, that will haunt you! There is a difference between being humble, an essential characteristic, and being vulnerable. In a long season, part of the process of camaraderie is definitely knowing when to roll with a situation so that you are the brunt of the players' humour – but you need to do so without becoming the team joker.

The reason I share this is that successful relationships with players are built upon mutual respect. This involves humility, in the sense that it is important to be modest, even politely submissive (to the needs of the players and the head coach). *Your* needs must come behind the players' wants, which is a hard lesson to learn, and which can take even the best a while to comprehend. With our knowledge base, why should we compromise what we know to be right? The answer comes down to being able to look at the world through a different lens than your own – then when you gain insight into the individual you are working with, you can be innovative in how you work with them to achieve the outcome that you want.

S&C and players have very different talents; our histories and educations are typically different, and our experiences vary from one another (even if we started on the same path as trying to make it as a professional athlete). I have never played in front of 80,000 people, I can walk down the street and not be bothered by fans, I can't afford a luxury sports car. However, the players have never sat for thousands of hours planning programmes and trying to work out how to make someone else better. As a coach said to me early in my career when I was working with a professional soccer team – "you spent seven years studying at university – most of these players finished school at 16 – don't try and understand them". It was a great lesson for me – humble people realize their understanding is limited and embrace it.

Developing ownership

In doing everything to make players better, and individualising every aspect of preparation within the context of the team's schedule, there are times when what you want them to do and what they want to do are different. As a young coach, this was initially a challenge to my ego – but ultimately with experience you realise that there isn't one way to do anything. To get the best out of a player I had to work with them without sacrificing the integrity or outcome of the programme. Humility teaches you to wisely look for answers outside of yourself, and this is where we need to work with the players so that we can marry what they like with what we need them to do: this enables them to own the programme, and thus achieve buy-in.

So, you develop suggestions based upon conversations with the player around "if that really works for you, why don't we adapt this to reflect that?" You achieve a balance that enables the player to have ownership of the programme, without compromising your objectives. This is both situationally and culturally specific. Many players are happy to simply do as they are told, trusting in the knowledge that the S&C coach knows what is best for them. Others will need to understand the 'why' a bit more, which we always need to be able to provide. Others, especially I have found in baseball, want more ownership of their programme and it truly is a partnership with the player to pull their programme together. This partnership doesn't typically extend to team conditioning sessions though, especially in a contact sport like rugby. Here, players want and need to be pushed, and to go through a common shared experience; knowing that those who seek short-cuts in tough sessions will likely do so in a game, and that this will cost the team. So these sessions are put together with the coaches with a view to identifying critical variables that will fatigue the team in a sport-specific manner through which players can be stressed. Such practices are designed to develop camaraderie through shared hardship, and expose physical and mental weaknesses to others who will line up alongside them on game-day and expect them to put their body on the line. This is where the S&C coach needs to be strong enough to look a player in the eye and tell them they aren't delivering, encourage them to stand straight, not look tired and so, penalise the team. When any player, regardless of who, takes the easy path, that will ultimately let everyone down. This doesn't mean shouting at the players though – they are professionals, and do not need to be disrespected. The feedback you provide should nurture their competitive spirit and inherent need to push themselves and their teammates to excel.

Game day!

Understanding the game-day routine of the sport and the team is hugely important. It is also essential that the S&C coach spends time understanding how each individual wants to be interacted with to enable them to prepare optimally. Team sport players are typically superstitious, and have set routines for everything, especially on game days. It is important that you know each player, and what they like to do, and how they like to be approached – and more importantly, what they don't like, as you don't want to disrupt their routine. As the S&C coach, you work through the pre-game routines with the players, whilst addressing individual preferences – who likes to talk, who wants to be left alone, who needs additional stretching work.

There are many who want to be in the dressing room environment prior to the game – personally, I have always found it easier to be 'around' the dressing room. This means I am available for anyone who needs me, but not in the way of preparation. So once I set everything up before the players arrive, catering for all their individual needs around equipment, supplements etc., I stay close enough so that I am there for anything a player needs, but I am not in the way of the players as they prepare themselves, until it's time for me to deliver the team warm-up.

Whether in training or prior to the game, the job of the S&C coach is to do everything possible to empower the player to be the best version of themselves that they can physically be. The challenge is to get past our own ego first though, and put whatever we are doing as secondary in nature: if an S&C coach is eating lunch, and a starting pitcher needs something, that is more important. We have to manage our own expectations around players, make sure that they know that we have their best interests at heart, and that they constantly understand 'why' we want them to do things in the way that we do – the key is to recognise that we have to put the player's needs first.

Essential relationships: the coach(es)

Explaining the structure and role of the coaching team around the players is typically pretty easy, and I can best do it using the analogy of a Formula 1 Grand Prix set-up. Consider the players as the multi-million-dollar sports car: this is what the fans come to see, the media want to speculate on the performance of, and definitely where the most money is spent. The manager or head coach (I will use these terms interchangeably) depending on the sports context is the driver. This person is directly accountable for the performance of the car in the race, and will make the key decisions during the course of the race (season). If the car doesn't perform, the media will first look to the driver!

In American sports, the general manager typically controls the playing staff roster, player transactions and bears the primary responsibility on behalf of the ballclub during contract discussions with players. They run the team on behalf of the owners – much like the team principle does in Formula 1. The assistant technical coaches, the strength & conditioning coach, sports scientists, medical staff and performance analysts are all the mechanics or engineers in the Formula 1 team. It is their job to set the car up exactly as the driver wants it so that it performs to maximum effect on whichever circuit is being raced that day.

Working with the boss

The context of the S&C role is very dependent upon the philosophy of the manager at the time – although the commonality is that it is ultimately the manager's programme. For example, at Widnes RLFC and the Toronto Blue Jays, I have a major role in planning the overall programme: this is because the head coach / senior baseball staff have valued my learned and experiential knowledge in workload management, and optimising learning and performance potential in the players through applied principles relating to skill acquisition, circadian rhythms, etc. This is common in many British teams where there is an experienced S&C coach, and this function has been hugely beneficial for my growth as a practitioner.

If it isn't the S&C coach, it may be a performance manager (my current role), sports scientist, or even another coach – it is more about who has the knowledge to map out all the requirements of the programme, develop an understanding of what methods might be used to achieve these objectives, and plan the loading cycle across weeks. In other models, the S&C coach is provided the time allocated to strength sessions, or conditioning work, and then left to programme this time accordingly. Fortunately, such situations are typically becoming rarer as the role of the S&C coach as an integrated member of the support team has evolved. Indeed, I suggest that a S&C programme written in isolation of the rest of the training programme is one that is destined to failure!

My experience is that, having been so involved in the detailed planning of the training week, the boss fully understands the 'why' of the plan, and therefore the need to follow structure and deliver the planned session. That said, there have always been days where the quality in the planned technical session wasn't what the boss would like, and the planned workload volume would be shelved in favour of technical practice. The benefit of me being involved in planning the overall programme is that adjustment becomes easy for the following sessions to avoid overloading players, and the balance of training inputs can be tracked. For me, it's important that the head coach has the ability to dictate practice schedules in this way and that staff are so well prepared that they can be adaptive in real time.

Balancing training and deconditioning loads is an essential role for data that can be shared with the coach in a way that is meaningful to him / her, and is a vitally important part of your relationship. Trust is such a big component, and your competence at skilfully and succinctly presenting relevant data in an impactful manner to the coach is a core part of that trust. The science has to be valid but, more importantly, accessible to the coach, who can then own the decisions that are informed by the interpretation of the shared data.

I have always encouraged the head coach to come into the weight room when sessions were being delivered. My feeling is that this has always empowered them to view the players working in all contexts, but it also highlights to the players that the head coach values the work in the weight room as much as on the field, and that (s)he is also interested in the work ethic of the players in this environment. This isn't always unproblematic however – when a head coach says to a player "don't lift too much, you'll injure yourself" it will cause a problem for the player in terms of confidence – so the discussion has to be had about why the head coach can't say such things, and that they have to trust me on what and how the player is lifting. Similarly, when the coaches use the weight room time to talk to the players about other things, and disrupt the flow and intensity of the session, this also needs to be addressed in an appropriate manner.

The medical team make me better

As well as a strong relationship with the head coach, the other key relationship to develop is with the medical staff. In all my roles, I have spent more time with the medical staff than any other person at the club: we would meet first thing in the morning, have multiple conversations throughout the day, and then speak after training or that evening to plan subsequent days. There should be no hierarchy between these professions in the context of the team – one role is inextricably linked with the other, and they are mutually beneficial.

In every instance, I have been involved in a player's injury management process from the moment of diagnosis – similarly, the medical staff have been involved in every player programming discussion, highlighting opportunities for protection against risk – either through appropriate strengthening of weaknesses or highlighting potential contraindications to a particular player with a movement. This means appropriate adjustment becomes possible.

Understanding that injury occurs where loading exceeds capacity (either through movement competence or tissue tolerance) predisposes the S&C coach to develop a close working relationship with the medical team. Similarly understanding that appropriate loading is protective against injury is also a fundamental first principle for both staff to accept.

One key learning is that the 'referral in' process is much more effective than 'referring out': the difference between sending the player to the medical team, as opposed to bringing the medical expert into my discussion with the player, is an important distinction. Referring someone in tells the player that I trust the medic's opinion to provide answers that I might not have, and that I am invested in the emerging story rather than dismissing the player to another's care.

The importance of exercise-based intervention in the treatment process cannot be overlooked. Therefore working together with the physio makes both professionals more effective at their role. My experience has been that working with the medical team to develop adaptive and challenging rehabilitation exercise patterns and loading programs has significantly enhanced both my understanding of human physio-mechanics but also of exercise progressions, and I have become a better coach for it.

My team-mates

There are other members of the support team who are highly important to interact with, and again the nature of this interaction depends upon the staffing structure at the club. The nutritionist is of paramount importance, for example. No player can out-train a poor diet, and their body composition is as much determined by their nutritional and lifestyle habits as the work they do with the conditioning coach. So the team nutritionist has always been someone I have worked closely with in order to establish goals for the player. Managing body composition requires a constant dialogue between me and the nutritionist in terms of the fuel in, energy burned and subsequent impact on performance output.

Mental performance coaches are also an important part of the support team, and I have found them an invaluable resource, especially around how to communicate with a player to get maximum impact. This has been especially important around issues related to adherence or avoidance behaviours, as players tend to work hard at what they enjoy. They have helped me understand players' situational motivation, to ask better questions of players as part of my feedback process, and have generally helped me influence the players and the environment more effectively, both at a team and an individual level. The ability to refer the mental performance coach into my role, so that we can improve the performance-health of the player, has always been an important process for me.

Essential knowledge and skills: what did I need to do the job?

Texts have been entirely dedicated to the undermining technical skills and knowledge requirements that it takes to be a S&C coach! It is hard to provide a summary of this without technical detail, but essentially it comes down to four main functions (which are not presented in any prioritised sequence):

- Can you understand the needs of the sport from a physical perspective?
- Can you integrate into the culture of the sport as part of the coaching team?
- Can you observe, analyse and provide mistake-contingent feedback in order to influence desired outcomes within group and individual settings – ie. can you coach?
- Do you have the required underpinning scientific and technique knowledge to maximise the desired physical adaptations whilst ensuring optimal recovery to fulfil potential in competition.

Delivering purposeful practice

There isn't scope to go into all of these areas within the context of this chapter, but I would highlight the importance of being able to coach and manage groups of players as being an important skill that many who come from a personal training or individual sport background often lack. Knowing how to organise a group, how to keep them engaged and focused, and how and when to feedback in group sessions are all key skills for the S&C coach. Even knowing when and how to provide individual feedback in a group context is important. For example, if you are in a group doing sprint work where you are the only coach, knowing where to position yourself so that you can observe movements, and being able to grab an athlete to provide feedback before their next repetition, is an important skill: Don't be the coach that just says "go!".

Workload management is essential

Prior to the session, planning is key. Your success in the role depends upon the ability to keep the players training and playing, and to effectively communicate the players' state of preparedness with coaches so that you can best drive effective outcomes. Having a knowledge of how to best manage training stress within an overall training process is important. There is a right time to introduce a training stimulus, and it is important that the S&C coach is able to manage that within their system. This means having the ability to quantify and control training volume load, and appropriately balance out how that is affecting the athlete's neuro-muscular system, muscular-skeletal system, neuro-endocrine system, and also psychologically.

Subjective response questions around sleep quality / quantity, or soreness, are really valuable as a means of stimulating conversation. Simply walking up to a player and asking "is the baby teething?" because I knew he had a young child and his sleep data was way down are great ways of showing players that you care. Similarly, one player in pre-season once said to me "You pay no attention to that data: I'm really sore and you haven't changed anything". I agreed with him, he was really sore, I told him what number he had given for soreness so showed I knew it, and that was exactly where I wanted him to be so, no, I hadn't changed anything! As long as players know that you are using the data that you collate for their best interests (which are also your best interests, as you have got the same common aim), then players will typically work with you on anything, once you have established a relationship built on trust (for an example of this, please see Figure 10.3).

Once the season starts, all of the models that you will see about various loading patterns are invalidated. There are no heavy, light, etc. weeks – simply game weeks. It is all about winning every game, and as such the S&C programme becomes about managing fatigue from one game and physical preparedness for the next. This has to be framed in the context of maximising the ability to be involved, not minimising it – these are very different philosophically. The factors around days between games, travel, time of the game are all primary determinants in the programme that you put together. The game week is simply about having all the healthy players in the squad able to put in a physical effort game day −3, be available for a team run-through game day −1, and be healthy for selection by the coaching staff.

There is no book learning that teaches you to manage cumulative training load and fatigue across the season. You need to have a firm grasp of how the body adapts to different stressors

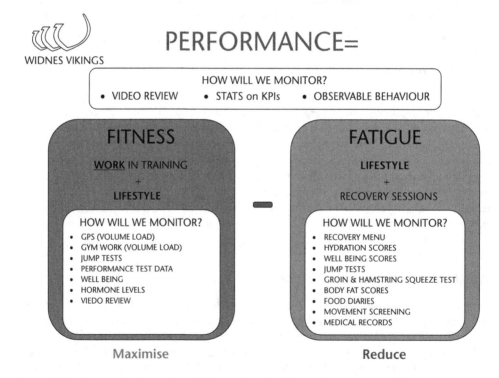

Figure 10.3 The poster we used at Widnes to remind players how we quantified performance, work done, and recovery/adaptation to that workload

Source: Used with permission of Widnes RLFC

around the various systems that comprise motor capacity and, equally importantly, how to manip-ulate training inputs in order to effectively impact these systems. To put together a sequential programme, week on week, that encompasses cumulative workloads and fatigue, is something that no academic learning will provide: this will only come from experiential knowledge, and having made many mistakes on the way that you can learn from. Theory will tell you about train-ing stimulus cycles and responses, experience tells you that every individual is different, and that there aren't fast times, or slow times, just the right time for that person. This is why it is important to have a plan developed, but also have objective criteria that will guide that plan to enable you to adapt it for each player. Without the appropriate stimulus, players can decondition or overtrain pretty quickly over a long season.

Understanding your office

Typically, the S&C coach is required to programme for and deliver group sessions within four specific environments

- Field based training
- Strength, power and speed programmes
- Promotion of recovery
- Team meetings

The ability to deliver a field-based session requires a delicate balance between being able to deliver a speed or conditioning session appropriate for the sport, and delivering a sports-specific session. Many of us transition between sports, as our expertise is in the S&C field. As such, I always plan the conditioning drills with members of the technical coaching staff. As there are elements of technique that are needed within the drills, I endeavour to have a technical coach assist me in the delivery. I don't have the expertise to be coaching say, a three-in tackle, so when this is part of the conditioning session, that needs to be appropriately coached. There are some S&C coaches who have graduated into the role as sports specific specialists, with either a technical coaching or playing background, and obviously they have different expertise: the key message here is that a definition of expertise has to incorporate knowing the extent of your sphere of knowledge, and not going beyond that. When a player knows that you don't know something, or a coach sees you coaching something that you don't know, people get upset!

Being able to control the variables of a drill is important in order to achieve the desired out-come. Motivationally speaking, players will always work harder (in a conditioning sense) than they realise if there is a ball involved! We have compared heart rate and work output (GPS) data from sessions based simply on conditioning drills, which players have rated as 9/10 in terms of RPE, with conditioning games where the players have worked harder, yet perceived efforts were at 7/8. As Figure 10.1 shows, it's about how we achieve an appropriate balance that determines the long-term success of the program. Ultimately, in-season, specific conditioning sessions with players who are starting games regularly are hard to achieve – this requires a col-laboration with the coaches to ensure that the work–rest ratios within the technical sessions are of sufficient intensity to prevent deconditioning.

So the S&C coach needs to have the technical knowledge to coach conditioning, speed mechanics, agility mechanics, plyometrics, and all forms of resistance training to be able to deliver. You will be required to coach all of these to groups and individuals every week. As well as the technical knowledge, you need to find a means to manage large groups in the weight room. I have always tried to maintain an absolute maximum ratio of 12 players to one coach, so if you haven't assistant S&C coaches, this needs to be factored into the scheduling. Then knowing how to supervise a weight room, where you stand to ensure you can see most of the work occurring, and how you can then prioritise which player needs help the most at any one time. For me it was always in a priority order of:

1   Safety
2   Movements with high levels of technical complexity
3   Movements requiring precise postural control or joint positioning
4   Anything else

This requires the weight room to be appropriately designed, with clear lines of sight, demarked space that enables weights to be dropped safely, and appropriate division of people throughout the area. This typically means having as much free space in the middle of the room as possible. This is your area to manage, and it is important that the weight room is designed to deliver sessions how *you* want them to run. This includes such fine detail as the sound system – who is able to put on music, do you tolerate players changing songs during the workout, etc. All these factors will dictate the rhythm of the training sessions that you supervise. Ultimately I have always expected the players to bring 'intensity' to a session, but there are key environmental factors that you can 'bake in' that will help.

In summary

The S&C coach is a unique role within the team sport environment; arguably the heartbeat of the coaching, medical, and performance processes. I have the training of a scientist and a S&C coach, but none of this has developed the interpersonal characteristics needed to be successful in the role. As a coach, there is a fundamental need for me to be able to develop relationships with the staff and players that are based on trust. This enables me to be successful in this role. I have also been nutritionist, sociologist, relationship counsellor, and kit man, without formal training for any of these. As with many coaching roles, the keys to success have been related to over-planning the delivery, being flexible at an individual level with the delivery and, within the overall culture of the club, creating a programme where players want to work hard. The head S&C coach needs to be accountable – as this empowers responsibility, which means that your programme matters and contributes to the bigger scheme of things. Being accountable means that every day I have to look at myself in the mirror and question what I can do better to make others better; with this honesty comes the selflessness to know that now is the players' time to achieve, and how we best get the most from them will determine the success of the athletic development component of the programme.

11

Performance analysis

Working in football

Christopher Carling

Editors' introduction

Christopher Carling has worked for over 20 years in elite sport and notably as a performance analyst and sports scientist. He has extensive experience working in several high-profile football settings including Manchester Utd, PSG, Olympique de Marseille, Lille OSC and the Clairefontaine National Football Centre. He has also previously worked for the French National Institute for Elite Sports Performance. Christopher is currently programme director for the Professional Doctorate Award at the University of Central Lancashire, UK. He has a PhD in Sports Science and has co-authored two books, six book chapters and more than 80 international peer reviewed papers.

Introduction

Performance analysis is used in football (soccer) to assess technical, tactical, and physical performance, both individually and collectively, and generally in the competition setting (Carling et al., 2018). Factual evidence derived from analyses provides an opportunity to critically appraise how players are performing through qualitative (e.g. video clips) and quantitative (e.g. data) assessment and is one of the foundations for providing feedback to coaches and players. The information from performance analysis can be used to identify positive elements of play that can be subsequently built upon in practice while those considered negative can be remedied. It can also help to analyse the effectiveness of training in line with desired outcomes and aid preparation for forthcoming opponents following identification of their strengths and weaknesses. Analyses play a role in team selection processes and choice of team tactics as well as informing the recruitment of prospective signings. Larger datasets derived from analysis can be mined to model trends in data across matches and seasons in order to provide a deeper understanding of how past and present performance have evolved over time. Figure 11.1 demonstrates the role of match-play analysis within the weekly coaching cycle.

Over the last decade in particular, performance analysis has grown in popularity and is firmly rooted at elite playing standards (McKenzie & Cushion, 2016). This is mainly due to a greater recognition within football circles and importantly by applied practitioners of

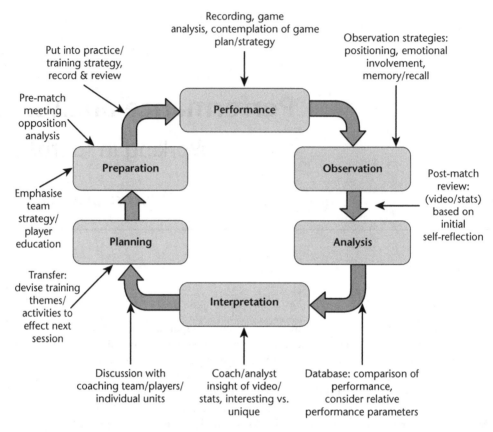

Figure 11.1 Match analysis within the weekly coaching cycle (Wright et al., 2014).

Source: Reproduced with kind permission from Taylor & Francis

its potential benefits to impact decision-making and prescription in the training and match lifecycle. This increase in popularity can also be associated with major advances in computer and video technology that enable comprehensive post-match and real-time analyses of performance. The latter notably provides opportunities for split-second evaluation and decision-making at any moment over the course of play. In addition, the emergence of a comprehensive mass of knowledge on competitive football performance through scientific research (Sarmento et al., 2014, 2018) and more recently, online social media sources and blogs, is providing clues to closer determine the winning formula associated with successful play. Finally, changes to coach education programmes by some of football's governing bodies to reflect advances in performance analysis have also improved the understanding, acceptance, and value of the discipline.

Reflecting this evolution, the majority of professional clubs (particularly in the UK) now formally employ performance analysts (PAs) to perform systematic ongoing assessments of match performance and to a lesser extent training. The perceptions and roles of the PA have evolved substantially over the last decade or so. PAs are no longer simply recording training sessions and match-play and providing edited video highlights according to the wishes of the coaching staff. They are reactively and pro-reactively handling, disseminating, and generating insights from video and data collected using sophisticated technologies to respond to the ever-changing demands of the game. This chapter provides an overview of the PA role and its challenges as well as exploring the knowledge and skillset required to work in contemporary elite football environments. Some of the insights are based on personal experiences of the author.

The contemporary PA: role and place in the team

Over the last two decades there has been a shift towards a more systematic scientific evidence-based approach to managing and preparing the contemporary high-level football player (Strudwick, 2016). There is a viable need for information and feedback from multi-disciplinary science and medical support services to aid the decision-making processes of coaching staff and impact upon player development and performance. Support in contemporary elite sport is ensured by a comprehensive backroom support team of physical conditioning and medical practitioners, physiologists, recovery analysts, injury rehabilitators, and nutritionists. These support staff are systematically implicated in collection, analysis, and interpretation of information on training, preparation, and competition and communicating findings. Recently, the creation of roles such as head of football analytics and football data scientist has confirmed the shift in the industry towards a more systematic approach to analysing performance.

Performance analysis personnel are generally employed to conduct analyses in first team, reserve team, women's teams and youth academy environments. Irrespective of their specific role, the analysis department essentially supports coaching staff by systematically collecting pre-, live-, and post-match analytical information (both video and statistical) on technical and tactical performance (Wright et al., 2013). The information generated is subsequently analysed and interpreted to make evidence-based judgements and provide feedback on individual and collective contributions. In turn, this should lead to prescription of informed coaching interventions in preparation for match-play.

Typically, there are three main contemporary PA roles: professionals working specifically to analyse first-team performance, those monitoring first-team opposition, and analysts within academies. Many clubs employ a 'head' or 'lead' PA (both for first-team and academy) who in addition to usual performing analyses has a managerial-type role (e.g., management and recruitment of other personnel). In this function the PA must ensure a high standard of work across their department (quality control at each phase of the analysis process) while simultaneously organising and constantly developing integrated, club-wide analytic processes. He or she must also monitor budgets and project expenditure and constantly look to improve policy implementation through building leaner, more flexible, and responsive processes. Some PAs can perform several key roles within a football club, whereas others focus on a solitary area. There can be a lack of uniformity in their key responsibilities and tasks across clubs and analysts can be deployed in various ways according to service demands and the culture of their organisation.

Over the last decade or so, there has been a gradual separation of technical, tactical and physical analyses. PAs mainly liaise directly with technical coaching staff and leave physical analyses to external workload specialists who liaise with physical conditioning, recovery, and medical staff. Hence, this chapter covers a more traditional technical/tactical PA role.

As contemporary performance analysis departments grow within football clubs, additional specialised roles have emerged. These roles tend to specialise in a subset of functions that were traditionally performed by a single PA and can include goalkeeper, set-play, and training analysts. Some of these roles are also performed on an external consultancy basis. Insights into the specific tasks performed by a traditional PA role within elite football settings were provided several years ago (Wright et al., 2013) and largely remain unchanged at the time of writing this chapter. In general, tasks traditionally performed are to:

- Record, edit and tag match and training footage
- Conduct pre- and post-match team and opposition analyses
- Produce video and statistical reports following analysis and interpretation of key points
- Dissemination of information and provision of feedback in de-briefs (coach one to one, presentations to group and individual players)
- Perform live match-day coding for half-time and immediate post-match de-briefs
- Update statistical and video databases for trend analysis
- Ensure the upkeep of filming and video capture equipment and storage of information.

Academy PA tend to produce content such as video compilations for development classroom sessions with youth players to provide a 'blueprint' of what is expected at the very highest echelons of play (McKenzie & Cushion, 2016). They also provide content and guidance relating to areas in which players could improve. Recruitment scouts use a combination of information from databases of video and statistics and subjective scouting reports to inform decision-making on player trading processes. Training analysts tend to film, code, and log daily training sessions. Irrespective of their title, all the aforementioned PA roles are strongly inter-related notably in terms of the technologies used and the ways in which data are collected, analysed, and utilised. For example, a recruitment analyst can share detailed information and knowledge from their online database on a team and its players that his or her club will compete against for the first time.

PAs are now considered an integral and indispensable part of the interdisciplinary support team (particularly in the UK). They can liaise with strength and conditioning and sports science personnel, sharing evidence-based insights on competitive performance. More recently, they are collaborating with heads of football analytics/data scientists to consolidate and develop data analysis and reporting techniques. PAs also work with other staff members, for example, welfare officers who may want to discuss off-field issues with a player that could be intertwined with training and match performance.

The skillset of a PA

For performance analysis to be a success, there is evidently need for provision of a high-quality service to coaches and players. This is intrinsically linked to an in-depth knowledge of the game and an abundance of craft skills acquired by the PA through education and chiefly hands-on experience. The working environment and skillset required to work as a PA within an elite football setting are subsequently discussed. The reader is also referred to two pertinent pieces (Carling et al., 2018; Jones, 2016) and to case-studies relating to practitioner reflections from football industry specialists (Gregson & Littlewood, 2018).

Working environment

Elite football is extremely results-orientated resulting in a high-pressure and non-stop working environment. PAs (particularly those involved with the first-team) are faced with long hours, weekend work, and must deal with a constant turnover of high-profile matches over extended periods. Some PAs also travel with their team, spending large amounts of time away from home. Maintaining motivation, passion, enthusiasm, and energy levels is essential. Although recognition of their value has progressed over the last decade (improvements in knowing who the PA actually is (!), what they offer, and the impact they are having), current salaries generally do not reflect the difficulties and pressures inherent to the role. When starting out, a PA can often be 'star-struck' and lack confidence. The ability to work through difficult situations is important as are self-analysis, reflection, and constant exchange. Several years may be necessary to build up to a sufficient level of confidence for working with both players and staff and coping with setbacks.

At the highest echelons of club football, performance analysis operations are mainly day to day and week to week. Medium- and long-term planning is extremely difficult particularly in an unstable and results-orientated setting. Research has shown that one of the biggest barriers to an efficient performance analysis service in elite sports settings is an all-round lack of time (Wright et al., 2014). In a 'usual' week, PAs are faced with two competing dynamics: planned tasks and ad hoc requests. The latter are usually top priority and require a rapid response to ensure reports are available in a timely fashion. For example, following a late Sunday away match, a PA spends Monday morning preparing a detailed statistical account of the match before presenting this to the coaching staff. Monday afternoon involves tagging and editing videos of the upcoming opposition's performance (Wednesday Champions League match) and compiling personalised opposition player video clips for downloading by players on their mobile viewing device. During this preparation, the assistant manager suddenly requests additional information on three of the upcoming opposition's players who habitually do not start games (apparently starting due to suspension and injury) for viewing during travel on the Tuesday.

Background: education, coaching and playing career

A background in performance analysis is clearly essential and can be acquired through educational and/or professional training courses. Initially, a general sports science degree provides holistic knowledge in a range of inter-related scientific aspects supporting sports performance (e.g., physiology, biomechanics). Learning the underpinning scientific principles and developing a strong understanding of the constructs associated with sports analysis is essential. A degree can be completed by a specific postgraduate analysis qualification such as a master's which combines academic, practical, and research-based performance analysis skills. Nowadays, a postgraduate qualification is often demanded when a PA job is advertised. Hands-on experience at the coal face is vital to enhance skills and can be acquired over the course of degree qualifications through work placements within club settings. Internship offers are frequent but generally unpaid and usually involve long hours and there may be little effort from the club to help develop skills. The reader is referred to a useful paper which critically discusses sports science internships (Malone, 2017) and another that explores experiences of neophyte internes with professional football (McKenna et al., 2018). A career can often be kicked off by performing voluntary work and part-time paid work (often at weekends and on a game to game basis) in lower level clubs to help gain experience and acquire and hone skills. It is worth mentioning that a representative body now exists to support medicine and performance practitioners working within professional football (The Football Medicine and Performance Association – www.fmpa.co.uk).

Performance analysis accreditation schemes exist (e.g. International Society of Performance Analysis of Sport – www.ispas.org) as do professional awards for provision of scientific support to high-performance athletes (British Association of Sport & Exercise Sciences – www.bases. org.uk). A range of professional training courses related to performance analysis are also available (e.g. Stats Ltd – www.stats.com, Catapult – www.catapultsports.com). Conferences on Sports analytics (such as that held at MIT) and football science are held annually and regularly include participation of high-performance practitioners. A plethora of blogs (e.g. analyticsfc, frontoffice.report, StatsBomb) and social media accounts (notably online infographics, see https://twitter.com/ylmsportScience) provide pertinent information and discussion around football analytics. Recently, clubs such as Manchester City FC and commercial football data providers have given open access to large datasets for research purposes and football analytics thereby providing useful learning opportunities. Online data science courses are also available and some are free. These aid PAs in developing their programming, modelling, and visualisation techniques skills to create advanced analysis reports using open-source programming languages such as R and Python.

Contemporary coaching awards frequently include elements of performance analysis. Although coaching experience is not essential, a recognised award can significantly aid the analyst in understanding some of the concepts, prerequisites, and philosophies that are part of both coaching and managing the contemporary elite soccer player. A coaching award can also help the PA gain in credibility with regard to coaches and players. Being solely a former top-flight player is generally insufficient within itself. However, long-term immersion and 'game' knowledge are crucial to developing expertise and are developed as a player, coach, and/or student. Taking additional sports science related qualifications (e.g., S&C awards) will complement current expertise in performance analysis. For additional and pertinent information on education and personal development programmes the reader is referred to The Video Analyst website (https://thevideoanalyst.com).

Working with technology

Technological advances in hardware and software now enable PAs to respond satisfactorily to the ever-evolving demands of elite football. Continual refinements in convenience, precision, and reliability of measurement tools have opened doors to optimise the entire process of collection, processing, and transmitting performance in training and competition settings. PAs frequently use a battery of equipment and computer hardware and software to respond to their needs. At the time of writing this chapter, a single solution that collects all the metrics required to cover the wide-ranging needs of PAs does not exist (although this is surely only a matter of time notably due to progress in smart clothing for example). Some solutions are developed in-house, some are acquired (rental or bought), while others rely on an external provider. Due diligence is necessary to provide a clear understanding of *needs* versus *functionality* versus *cost* of the different technologies and ensure the service functions efficiently. Systems must ideally be able to provide data and information to respond to needs as and when, and across the board (e.g. training, matches, academy, women's, first-team). They also need to be user-friendly, tailorable, quality-controlled, stable, and secure. For additional information and advice on due diligence in adopting match analysis solutions, the reader is referred to Carling (2016).

It is important that PAs are literate with the many forms of contemporary hardware and software technology. For example, expertise is required in software and/or applications including mainstream (e.g., Excel, Powerpoint) and performance analysis (e.g., Sportscode, NacSport, Performa Sports – see Figure 11.2). PAs evidently need to be comfortable with digital video (equipment such as digital cameras and editing software) to ensure provision of high-quality recordings of training sessions and/or competition. Contemporary smartphones and tablets with wide angle/fisheye lens attachments now offer practical means to capture high-quality video. Knowledge of the workings of electronic tracking devices such as GPS receivers, local positioning systems and technology embedded in the local environment (e.g., multiple camera tracking approach) (Linke et al., 2018) is useful. PAs must be able to use a range of contemporary commercial handheld mobile devices with different operating systems (e.g., macOS, Android).

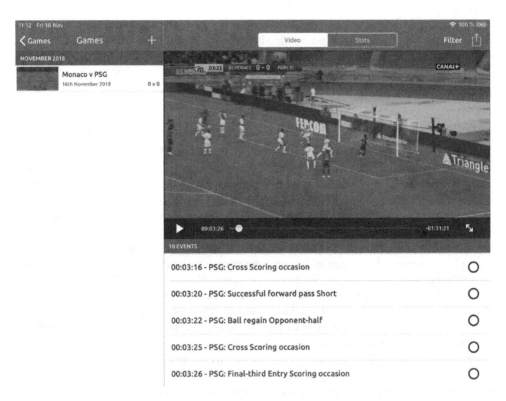

Figure 11.2 Example of coding using the Performa Sports' iPad application

Source: Reproduced with kind permission from Performa Sports Ltd (performasports.com)

PAs are now required to have expertise in business intelligence software (e.g. Tableau for data visualisations: see www.tableau.com, Microsoft BI) and advanced graphic telestration tools such as Coach Paint (chyronhego.com) and KlipDraw (klipdraw.com). The latter provide a range of options to dynamically enhance vision of video clips of play such as player cut-out, spotlight, zoom, player tracking, zone tracking, distance measurement, trajectory marking, and team formation tools. Knowledge of design and experience in using traditional database (e.g. SQL) and/or sports data management platforms for both cloud or local storage, analysis and visualisation of data is necessary as is familiarity with raw data formats (e.g. CSV, XML) commonly provided by commercial match data provider companies. At the time of writing this chapter, many PAs are developing advanced computer skills such as the ability to code using R and Python and creating API's to manage and exploit data flows. Some are also acquiring knowledge in machine learning techniques and big data storage and exploitation processes.

Finally, it is important to mention that although PAs are not IT technicians, they must be aware of solutions for dealing with any logistical and technical issues that might occur when collecting and presenting information. A seamless service is essential as coach and player buy-in may come under threat if there are recurring operational problems. Similarly, the PA is partly accountable for the intellectual property, confidentiality, and sensitivity of the information and its storage and security. All procedures must be in accordance with national and international privacy laws (e.g., GDPR). A contingency plan is necessary to ensure there is no loss or corruption of data. A close relationship between the performance analysis sector and their organisation's IT department is evidently essential.

Working practice

Working with video and data

The PA must translate the coaches' agenda into performance-related questions and conceptualise the information that is to be analysed. For this, there must be an organisation-wide accepted framework on which PAs and coaches are agreed upon. A key issue is the definition of events (McKenzie & Cushion, 2013) to help ensure consistency, clarity, and impartiality in data collection and that the data is fit for purpose. It is essential that pre-selected performance metrics (agreed upon in accordance with coaches) encompassing technical and tactical play are appropriate, insightful, and actionable. PAs must consider to what extent the information is simply providing a description of what is happening, i.e. 'nice to collect or nice to know', rather than providing a distinct performance advantage (Wright et al., 2014). The old adage of too much information, not enough knowledge is relevant. On the basis of the evidence, the PA must be able to formulate solid conclusions and make these positive and impactful. For this, they must be performance data literate with strong analytical skills to efficiently cleanse, collate, explore, select, synthesise, and present data and video.

In tactical and technical analyses of play, a combination of both qualitative and quantitative techniques is generally employed. Although top-level clubs receive comprehensive datasets post-match from third-party service providers, the majority nonetheless conduct their own analyses. This is frequently done to complement the third-party information, ensure provision of data that is unavailable, and provide in-house defined events in line with the coaching staff's needs. PAs frequently conduct in-house live analyses to deliver statistical summaries or clipped videos at half-time and immediately post-match. Following play, the PA will pre-tag events on the match recording and subsequently produce video compilations synchronised with the indexed data. They embed graphics (often using the aforementioned telestration tools) into video clips and complete with annotations and comments. These inclusions generally relate to pre-defined match objectives and coaching points in order to highlight and enhance key issues they and/or coaches have identified. At elite standards, digital video is of broadcast quality with multiple wide angles available enabling close-up analyses of behaviour during on and off the ball actions. Video is useful as it enables coaches to subjectively analyse additional behavioural aspects such as determination and aggression, factors that might not be clearly reflected in a typical statistical summary. Birds-eye view 2-D animations generated using positional data from tracking systems are employed for viewing of each player's positions and movements simultaneously throughout play.

For quantitative analyses of tactical and technical performance, game events are coded to provide information on four key factors: the player involved, and the type, position, and time of events. Collection of these four elements provides raw counts of match events commonly known as key performance indicators, or KPI (McKenzie & Cushion, 2013). The raw information can be aggregated and visualised in numerous formats including time (e.g. total time spent in ball possession), frequency counts (e.g. total number of ball regains), percentages (e.g. proportion of shots on target) and ratios (e.g. number of set-plays in relation to goals scored directly from set-plays). Statistical information can be accessed with the corresponding video clips to enable simultaneous visualisation and evaluation using both forms of analysis. Data can also be presented in formats such as graphs and charts represented by heat maps and radars. PAs can develop dashboards which are a visual display of the most important information, consolidated and arranged on a single screen/sheet. This enables the overall performance picture to be examined at a glance while permitting additional exploration of data through filtering and highlighting turning masses of information into a powerful and engaging story (Lacome et al., 2018b). For further discussion around visualisation of performance data, the reader is refereed to several recent papers (Buchheit, 2017; Lacome et al., 2018a, b).

Generally, KPI relate to frequency, efficiency, errors, and/or success rates in events such as turnovers, ball possessions, passes, crosses, set plays, final third entries, and goal attempts. For example, the ratio of crosses completed to goals scored from these actions, the percentage of 50–50 challenges won or number of turnovers made in the final 15-minute period. Using simple descriptive summary statistics, these indicators can be used to evaluate attacking and defending play and provide a quick snapshot of team performance. The summary data can then be fine-grained to examine links with playing position, individual players, and other game items. For example, the percentage of the total number of ball regains achieved in the final third of the pitch by forward players which subsequently led to creation of a scoring occasion.

Any sports performance indicator must represent aspects of play that are relevant and important (O'Donoghue, 2010). However, isolated KPI only provide a rudimentary understanding of performance and contribute little information about techniques and behaviours underpinning the outcome measure and analytical focus should be on performance not just outcome. Recently football analytics has developed advanced metrics such as expected goals (xG), expected assists (xA), total shots ratio, speed and directness of attacking actions, expected saves, intensity of defensive press and sequences of play (see Figure 11.3). xG for example, assigns a value to the chances of a shot resulting in a goal and rates the quality of a chance rather than its actual outcome. It is based on several variables such as assist type, shot angle and distance from goal. Totalling up xG can give an indication of how many goals a player or team might reasonably be expected to score or concede, given the particularities of shots they have taken or conceded. In elite football analytics circles, this metric is acknowledged to be a key indicator of successful attacking/defensive performance. For more discussion on these analytics, the reader is referred to optasports.com and statsbomb.com.

Contemporary PAs are taking an interest in combining data from optical tracking systems and GPS with artificial neural network (ANN) and machine learning techniques to quantify tactical and technical behaviours through analysis of dynamics, space, time and interaction between players (Rein & Memmert, 2016). Information can be provided on collective system behaviours such as team centroid (geometrical centre of a set of players), team dispersion (quantification of how far players are apart), team communication (establishing networks based on passing sequences), and sequential patterns (predicting future passing sequences). Work by STATS (stats.com) has attempted to measure unmeasured statistics in soccer such as defensive balance, numerical dominance, player space, and vision. Recent research using ANN and machine learning techniques is also impacting upon recruitment processes and prediction of elite player career trajectories (Barron et al., 2018). The present challenge remains for PAs and researchers to align and integrate these and future measures with the needs of coaches to systematically produce practical and actionable information (Sarmento et al., 2018). Nonetheless, the PA must recognise that analytics tools are slowly evolving from the generation of data which provide a rudimentary description of *what has happened* to intelligent systems that attempt to answer *why it happened*, then predict *what might happen* and inform prescription *to make it happen*.

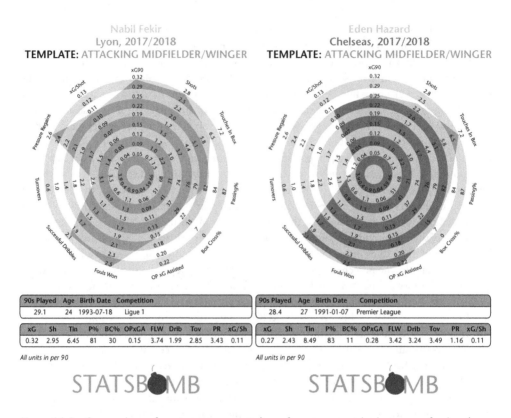

Figure 11.3 Comparison of contemporary match performance metrics in two professional soccer players using radar diagrams

Source: Reproduced with kind permission from Statsbomb (statsbomb.com)

Professional players participate in many competitions, and with tour and pre-season matches and international obligations, this can push the total up towards 70 games in any one season. Accordingly, PAs use spreadsheet software (frequently Excel) and databases (developed in-house or commercially available) to store, search, cross-tabulate, compare, and display longitudinal data. They create benchmarks for comparison and explore trends in performance during selected in-match periods, over recent matches and periods of fixture congestion while intra- and inter-seasonal analyses can easily be performed. Analysis might attempt to quantify variations or, conversely, look for consistency, or detect improvements in certain areas of performance over a number of matches following a training intervention. The dataset can also be broken down to identify statistical trends such as how a team or player performs when winning or losing games, according to changes in scoreline, when playing against top six teams and following mid-week European matches. Similarly, online databases dedicated to player recruitment (e.g. Wyscout. com, info.scout7.com) allow comprehensive online mining of technical and tactical data and video. Performance data on a potential recruit can be compared against benchmarks for a club's own players or against league averages internationally for players in the same playing position. Companies such as 21stclub provide asset management tools for managing player portfolios and supporting squad administration, performance intelligence, strategic planning, and recruitment (see www.21stclub.com).

Match performance data are often 'noisy' in nature and are affected by the random and natural variations across games. At professional standards, high levels of variability in technical performance occur across matches as numerous extrinsic and intrinsic factors potentially influence results (Bush et al., 2015). As such, PAs must always 'contextualise' their data whether this is generated in-house or supplied by a third-party. There are numerous external factors that must be systematically accounted for including current form and results, matches that are home or away, cup or derbies, travel, recent national team obligations, and return from injury/suspension. Environmental conditions (e.g. temperature, pitch quality), effective playing time, changes in team formation, substitutions, and scoreline also influence performance. One or a combination of these factors can partly explain discrepancies in results, for example a substantial difference in an outcome measure in the latest match compared to a mean score generated across previous matches. Finally, raw summary statistics do not always accurately represent the bigger performance 'picture'. Teams can 'statistically' underperform against an opponent but win leading to a false idea of how well it performed individually and collectively. The marriage of quantitative and qualitative methods (especially video) provides a greater understanding than either approach can achieve alone.

Working with coaches

The environment of an elite football club has a very specific culture and identity, and is unlike many other work settings. The PA and their department have to be culturally 'in tune' with this environment and especially with coaches who have variable levels of experience, expertise, and interest in performance analysis and who are constantly under pressure to obtain results (Carling et al., 2018). Collaborations might be with practitioners who have totally a different vision of the game and prefer to rely on opinions, perceptions, and analyses founded on tradition and personal experience.

Balancing workload in these settings is therefore crucial and the analyst must be seen to anticipate by organising and managing multiple tasks efficiently leaving space to respond to any unplanned requests. The ability to manage time and organise workload and adhere to deadlines are essential skills. A proactive attitude is necessary to anticipate the questions and requests of coaching practitioners and stay one step ahead, particularly in relation to current form and forthcoming opposition (which constantly require a switch in focus and attention). For example, research has shown that elite coaches can change their choice of KPIs from game to game (Wright, 2012). Whenever there is time to spare, this is an opportunity to plan for upcoming games and produce additional content if the PA feels this will complement their usual outputs. It is also important to stay abreast of industry developments through keeping an eye out for emerging tools and technologies.

PAs working in international football generally have more time than peers in clubs allowing them to produce more in-depth reports. However, as McKenzie and Cushion (2016) highlight, the provision of performance-related feedback to players is difficult in this context, as players tend to re-join their clubs immediately after the final match in the international break. Also interpreting players' true level of performance at international standards can be difficult as they frequently operate within a playing system or a style of play that are different to those employed in their club.

It is the coach's role to give clear and detailed guidance and direction to the analyst on what they are looking to get out of the analysis. In return, it is the PA's role to ensure the coach understands in detail what they're planning on delivering. This will help ensure there is consensus on the information gathered and that it is meaningful while accurately reflecting their needs and approach. The PA is accountable for ensuring that the user understands the data they receive to enable them to make effective decisions. There is a clear need for PAs to understand the coach's personal philosophy and objectives, their strategic and tactical vision, and the individual roles and responsibilities they designate across the team. For this, an open line of communication, visibility, and a close working relationship are evidently necessary; all framed within the language of coaching, not that of analytics. Where possible, the PA must always 'tap in' to the craft knowledge of coaches and take advantage of their subjective perceptions of performance. Concomitant subjective and objective analyses enable provision of a complimentary balance of information with greater real world meaning. In an ideal world, the PA will observe training sessions pitch side (evidently in agreement with the head coach). Observing the types of sessions conducted and getting a day to day feel of how players are performing are extremely useful in informing the analysis process. When travelling with the team to away games, it is common for coaches to informally discuss past and present performance with the PA. This is often a useful opportunity for less formal exchanges with coaches as is sharing coffee breaks and meals. In these situations, there is always a need to have supporting information to hand.

PAs must always remain objective in their approach to data collection, analysis, and interpretations. They should not provide information only relating to what they think coaching staff would like to see or hear! In theory, analysts should be able to give an objective opinion they have formed using their analyses and provide practical action-focussed recommendations. Indeed, as perceptions of PAs have improved, some coaches seek an 'opinion' following presentation of data and key findings. However, the relationship between PAs and certain coaches may still be a give-and-take affair despite the great strides contemporary analysts have made in deepening their knowledge of the game and understanding what is important to high-performance coaches. Performance analysis can only be truly effective if coaches and the organisation generally are fully committed to an evidence-based approach.

PAs require excellent written and communication skills along with the ability to present results clearly and concisely to staff. They might work with foreign coaches who are possibly coming to grips with a new language. Scientific jargon and academic terminology should be avoided (Martindale & Nash, 2012). Inter-personal skills are highly important, yet there is no training offered to develop these before integration into an elite setting: nothing replaces experience, high personal standards, and humility at this stage, skills which are developed over time (Buchheit, 2017). Adaptability is also compulsory as PAs regularly engage with new coaching staff (generally following a change in manager) who have substantially different analytic needs and philosophies.

Some coaches entrust player debriefing sessions to the PAs, whether on a group or one on one basis and might not always be present. In contrast, it is not uncommon in football clubs on the continent for PAs to have no or limited interaction with players (Wright et al., 2017). Gaining the respect and trust to perform debriefs alone is as much a matter of personality and communication ability than scientific knowledge and skills. Nevertheless, it is important that the coach is always aware of the presentation content and given feedback on the session.

Probably the biggest challenge faced by PAs is to evaluate the real-world impact of their work through integration (or not) into practice by coaching staff of the evidence base generated. In general, they have little or no input in the field and do not observe training interventions conducted by coaching personnel. The general lack of information on the application of performance analysis is linked to the reluctance of coaches and clubs to reveal their 'trade' secrets alongside an insular culture to try to maintain competitive advantage over the opposition that precludes access by other organisations (McKenzie & Cushion, 2016). The analyst can however, up to a certain extent, evaluate whether there is evidence of progress (or not) in the competitive setting. For example, by comparing performance data collected before and following an intervention whilst relating this to desired outcomes outlined by coaching staff. Some useful examples of training practices developed through statistical evaluations can be read in a piece by Smith (2016). The reader is also referred to more generic articles exploring the impact of evidence-based practice in high-performance settings (Drust & Green, 2013).

Working with players

There are many social and pedagogical complexities involved in providing performance-related feedback to the professional football player. PAs will encounter large discrepancies in learning style and ability and buy-in amongst a squad of players. Many players might not be native speakers and this must be considered. Their prior experiences, thoughts, and perceptions of match analysis can greatly affect how they receive feedback. Indeed, debriefs can unfortunately be ad hoc, results-focused, hostile and 'punitive' in nature with little opportunity for exchange. Some players have a positive approach to match analysis while others are sensitive to criticism even if results and feedback are presented 'constructively'. In this case, care is needed not to alienate the player. It is important to consider the role of 'None Stat All Stars', players who play a pivotal role in the success and even failure of a team, but whose contribution might not be fully appreciated within the game analysis (Wooster, 2013). Recent research in elite football has identified a need for greater appreciation of the psychological responses engaged during delivery of feedback and the impact of the delivery climate surrounding practice (Middlemass & Harwood, 2018).

Analysis debriefs can be coach-led. In this case players are frequently passive receivers of information and are expected to seamlessly transfer this into improved performance (Mckenzie & Cushion, 2016). It is important that players also engage (coach permitting), take initiative and ownership of their own analysis so that it has greater meaning to them allowing development of their own decision-making capabilities. The post-match debrief must be inclusive – players can rapidly lose interest and become less attentive if they feel that much of what is being described does not concern them. Post-match debriefs are commonly performed the day after the game itself while performance is still 'fresh in the memory' of coach and player. Player self-analysis and reflection prior to meeting should be encouraged through viewing and analysing video footage, for example via an online analysis sharing platform. During the ensuing debrief, they can even lead the session and highlight various points and share their opinions on what aspects they felt were positive and negative. For more information on elite football player engagement with performance analysis, the reader is referred to research by Wright et al. (2016).

When the session is coach- or PA-led, it is vital that the message from the deliverables is conveyed in a clear, concise, logical, and direct manner – players must not be over-burdened with complex terminology, endless lists, or unclear graphics. The information may be clear to the person leading the session but not to players and must be set out in an unambiguous manner for ease of understanding and offering no doubts regarding interpretation. Visual information can help convey a message more clearly than only verbal/textual content. Presentations should be based around transmission of the most essential messages derived from the analyses while having additional detail to hand. Content must have value in terms of objectives and results within the current playing context. Duration of debriefs should be under 30 minutes (Wright et al. 2016) and systematically finish on a positive reinforcing note – for example, presentation of instances of successful performance or drawing attention to a play subsequently practised in training and successfully implemented in competition. When performing sessions related to forthcoming opponents, a balance needs to be struck between emphasising their strengths and weaknesses – the aim is not to make the players feel it will be either too easy or too difficult.

Conclusion

This chapter has provided an overview of the challenges faced by PAs and the wide-ranging set of skills required to work in contemporary elite football settings. Simplified, the role of the PA is to deliver key performance insights that can be assimilated by coaches and used to drive coaching processes and impact upon competitive performance. It is clear that performance analysis has seen significant growth regarding its recognition and utilisation in elite football. Testament to this is the requirement for top youth academies in England professional soccer to have two PAs. While managers, coaches, and players have a greater understanding of and are engaging with the discipline, many PAs have arguably made greater progress in the other direction, deepening their knowledge and understanding of the game and factors that are essential to maximising performance (Carling et al., 2018). From a coach's point of view, the next decade will see improved education, knowledge of sports science and player management within a high-performance setting based upon systematic performance models and increased accountability (Strudwick, 2016). At the same time, the hallmark of a progressive PA will be to remain at the forefront of developments in technology and tools while maintaining best practice in exploiting the knowledge base they generate.

References

Barron, D., Ball, G., Robins, M., & Sunderland, C. (2018). Artificial Neural Networks and Machine Learning to Predict Career Trajectory Using Key Performance Indicators in Professional Soccer. *PLoS One*, **31**, 13(10):e0205818

Buchheit, M. (2017). Want to See My Report, Coach? *Aspetar Sports Medicine Journal*, 6, 36–43

Bush, M. D., Archer, D. T., Hogg, R., & Bradley P. S. (2015). Factors Influencing Physical and Technical Variability in the English Premier League. *International Journal of Sports Physiology and Performance*, 10, 865–872

Carling, C. (2016) Match Evaluation: Systems and Tools. In Strudwick, T. (Ed). *Soccer Science*. (pp. 545–559). Champaign, IL: Human Kinetics

Carling, C., Wells, S., & Lawlor, J. (2018). Performance Analysis in Professional Football. In Gregson, W. & Littlewood, M. (Eds). *Science in Soccer: Translating Theory into Practice*. pp. 213–239. London: Bloomsbury Publishing

Carling, C., Wright, C., Nelson, L., & Bradley, P. S. (2014). Comment on 'Performance Analysis in Football: A Critical Review and Implications for Future Research'. *Journal of Sports Sciences*, 32, 2–7

Drust, B., & Green, M. (2013). Science and Football: Evaluating the Influence of Science on Performance. *Journal of Sports Sciences*, 31, 1377–1382

Gregson, W., & Littlewood, M. (2018). *Science in Soccer: Translating Theory into Practice*. London: Bloomsbury Sport, UK

Jones, W. (2016). Performance Analysis Employment. accessed on https://thevideoanalyst.com/performance-analysis-employment-will-jones/

Lacome, M., Simpson, B. M., & Buchheit, M. (2018a). Part 1: Monitoring Training Status with Player-tracking Technology – Still on the Road to Rome. *Aspetar Sports Medicine Journal*, 7, 54–63

Lacome, M., Simpson, B. M., & Buchheit, M. (2018b). Part 2: Monitoring Training Status with Player-tracking Technology – Still on the Road to Rome. *Aspetar Sports Medicine Journal*, 7, 57–66

Linke, D., Link, D., Lames, M. (2018). Validation of Electronic Performance and Tracking Systems EPTS Under Field Conditions. *PLoS One*, **23**, 13(7):e0199519

McKenzie, R., & Cushion, C. (2013). Performance Analysis in Football: A Critical Review and Implications for Future. *Journal of Sports Sciences*, 31, 639–676

McKenzie, R., & Cushion, C. (2016). Player & Team Assessments. In Strudwick, T. (Ed). *Soccer Science*. (pp. 541–543). Champaign, IL: Human Kinetics

McLean, S., Salmon, P. M., Gorman, A. D, Read, G. J. M., & Solomon, C. (2017) What's in a Game? A Systems Approach to Enhancing Performance Analysis in Football. *PLoS ONE*, 12, e0172565

Malone, J. J. (2017). Sport Science Internships for Learning: A Critical View. *Advances in Physiology Education*, 41, 569–571

Martindale, R., & Nash, C. (2012). Sport Science Relevance and Application: Perceptions of UK Coaches. *Journal of Sports Sciences*, 31, 807–819

McKenna, M., Cowan., D. T., Stevenson, D., & Baker, J. S. (2018). Neophyte Experiences of Football (Soccer) Match Analysis: A Multiple Case Study aApproach. *Research in Sports Medicine*, 26, 306–322

Middlemas, S., & Harwood, C. (2018). No Place to Hide: Football Players' and Coaches' Perceptions of the Psychological Factors Influencing Video Feedback, *Journal of Applied Sport Psychology*, 30, 23–44

O'Donoghue, P. G. (2010). *Research Methods for Sports Performance Analysis*. Routledge: London

Rein, R., & Memmert, D. (2016). Big Data and Tactical Analysis in Elite Soccer: Future Challenges and Opportunities for Sports Science. *SpringerPlus*, **5**, 1410

Sarmento, H., Marcelino, R., Teresa Anguera, M., Campaniço, J., Matos, N., & Carlos Leitão, J. (2014). Match Analysis in Football: A Systematic Review. *Journal of Sports Sciences*, 32, 1831–1843

Sarmento, H., Clemente F. M., Araújo, D., Davids, K., McRobert, A., & Figueiredo, A. (2018). What Performance Analysts Need to Know About Research Trends in Association Football (2012–2016): A Systematic Review. *Sports Medicine*, 48, 799–836

Smith, R. (2016). Statistical Evaluations in Soccer. In Strudwick, T. (Ed). *Soccer Science*. (pp. 545–559). Champaign, IL: Human Kinetics

Strudwick, T. (Ed). (2016). *Soccer Science*. Champaign, IL: Human Kinetics

Wooster, B. (2013). Football Analytics.The MIT Sloan Sports Analytics Conference. Boston, March 2013. Available online at: www.youtube.com/watch?v=2Ye-mvV9ELI

Wright, C., Atkins, S., & Jones, B. (2012). An Analysis of Elite Coaches' Engagement with Performance Analysis Services (Match, Notational Analysis and Technique Analysis). *International Journal of Performance Analysis in Sport*, 12, 436–451

Wright, C., Atkins, S., Jones, B., Todd, J. (2013). The Role of Performance Analysts Within the Coaching Process: Performance Analysts Survey 'The Role of Performance Analysts in Elite Football Club Settings'. *International Journal of Performance Analysis in Sport*, 13, 240–261

Wright, C., Carling, C., Lawlor, C., & Collins, D. (2016). Elite Football Player Engagement with Performance Analysis. *International Journal of Performance Analysis of Sport*, 16, 1007–1032

Wright, C. M., Collins, D. J. & Carling, C. (2014). The Wider Context of Performance Analysis and its Application in the Football Coaching Process. *International Journal of Performance Analysis in Sport*, 14, 709–733

12

Working with psychology in professional football

Geir Jordet

The interest in psychology is high among people in professional football. With some colleagues, I recently surveyed 75 professional football coaches in the Netherlands about their interest in sport science topics, and the results showed that mental skills was the number one topic they wanted to know more about (Brink et al., 2018). However, in the same survey, conservatism in these coaches' clubs was perceived as the major barrier to applying the sport sciences in their work.

In this chapter, I will rely upon 20 years of experience as a sport psychology consultant working with many different professional European clubs and associations, to explore some of the specifics of applied performance psychology in professional football. Kicking this off, I want to briefly discuss some parts of the professional football culture, and how this might be relevant for the practice of psychology.

The paranoid game

We often call football "the beautiful game", a famous statement popularised by Brazilian football legend, Pele. The game is indeed beautiful, with its sometimes breathtaking displays of dynamic and sophisticated skills, its deep and complex tactical patterns, and its intense and vibrating excitement. Another type of beauty can be admired when a group of ten-year-olds clash together in a pickup game on the street, with raw and immature skill, but tons of passion and effort. Or, when fans from opposing teams at a World Cup join each other at a fanfest outside the stadium before a game, where the joy and shared love of football are so much larger than the rivalry and subsequent outcome of the match. However, zooming in on performance, at the professional level, football is also a massively competitive, 'winner takes all' business. The rewards for winning are immediate and immense, and this is attractive to many people. At the same time, the public downsides of defeat are more dramatic, appalling, and potentially life-changing than ever, with the consequence being that many people in football live with a perpetual fear of failure and deeply embedded paranoia. Football is also a game for the people, a working-class sport. The primary decision-makers (i.e. sport directors, managers/head coaches) are recruited internally or from a pool of previous pro players, so old, experience-based wisdom is re-produced, sometimes wisely and other times foolishly or at least naively. Personal bonds are heavily depended upon. Managers/head coaches come in to a new club and they often want to bring with them their own staff. Trust is vital, and loyalty is valued and rewarded. All these seemingly contradictory aspects of football create a very unique culture, which puts constraints on all types of professional work with teams, coaches, and players. Although the specific culture obviously varies from club to club, I would argue that the general culture in professional football gravitates towards being:

- Conservative and traditionalist
- Anti-academic and anti-intellectual
- Protective
- Paranoid
- Masculine/macho
- Emotional
- Loyalty-driven
- Short-term-focused

Note though, this is about men's professional football. Women's football, although it also shares some of these characteristics, because it still sees less global interest, is somewhat different.

Why would anyone then, who likes to think of themselves as both rational, educated, and progressive, want to work in this type of insecure, skeptical, and seemingly chaotic culture? For me, personally, one reason is my own roots in the game and my ongoing fascination for it. But there is another aspect, and one story may illustrate it. Once, after a presentation I gave for a mixed audience of students and practitioners, where I had shared some of these cultural obstacles that seem to permeate the world of football, I spoke with a young and newly graduated sport psychology practitioner. He proudly and enthusiastically told me that in his sport (I think it was volleyball), all the coaches and athletes would immediately put to practice the different psychological training regimes and techniques that he suggested, with no hesitation and no questions asked. Surely, he found, this was much better than knocking your head against the walls set up by those defensive, distrustful, and stubborn people in the football world that I had just described. My immediate reaction to him, which I later regretted, as it could have been received as both disrespectful and demotivating, was "that sounds so boring!" I did then try to explain, that to me, the joy is in trying to operate and perform in a world that is dense with challenge, skepticism, and paranoia. This work is incredibly difficult, on many levels, but also incredibly captivating. With this said, the goal with my work is not necessarily (although sometimes it may be) to change the culture of football i.e., eliminate the 'paranoia', rather it may be to help people respond better to it – i.e., develop, stimulate, or inspire *"productive paranoia"* (a term borrowed from Collins and Hansen, 2011).

My journey

Growing up I always wanted to be a professional football player. My career progressed as I had hoped until I was 18 and I got a contract with a semi-professional Norwegian team. However, in our first pre-season game that year, I picked up a serious injury. This effectively ended my playing career, and I never played again, competitively. My major coping strategy became to channel all the passion, energy, and time that up to that point had been focused on becoming a player, into my studies, and my newfound passion, the psychology of football. At the same time, I took my football coaching education, and worked as a coach. However, I cared much more about the psychology side than team tactics and staff management, so I left coaching and continued to specialise in performance psychology, specifically in football. I started working as a psychology consultant in football in 1995, begging one of my friends who was coaching a fourth-tier team in Norway, to do pro-bono work with his players. Since this, in summary, I have done long-term one-on-one applied work with more than 120 senior professional players; conducted more than 55 group presentations/sessions with professional teams; and given more than 150 presentations to professional senior or academy coaches. This work has taken place in 12 different countries.

At the same time, I have pursued an academic, research agenda, although this has always been practically motivated. Among the topics I have focused on are football players' ability to cope with (or choke under) extreme pressure moments, elite player development (including deliberate practice, effective learning, self-regulation of learning, and self-control), and the perceptual and cognitive processes that underpin in-game decision-making.

For this chapter, I have reflected on what would have been useful insights for me to receive earlier, as I progressed through my career. Thus, here, I will try to provide some descriptions and lessons that I would have loved to receive myself. Specifically, I will outline my basic applied sport psychology work philosophy, describe the nature of this work in football, and explore some of the more specific lessons I have learned.

Philosophy

There are many philosophical foundations of my practical work. Here are three.

Context-specific

I am a big proponent of using sport-specific knowledge to guide your psychology interventions. Conceptually, this view is couched in ecological psychology (e.g., Gibson, 1979; Bronfenbrenner, 1979), which holds that psychological processes are best described as the dynamic between a person and his/her environment, rather than decontextualised and disembodied structures within a person. Further, the sport environment contains information, meaning, and value; and psychological work is about helping athletes in exploring, discovering, and utilising these (see Jordet & Pepping, 2019, for more on the philosophical and theoretical foundations of this view). Trusting and building upon context specific insights means to let sport knowledge direct interventions to target the most critical drivers and/or obstacles of performance in a sport. However, professional football, as the global, intensely competitive, and sometimes (as described in the introduction) fairly conservative, macho-oriented, and paranoid sport may psychologically have more in common with a high-paced hospital emergency room, a commission-driven stock exchange filled with men with large egos, or the intensely publicly scrutinised entertainment industry, than it has with most sports. Psychology practitioners in football can learn loads from practitioners in these contexts, as they can from those in other sports. Thus, the context-specific approach does not mean that psychological knowledge is not at all universally applicable across contexts and sports. It does mean though, that deliberately using knowledge about a specific sport, in my case football, can make psychology a potentially more effective and immediate problem-solving tool for athletes. Working with professional players and coaches, the primary focus is on solving a practical problem that has arisen between the person and his/her context, and the secondary focus is whatever psychological process that needs to be activated or put into play to make problem solving happen. Targeting these problems directly, where the focus is to help an athlete activate a series of different types of mindsets, psychological mechanisms, and methods to alleviate or solve them, has the potential to add immediate value, even to players or coaches who are not necessarily so open to more traditional, psychological skills-based approaches. This type of immediate, functional problem-solving can then provide a bridge, or a Trojan horse so to say, to deeper and more psychologically sophisticated types of work. Advice can be offered based upon insights from experience in how to cope with this given specific situation in this sport. The traditional alternative would be to take a detour via generic psychological processes and generalise from these. The same goes for language. Although psychology operates with specific psychological mechanisms (i.e. mental states, cognitions, and emotions), the language used needs to be effectively communicated to players and coaches, and there is a major benefit if it can be adapted to the existing language and jargon in a specific context.

Behaviour-oriented

What are athletes and players actually doing? Psychology is often defined as the science of behaviour, but the standard methodology in the field of sport psychology is not to measure behaviour, rather it is self-report questionnaires or interviews. Thus, in a way, ratings on a scale and verbal descriptions can easily take precedence in a psychologist's world, over what these athletes in fact do in games and on the training pitch, in their sport. In sport psychology, which naturally is about goal-oriented movement behaviour, this is not only odd, it is highly unfortunate. This paradox was clearly pointed out by Anderson et al. (2007) in sport psychology, and similarly, by Baumeister et al. (2007) in social psychology. They both showed how almost the only behaviours now being studied, as evident from publications in these fields' primary research journals, are pen strokes (on questionnaires) or lip movements (in interviews). In my practice, I make a deliberate and concerted effort, always to focus on behaviour; what do professional players do in games and in training? This is the starting point.

Autonomy

Developing autonomy in the people you work with is key, helping them become more self-determined in their motivation and more independent of you in their problem-solving and learning. Thus, I rarely speak with players on game day. The player has to eventually perform alone and I find that leaving them to this gives better results, with my way of doing this. However, before game day, we can have good conversations about what to think about, and what to do, on that upcoming day. When the day arises though, the player needs to take full responsibility himself. Generally then, I use a very indirect, player-centred approach, where I guide using questions. This style is consistent with Corlett (1996), who argued that sport psychologists, rather than relying on a sophist technique-oriented way to achieve psychological control, should consider a Socratic approach where questions are posed to influence athletes to reflect and ultimately reach higher levels of knowledge about oneself. This also touches upon what philosophers do when they sometimes engage clients in philosophical counselling, where they explore the world views of their clients, to ultimately gain an authentic and better life (for more on application to sport, see Jordet & Moe, 2002). With that said, I am also mindful that the player's personality and/or the situation may call for a much more direct approach, at least at times, and it is important to be able to flexibly adapt your style to this.

Nature of work: management consulting

Sport psychology work in professional football is rarely only with players. People who make senior decisions in football clubs, such as managers/head coaches, sport directors, and CEOs are all required to perform under immense levels of pressure, and under tremendously fluid, complex, and sometimes even chaotic conditions. Even if you may be brought into a club to work with players or a team, you will quickly find yourself in conversations with managers and directors at the club, and it is expected that you add value to these conversations, based on your knowledge and competency. Quite often you are also asked to contribute more formally with presentations or workshops, to the board, club administration, and to sponsors, and ultimately, they may approach you and ask if you can consult or support them on a more formal basis. In the majority of this chapter, the focus will be on the more technical, sport, matters, but because consulting with management is such an integral part of this job, I will first quickly touch upon some of the major issues here.

Topics

The topics vary a lot, based on role (CEO, sport director, or manager/coach), person (personality, age, experience, etc.) and situation (type of club, culture, time of season, etc.). Everyone in these roles are under intense scrutiny, not just internally from people at the club (players, coaches, performance staff, administrative staff), but also from fans and media. Some of the topics a CEO will typically address with you can be organisational culture, staff decisions, financial constraints, media pressure, and difficult conversations. A sport director will want to address some of the same topics, in addition to the specific relationship with the manager/head coach, general coaching/performance staff issues, everything related to player transfers (transfer targets, agents, scouts, negotiations, etc.), and questions about the psychology of specific players. The manager/head coach will typically focus on the next game, what it takes to win it, selecting the right team, communicating optimally with the team leading up to the game, and getting more out of certain players. Moreover, they will want to talk about their media appearances, relationships with their bosses and their staff, all types of issues related to individual players, general injury and fitness concerns, training planning and periodisation, and the structure of their training sessions (including specific exercises and drills).

In addition, everyone in these three types of roles is constantly trying to do a better job with themselves. This can be about coping with pressure, keeping focus on their primary tasks and away from distractions, and trying to manage their energy and maintain work-life balance. Ways to deal with personal stress is a big topic, and although these people have lived most of their lives in this highly stressful industry, and know the mechanisms well, they do not all have healthy stress management strategies. Sometimes this work will be about helping them replace coping techniques that they know are destructive and not sustainable (e.g. extreme and complete absorption in the job, medication, or alcohol) with more constructive strategies such as a healthy mindset, daily meditation, a minimum of 'regular life' activities, and/or daily exercise.

Process

These people are incredibly busy, with a lot happening in their work day, and things change all the time. Thus, it tends to be difficult to set up formal meetings, and a lot of this work tends to be informal. If I am at the club, you find pockets of time, if and when there is time. If you are lucky you can get a half hour of uninterrupted conversation, but more often you grab a quick coffee or lunch together. A phone call while the person is in the car is equally common. Confidentiality is as important with these people as it is with players. If information from a conversation were to be exposed it not only makes them personally vulnerable, but performance or business may instantly suffer as conversation topics can be related to strategy (e.g. what team to play in the coming weekend) or major business-related decisions (personnel changes and transfers in and out) (for more on confidentiality, see below). Boundaries of competence is also an issue. Because you are a sport psychology specialist, you are often expected to have competence on all related areas, including leadership/management and organisational/occupational psychology. It is important to be up-front about the questions that you can professionally and competently deal with, and which you can not.

Nature of work: team presentations

When working with psychology in football, requests to present something for a team are common. I sometimes feel that colleagues in sport psychology talk down the 'team presentation', and hence give it an undeserved bad reputation. Of course, there are limits to what can be achieved in a group presentation: time constraints (it is hard to keep a team's attention for very long), the lack of personal connection (when talking to everyone, it is difficult to really connect on an individual level), and impact – how influential can a single session lasting only half an hour really be? With that said, this format remains a time-effective manner to get a message across (and actually create an impact, if it is done well), it is an effective way for a team to get an important first taste of a topic or a person (you), and a successful session might also provide a welcome and entertaining diversion from their everyday routine. In my experience, and possibly for these reasons, sport directors and managers/head coaches in football are quite comfortable asking a sport psychology specialist to give presentations for their teams. Personally, I love and cherish these moments, and I put a lot of pride and countless hours of preparation into making these sessions as first-rate as they possibly can be. Here is how I do it, as well as some of the things that I have learned.

Topics

There are some standard or popular topics. The classic is when the team is struggling with a string of poor results, and the belief sneaks into the coaches' (and players') heads that there may be psychological reasons for the substandard performance. Sometimes coaches ask for this as a last resort, when they have tried almost everything else. Other times (which is absolutely preferable), they may proactively see where they are heading over the next few weeks (perhaps they have some key players out with injuries or suspensions, or that they are about to encounter some high-quality opponents) and they set up a session like this before they actually are in a bad period. I have experienced several times that a well-timed group session can contribute to a team not ending up in a slump, when all the odds suggested they would. Another topic coaches tend to ask about is everything related to the team, such as improving team cohesion, communicating more or better, and helping some of the team leaders have more impact. Then there is dealing with pressure – e.g., helping the team sustain their level of performance in a very important game (could be a cup final, a decisive play-off game, or the end of the season where the results will determine medals, European qualification, and promotion/relegation) or something that could combat the tendency for a team to give away games in the last minutes. Finally, occasionally coaches may not have a specific performance topic in mind, but they simply want another voice in front of the players and they are open to whatever you could bring to the table.

Collaboration

If possible, you want to work as closely as possible with coaches and other staff, to help prepare the presentation. Coaches are very different here. Some will ask you to give a presentation, but there is no discussion beforehand, and they may not even take the time when you ask to talk about the session. Other coaches will work with you at length beforehand. This can vary from them setting a topic, then wanting to see slides and other material that you have prepared, and ultimately giving comprehensive and detailed input on what they like, what they want cut out, and what they might want to see more of. Others can quite cleverly ask you to speak about very specific issues that are an integral part of what he or they already have addressed, so that your presentation is not a stand-alone event, but rather an integrated part of a well-planned holistic setup. Sometimes, a psychology presentation can be about more than just a message being delivered to a team, and here is an example of that: on several occasions, with different teams and different coaches in charge, I have arrived at a professional football club's training facilities to give a presentation to the team and found journalists waiting for me outside. This has always struck me as very odd. An obvious professional foundation for all this type of work is that you conduct it discreetly, without talking to any outsiders about it, and certainly not involving any type of media. For all ethical and professional reasons this is a given. Sometimes though, a coach may see this differently. In all those cases where the media were there, waiting, they have been informed by the coach that "a psychologist would come to talk to the team", and they were ready to write about it. Although my professional code of conduct is very clear (do not say anything, unless unmistakably agreed upon with people in charge), these situations can be challenging and it took me some time (and some of these experiences) before I fully understood the mechanism at play. In most of these instances the team had been struggling with poor results, and everyone at the club, particularly the manager/head coach were under severe pressure by fans, media, and their own owners/board. Also, often, media had over time asked questions about the mental state of the team, and whether it would be time to bring in specialists on that topic. Thus, bringing in a psychology person can be a way for the coach to communicate a few impactful messages not only to people internally at the team and at the club, but also to media, and fans; such as: 1) "I am doing something, not just passively more of the same"; 2) "the reason we are under-performing is not what I am in 'charge of' – it is something outside of my control – psychology, and I am bringing in someone who can help us"; or 3) "I am a progressive coach, as I bring in psychology". This invitation to the media might then buy the coach some time in a very critical period. Of course, suddenly the pressure is now put on you, and although if played right, this could take pressure off the ones who actually have to perform on the pitch, which could have positive consequences. I, now, always address this issue up front and the default position, regardless, is to go under the radar and keep media away.

Style/format

Ideally, you choose the format based on the agreed-upon purpose of the presentation. It can range from highly interactive, where the whole session is a conversation, and players are actively involved and called upon, to the opposite – a one-way, 'Ted talk'-like presentation, where players sit back and listen to you talk. Even with the latter, there needs to be some type of interaction for it to be effective with such groups, for example by regularly 'checking in' with the players about relevance and understanding (more on that below). Also, content and format are very related. Over the years, I have systematically accumulated examples, videos, images, quotes, stories that can be used to add clarity, life, flavour, and a laugh to these types of presentations. Most of these are highly visual, as I have always had the belief (which quite possibly is biased by some of my earlier very unsuccessful presentation experiences) that football players prefer visually strong material. Lately, I have combined the lecture format with a highly interactive style, where I call upon specific players in relation to some of the sub-topics, by challenging them in the group setting on issues that I have pre-prepared in collaboration with other staff because they are particularly important for this particular player. This style is extremely demanding, as it requires both an insane level of detailed preparation, and a sharp mind during the presentation itself, as you have to simultaneously drive two agendas – the general topic, team-oriented agenda and the specific, individual player agenda. Also, there are risks involved, players may respond negatively, and this can happen both because you were wrong about something with respect to them, and/or the opposite, that you hit the nail right on the head, but they might not approve of this very public exposure of something pertaining to them, in front of their teammates. It is critical to add that I, in this setting, would never use information gained in confidence from a player, and I am always very sensitive to what players are likely to accept and approve of.

Location

The choice of location needs to be based on a combination of considering the purpose of the presentation and what is comfortable and convenient for the group. Most professional teams have rooms they tend to use for team meetings, and typically, you are asked to use the same room when addressing the team. However, there are instances where other spaces may be more beneficial. Much can be said for doing a presentation in the dressing room itself, particularly when a comfortable and intimate atmosphere is important. Typically, the coaching staff will be a part of these meetings, whereas other times, it may be desirable to include the extended support staff. In certain major clubs, this could mean a total group of 60–70 people, and alternative locations are necessary. Of course, this is also related to the content of the presentation and your preferred style, where sometimes it is critical to have a good audiovisual setup (screen, loudspeakers etc.), while other times it is all about creating a personal, intimate connection with individuals.

Language

Professional football is now inherently global, with expatriate players being the norm, rather than the exception. I have given presentations for teams in Norway, Sweden, Denmark, England, Netherlands, Belgium, and the USA. Which language you speak is always important, and there are several factors to consider. Fundamentally, you need to know languages, and because these players come from all over the world, the more you know the better. Then, it is about adapting to the specific country and context, and this can happen in multiple ways. Even when giving a presentation for a team in a country where my Norwegian mother tongue would be understood (i.e., in Norway, Sweden, and Denmark), English is quite often the preferred language, because there will be a number of non-Scandinavian players on the team. When I present to a team where I have a certain command of the language, but will be much more effective in English (e.g., in Netherlands or Belgium), I will always start with the local language, to establish some rapport with local players, then proceed with English. The initial section in their language is important as I tell them (with both the words and the fact that I have some vocabulary in their language) that they are welcome to ask questions and give comments in their most comfortable language, even if the rest takes place in English. It is also quite common to have a few players in a group who do not deal so well with English, and I always prepare for this, and make sure to repeat a (limited) number of key words and phrases in those players' specific language (e.g. Spanish or Russian). Some teams also have interpreters for select players, while in large clubs they may have a whole team of interpreters. One of the more surreal experiences I have had was giving a presentation to a team where no less than four interpreters were present, simultaneously translating to four different languages. They all were located in individual booths at the back of the room, speaking into designated microphones that the players could tune in to on their individual listening devices placed on all chairs.

The dynamic

Professional football players are not students. Most of them are not so keen on long theory sessions. They are impatient, and they are critical. At the same time, they are curious, most of them are open for new input, and they want to listen to people who can give them something that can help them or give them an edge. My experience almost always is that the best and most accomplished players in the room are the ones who come up to me after the talk to discuss some of the issues more at length. At the same time, there are always players in the room whose default stance is to be skeptical, and the truth is that you don't have much time to make an impression. If you have a half hour with such a group for the first time, above all you need to show humility and respect for them. This can be achieved in different ways, one of which is to relate to something they are likely to think about or feel at that particular moment. However, at the same time, they will respect you for unapologetically, proudly, and boldly standing before them with knowledge and information that can mean something for them. With this said, now and then, you may not get it right. A few times, I have missed, and sometimes badly. Once, I wrongfully interpreted a football situation on one of my videos, and a strong and internationally accomplished, but also very opinionated player sitting in the first row, quickly corrected me, with a clear undertone of dissatisfaction. I made several attempts at revising my initial observation while keeping true to the overall message I wanted the video to illustrate, but because I still had not understood his interpretation, his contempt for me grew stronger and the hole I was already in just became deeper. At this moment, I was seriously on my way to losing the respect of an entire group of players. As luck had it though, the next slide I had lined up featured a video with a very surprising ending. Before I describe what happened, let me try to explain the video – it started with a close-up image of a famous player (let's call him Player A); and once I click on the image and the video starts, Player A immediately makes a mistake, but straightaway, after just one to two seconds, another player (Player B) makes a remarkable appearance where he instantly corrects Player A's mistake. Hence, back in the room with this team, I click to this slide, and I loudly announced it as an example with Player B. Everyone in the room saw that the player in the close-up was Player A – not Player B. At this point, the opinionated player in the first row literally fell off his chair in frustration with my complete cluelessness. Regardless, I started the video, pretending as if I didn't hear them correcting me. When then indeed Player B came crashing the scene in the video, showing fantastic ability to recover from failure, everyone recognised the brilliance of what he did, and that it's not about whether you make mistakes or not, it's about how you recover from them. I had won the room back. And even though the dissatisfied player in the first row never became a great friend, his teammates were sufficiently persuaded for the session to overall become a positive input for them. Since then, I've always had that slide lined up, so if in trouble, I could access it and pull the same stunt. For more information on how to navigate the dynamics of a room in a general group presentation, there are several excellent resources out there, covering everything from structuring a story (Duarte, 2010; Heath & Heath, 2007), connecting with people (Reynolds, 2010), to the specific techniques used by experienced speakers to engage a group (Greatbatch & Clark, 2005).

Nature of work: one-to-one

Not all coaches are open to having their team meet with a psychologist as a group (e.g. see Egil Olsen's chapter in this book), but most coaches seem to be open to players doing individualised psychological work. Consequently, more and more professional clubs have internal psychology specialists in place around their first teams, where one-to-one work with the players perhaps is the most important task. Sometimes however, players prefer the person they work with to come from outside of the club, for a few reasons: 1) this service is very personal, and the players want someone who knows them well, cares about them personally, and who is not a part of the day to day coaching staff; 2) club bonds are not forever, and with players' careers taking them from club to club, it makes sense to have someone who can follow the player around, instead of starting from scratch, with a new person, at each club; and 3) many expat players, who play in a foreign country, prefer to work with someone who knows their own language and culture, thus making it easier for them to express themselves and feel understood. Here are some of the ways this work has been for me.

Location

When I have the role of internal consultant, I always see players at the club, and formal meetings can take place in assigned meeting rooms or offices. In addition comes all the informal meetings, at lunch, in or around the dressing room, on the pitch at practice, on a bus, at an airport, etc. When I am an external consultant, either hired by the player himself, or his national team, I will typically travel to meet players once every five to six weeks. The physical meetings will take place either at the club, at a public local cafe or hotel lobby, or at the player's home. If possible, I prefer to do this at the club, as this is the player's professional context and it will send the signal to him and others that this is work done as a part of his role as a football player. This also makes it possible to connect with and have conversations with staff at the club, where I will get a lot of useful information on the player from their viewpoints. Additionally, I can watch him in practice, and first-hand observe some of the interpersonal and group dynamics in and around the team. Between these personal meetings, we will have phone conversations and even more frequently communicate via text messages. With respect to the latter, players are very different, with some being very comfortable about having long text message conversations. If so, this can be a powerful tool as it will be able to facilitate a deeper level of reflection than the more fleeting personal conversation might do.

Topics

At the professional level, much of this work is about problem-solving, where some or several types of practical challenges decide the topic at hand, and the consultant becomes an active part of the problem-solving process. The topics that are typically addressed in these conversations range from highly performance- and match-oriented to highly personal. On the performance side, the primary direction always revolves around the performances in the last match and the plan and goals for the next match. Individual tactics, skill development issues, and priorities in training are common aspects to address. However, these discussions are always related to one or more psychological mechanisms involved in effectively solving the performance issue. These sub-topics could be cognitive processes involved in decision-making (e.g. visual perception, visual exploration, and cognitive flexibility), learning related processes (e.g. self-regulation of learning, planning, reflection, and evaluation), social psychology processes (e.g. leadership, followership, and communication), and motivational-emotional processes (e.g. sources of motivation, self-confidence, resilience, and coping strategies). Equally frequent are topics related to typical challenges arising in the life of a professional football player, such as being injured, being benched, being selected for the national team or not, having a conflict with a coach or a teammate, transitioning between clubs (which often requires a move to a different country, and sometimes to a completely different culture on and off the pitch), and dealing with media. Finally, purely personal issues are also a part of these conversations, and this could stretch from identity issues, relationships, homesickness, and worries about life after one's career to heavier clinical topics such as obsessive-compulsive behaviours, health anxiety, and gambling or alcohol problems (see below for a discussion on how to handle topics that are outside your professional competency).

The process

If I work individually with a player, I will see all his games. When they are not aired live on TV (which often is the case with players abroad, as it is hard to get access to broadcasts from other countries) there are online video platforms offering video recordings (after one to two days). The games are the natural starting point of these conversations, and sometimes we can check in a day or two before and/or immediately after the game to provide a natural routine for this. I try to set up a frame in our conversations, where there is a certain routine with respect to what we address and how we address it, at the same time that I am cautious of this becoming static and boring, so I try to vary up some of the exact wordings. The conversations are always aimed at helping players find solutions to whatever ongoing performance agenda they have. The consultant becomes an active, constructive, and supportive person to aid in the process the player is already in. One of the aspects that sets this type of work apart from that of a coach, a physiotherapist (who would happen to have good conversation skills), an agent whom the player trusts dearly, or even friends or family members is that a psychology consultant will tend to focus on the specific cognitive, emotional, or social mechanisms that can trigger or perpetuate a problem, and the equivalent mechanisms that can cause change and facilitate solutions to a problem. Specifically, in addition to brainstorming, suggesting, and discussing specific short- and long-term solutions, this work will be about reaching self-insights, understanding and strengthening the player's identity, and exploring the behavioural implications of this going forward. Reflection, planning, and evaluation are used as primary tools. Secondary are the behaviours that we identify as next steps for the players, on or off the pitch. We set training-related, process goals, such as staying behind after every training session to work extra on specific details, addressing a specific and perhaps difficult issue with a teammate, doing at least ten minutes of mindfulness meditation every day, etc. The classical sport psychology tools (e.g., imagery, self-talk, etc.) can also be introduced and relied upon, but they are never the first resort.

Confidentiality

For this work to be effective, it is paramount that players have trust in you. In my experience, trust is gained from the consultant genuinely caring for and being there for the player, being reliable, holding your promises, checking in (especially in periods where they struggle), and being professional. Always. Related to this, confidentiality is not only an ethically unwavering principle, it is an imperative ingredient of trust and it can also be a powerful tool in the relationship with these players. Players do not really have these types of relationships, in the club or outside the club, so to be able to relate and communicate to someone whom they know is obligated to not convey information further, gives a security that in itself can be liberating and impactful. That said, you may have to educate them about confidentiality as they will not necessarily know exactly what this entails. As I start to work with a player, I explain what this means, which basically is that I will not tell anyone about the two of us working together, and/or about what we talk about. If indeed there is a situation where I think it would be beneficial in one or more ways to share with someone what we speak about, I will always ask the player's permission beforehand. Although this sounds easy to follow, and in a way it is because there is simply no way around it, it can be tested in different ways (e.g., in relation to teammates, family members, coaches or other staff, media, etc.). In these situations, it is critical to err on the side of caution. As a rule, I proactively address with players, whenever something comes up that could be or turn into a confidentiality issue. And, if I am suddenly in a situation where information is required of me and I have not addressed it beforehand, even if I strongly think that the player would have been ok with me giving away information, I do not say anything. Over time, and especially as a result of frequently and explicitly addressing some of these situations with the player, you learn more about their boundaries, and trust between you is strengthened. It is then easier to agree on some general rules, pertaining to disclosing certain types of information to other people at the club or around the team. Examples of such rules could be: this particular topic can be talked about to this and this type of person; you will tell me if something should not be talked about; I will use my knowledge about you and my care for what I know you want and do not want, and share information accordingly if this is required.

Professional boundaries

Another major ethical issue is recognising the boundaries of your own competency or role, and adhering to this. For me, there are two aspects that I must constantly consider.

The first aspect relates to the football-specific, game-based philosophy I have for my psychology work, where so much is connected to what happens on the pitch. There is a risk that my work crosses the border to become a type of football coaching. I deal with this risk in a few ways. First, above all, I am very clear with the player, from the outset and moving forward, that my role is that of a mental consultant, not that of a coach. Further, even though I see all games, and will have both knowledge and thoughts on what the player might do differently or better from a coaching perspective, my approach to this is extremely player-centred, so we talk about issues that he brings up. With that said, a perpetually surprising insight for me when working with some of these players (often in major European clubs), is how little feedback and information they are getting from coaching and analytics staff about their own performance in a game. Even in clubs with large coaching staffs (up to seven to eight coaches affiliated with a team) and even larger analytics departments, there is a clear reluctance about providing feedback and disclosing information to players. There is obviously a lot of information, commentary, and discussion in media and particularly now, on social media, about individual players. But players do not get much information from people with insight into their performances, whom they know will be honest, and whom they can trust. To some extent then, I will be in the position to engage the player in a discussion about events in the game, but always player-centred and always with a view on how this relates to different psychological mechanisms that can be worked on.

The second aspect is related to issues that are more on the clinical side of psychology, when the player struggles with some type of psychological disorder or pathology and the competence of a clinical psychologist is needed, not that of a performance psychology specialist like myself. Here, I use my professional network and will typically, in an early phase, consult with a specialist in clinical psychology on what I can do, if anything, given my limited formal expertise in this realm. Sometimes I will continue to do very basic work with a player on some of these topics, while being guided by a clinical specialist. I have found this to be possible and effective in instances where the issue is relatively light and the player for different reasons (e.g. trust or logistics related to travelling) does not want to introduce another person into his circle. With that said, if the issue is serious, there is a specialist readily available, and no trust/logistical concerns, I have many times gone to the step where I have referred players to work directly with a clinical specialist. This can be with me as part of the process, or where we just identify this as something separate to the work I am currently doing. As such, I have referred players to specialists with issues related to obsessive-compulsive disorders, depression, alcohol or substance abuse, gambling, other addictions, health anxiety, and relationship issues, to name a few.

Regarding clinical referrals, it has been important for me to put together a team of available clinical psychologists with various types of expertise, whom I trust to be both ethical and competent and whom I can refer players to when needed.

Nature of work: academy

Although there are more and more competent sport psychologists operating as integrated members of staff in professional football academies across European elite clubs, I believe the best use of resources invested in psychological development of players at the age from six to 21 is to educate and support their coaches to better use psychology in their interaction with players. Sometimes, of course, clubs employ sport psychologists with that specific purpose as their primary task. The general aim of my work in this sphere, being an external consultant, has been to equip professional academy coaches with knowledge, frameworks, and tools, as well as to inform, inspire, and support them to develop their own curiosity, respect, and confidence, so they can more effectively address psychological aspects in their roles working to develop young football players. More specifically, this work in academies has focused on either consulting with academy leadership (i.e. the academy director), on ways to most effectively set up different aspects of a psychology programme, and/or to provide different types of programmes, courses, and workshops in psychology in coach education/development. I will say something about each of these two here.

Integrating psychology in an academy

Some years ago, I listened to a presentation by Hugo Schoukens, the CEO and founder of the Belgian company Double Pass. Double Pass is or has been heavily involved with the quality control of the academies in all the clubs in First and Second Bundesliga (Germany), Premier League (England), the Jupiler Pro league (Belgium), Major League Soccer (USA), and many more. Needless to say, Schoukens has a good overview of how leading clubs across the world have structured their player development academies. In this talk, Schoukens expressed one thing that stuck with me: "We have not seen one single club with an effective and football specific program for psychological support in their youth department". Since hearing this, I have been thinking, surely it is possible to create such a programme, particularly in an academy that has some resources. A comprehensive way to do this must involve leadership, structure, systems and processes, competency, testing, training plans, and clearly placed responsibilities, to name a few components. To give a full and detailed overview of it all is beyond the scope of this chapter. Rather, I will quickly describe an approach I've taken several times (partly in collaboration with Tynke Toering) to help an academy set up a football- and club-specific model for psychological performance, that they can then structure their subsequent psychology work around. The starting point is a summary of what we know from research on performance psychology in elite (youth elite and senior professional) football players, which can be summarised in a model focusing on the behavioural and functional outcomes of positive and constructive psychology mechanisms (see Figure 12.1, an updated version of what was first presented in Jordet, 2016).

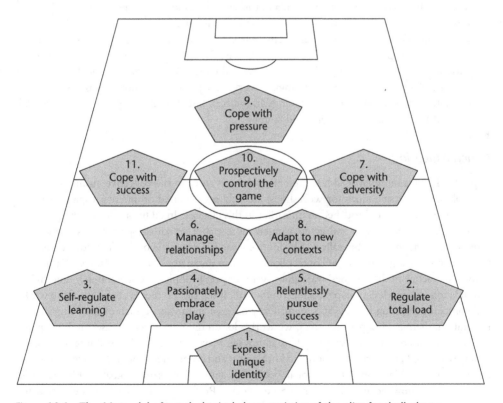

Figure 12.1   The 11-model of psychological characteristics of the elite football player

Source: Adapted from Jordet, 2016

Given that this model attempts to cover the incredibly dynamic and complex interplay of different psychological factors upon which football performance rests, I am under no illusion that this is an optimal model. However, for the purpose of facilitating and supporting practical work for coaches in an academy setting, the model provides a sufficient foundation for more focused work with players. Hence, to accompany this model, we have developed a practical set of items – which can be used as a self-report tool, a behavioural observation checklist for coaches, and above all, a conversation starter to trigger self-insight and communication between a coach and a player. For each of the 11, we have about 15–20 such items, and in Figure 12.2, there is an example of this; based on Factor 7 – Cope with adversity. Part of this work is done using self-report checklists, where players rate themselves and fill out the extent to which they agree or not with statements related to different psychological topics.

At clubs where this is put in place, we start by systematically interviewing ten to 15 key people (e.g., the CEO, sport director, head coach, academy director, academy coaches, mental coaches, physical coaches, senior players, youth players, and former players/club legends) about what they see as the culture and mentality that permeate their club. For these interviews, we initially attempt to obtain the interviewees' raw and unbiased reflections on the psychological factors they think characterise elite players. Then we probe into the specific psychological demands of making it and playing for their club, incorporating both the specific club history and culture, as well as the national and/or regional mentality and culture in the country. Finally, we present the 11-model, and obtain their responses to which of these points they find important, and which they find less important. A detailed report from these interviews is handed over to the academy director, discussions are had, and this culminates in a club-specific model for psychology in the club. Typically, this model is structured, visually, to look a bit like the 11-model. Following this, we then create checklist items/self-report questions that connect to each of the factors in the club specific model. For this work, we rely on the data bank of football specific checklist items/questions that we already have created (connected to the 11-model). This then becomes a club-specific tool for psychological work with players, that not only is based on the current state of knowledge about psychology in football, but also on the specific mentality and culture in that particular club, region and country.

Coach education

Typically, I give a number of ad hoc presentations every year, to the collective group of coaches at a club. These presentations (or workshops) are held on a myriad of different topics, many of which are mentioned and touched upon earlier in this chapter. In addition, during the past four to five years, I have created and given a much more elaborate course specifically designed for elite football academy coaches called "The football coach as a mental coach". The course has four levels, involves a large number of contact hours with an instructor, but also requires a lot of self-study and practice in the coaches' own clubs. With respect to topics, we spend much time laying a foundation of knowledge on psychology in football, using the 11-model above as a framework, and constantly pointing to ways to systematically observe and measure each of the components. In addition, there is a big part on ethics, we work a lot on different practical cases, and we spend time on typical coaching scenarios such as addressing players before and at halftime at a game, having structured player conversations, and behaviour and communication in practice. In collaboration with the Norwegian Professional Football League ("Norsk toppfotball"/"Eliteserien"), this course has now been included in the Norwegian Professional Football League's academy certification criteria (the Norwegian equivalent to the English Premier League's Elite Player Performance Plan (EPPP)). With this, the clubs need to have a certain number of their coaches

Cope with adversity

	Never	Sometimes	Often	Very often	Always

I am a player who. . .

1. . . . does not let my game be negatively affected when I have made one or several serious mistakes, that for example lead to a goal against us. ☐ ☐ ☐ ☐ ☐
2. . . . does not let my game be negatively affected when I have made several passing errors. ☐ ☐ ☐ ☐ ☐
3. . . . does not let my game be negatively affected when I have had several bad games in a row. ☐ ☐ ☐ ☐ ☐
4. . . . continues to work hard and focus in practice, even though the level is somewhat too high for me, so I don't play particularly well. ☐ ☐ ☐ ☐ ☐
5. . . . is able to continue to focus and play even though I have small pains and nuisances (when they will not lead to more serious injuries). ☐ ☐ ☐ ☐ ☐
6. . . . works hard with myself in training to quickly get well after illness and injury. ☐ ☐ ☐ ☐ ☐

(Cope with adversity on the field)

7. . . . works really hard with myself and what I can do something about, when I am on the bench. ☐ ☐ ☐ ☐ ☐
8. . . . works really hard with myself and what I can do something about, when I am on the bench, even if I would feel that the coach is not treating me fairly. ☐ ☐ ☐ ☐ ☐
9. . . . maintains my performances even though the coach's feedback and support in periods are missing. ☐ ☐ ☐ ☐ ☐

(Cope with limited playing time)

10. . . . maintains my performances even though I in periods struggle at home. ☐ ☐ ☐ ☐ ☐
11. . . . maintains my performances even though I in periods am not doing so well outside the field. ☐ ☐ ☐ ☐ ☐

(Cope with adversity outside the field)

12. . . . takes charge of what I can control in adversity, and is less preoccupied with what I can not control. ☐ ☐ ☐ ☐ ☐
13. . . . focuses on myself and what I can do in adversity, and avoids blaming others. ☐ ☐ ☐ ☐ ☐
14. . . . uses adversity to motivate me to give more energy, focus better and do more hard work. ☐ ☐ ☐ ☐ ☐
15. . . . takes responsibility and contributes positively to my teammates when the team has lost a lot or is badly positioned in the league table. ☐ ☐ ☐ ☐ ☐
16. . . . seeks out coaches and other staff to get help when I struggle. ☐ ☐ ☐ ☐ ☐
17. . . . seeks out people outside the field when I struggle, when they can help me to work harder on myself and focus more on what I can control. ☐ ☐ ☐ ☐ ☐
18. . . . AVOIDS, when I struggle, to listen to people who give me a <<wrong>> focus (by letting me blame others and think about things that I can not control, and less on what I can do something about). ☐ ☐ ☐ ☐ ☐

(Resilience, general)

Figure 12.2 Factor 7 – Cope with adversity, self-report checklist for coach–player meetings

having completed certain levels of this course, to be able to get different degrees of central funding for their development activities every year. Note that an important part of the course is to equip coaches with knowledge and insights about ethical and responsible use of our self-report/checklist tools to approach elite youth player development as a psychological process.

Nature of work: recruitment and scouting

Making the decision to sign a new player can be a very fluid and complex undertaking, and it is logical that people with knowledge about psychology are around the table where those decisions ultimately are made. My experience is that heads of recruitment and scouts are curious and open to discussions about the psychology of elite performance in football, and about the psychological characteristics of potential new signings. A sport psychology specialist can play an important role in these discussions. However, when assessing specific targets for the club, there is an inherent limitation with the traditional psychological methods such as questionnaires and interviews, given that clubs typically will not have the direct access to players that these methods will require (unless they are assessing their own players). Consequently, there is a need to use alternative methods, such as behavioural (video) observation and social media feed analysis.

Another relevant area is the manner in which psychological processes influence the scouts themselves. One way to address this is to educate scouts on the research about how we make systematic errors in our decision-making. This is known as biases, and the Nobel-prize winning psychologist, Daniel Kahneman, is the world-leading authority. We know from Kahneman (2011) that people quite frequently and systematically make all kinds of judgement and prediction mistakes, and we are particularly prone to make mistakes when:

- We have to assess many different types of information at the same time
- We make automatic decisions based on intuition, with little or no effort
- We make decisions fast
- We are under stress or are tired
- We feel that we are authorities in the area

Recruitment departments can take proactive measures to prevent such mistakes. Simply addressing and discussing known biases that logically will impact scouting is a way to do this. There are literally hundreds of known biases, and here are just a few tastes of some of the biases that most likely will affect the scouting process:

- *Confirmation bias*: the tendency to notice information that confirms your beliefs and to ignore contradictory information – when you like a player, and you only notice information about him that confirms he's a good signing for you.
- *Halo effect bias*: the tendency that an observer's overall impression of a player influences feelings and thoughts about other aspects of that player (e.g. elegant players viewed as better than inelegant ones).
- *Race stereotype bias*: the tendency to assign players of a certain race/skin colour specific traits (beware that these biases can be implicit, hence you are likely to not think that you are racist, but you still may be vulnerable to race stereotype biases).
- *Anchoring bias*: the tendency to let the first information received overly decide subsequent judgement – when the first statement given about a player in a recruitment meeting becomes more important for the discussion than any subsequent (and equally or more valid) statements.

- *Recency bias*: the tendency to over-estimate the significance of recent events for the outcome of (long-term) future events – when the last statement becomes most important.

Based on Kahneman's (2011) suggestions for how to reduce the harmful effects of biases, the following guidelines can be formulated:

1   Cognitive biases can NOT be fully eliminated, but the harmful effects can be minimised and controlled.
2   Be aware the potential effects of cognitive biases, and recognise when you are in a "Cognitive bias minefield".
3   Slow down, and take time to process information.
4   Be slow and careful in the decision process, but optimistic and decisive in implementation.

Normally, I have worked with scouts on these topics in designated workshops, where I present some of the general evidence, and we all discuss the extent to which they are susceptible to the effects of biases and how we can minimise them.

Conclusions

At the 2010 Leaders in Performance conference in London, previous Arsenal FC manager Arsene Wenger expressed:

> In the last 10–15 years we have been in the physical and in the technical area; the next 10–15 years, we will certainly move forward in the mental area. This is not only linked with desire to win, but with vision and speed of understanding of the game, and that's certainly the new area of development of our sport.

I would say Wenger has been right in his predictions, given that the interest in psychology seems to have dramatically grown in football in these past years. It is also true that more and more people are hired in this area, with both leading clubs and associations now staffing up on psychology. With this said, there is still a question whether we have made real, significant, and tangible moves forward in the quality of psychological practice, and as a result whether players and teams now show stronger mental performance than before. For the near future, I think it will be critical that we continue to push this side of the game, and here are three areas that I think will be of utmost importance:

1   *Football specific psychology.* For psychology to truly be accepted, integrated, and hence be effective for football players, it will need to be based on a football-specific knowledge base, and be driven by football psychology specialists. There will always be highly competent and effective exceptions to this, but for the field to grow, I believe specialisation is critical.
2   *Psychology analytics.* As sport science and game analytics progress, and the use of different types of data becomes more and more prevalent, there is a need for more valid and reliable psychological data. Personally, I think the major leap with this will be in the use of video observation, where players' psychological behaviours in games and practices will be analysed in the same way that physiologists now analyse the distance and intensity of running.
3   *Technology.* I'm convinced that going forward different types of technology will facilitate and support psychological practice in football. We have already started to see sophisticated

cognitive assessment and training software where the game is simulated, and practitioners can measure cognitive improvements, structure individualised cognitive training, and provide an alternative mode to train and improve football skills with low physical load. In addition, there is now a big growth in analysis software literally knocking on the doors of football clubs, featuring everything from advanced facial and bodily feature recognition to algorithms detecting psychologically meaningful patterns in all types of data. It's hard to predict exactly how technology will impact psychology in football, but it is certain that it will.

In sum, in this chapter I have tried to present and discuss some of the ways that I am working with psychology in European professional football, focusing on some of the specifics of 'how' this practical work is carried out. Hopefully the text can be a small contribution to help leaders in the field embrace performance psychology and progress it even further, for the benefit of everyone involved in professional football, and professional sports as a whole.

References

Anderson, M. B., McCullagh, P., & Wilson, G. J. (2007). But What Do the Numbers Really Tell Us? Arbitrary Metrics and Effect Size Reporting in Sport Psychology Research. *Journal of Sport & Exercise Psychology*, **29**, 664–672

Baumeister, R. F., Vohs, K. D., & Funder, D. C. (2007). Psychology as the Science of Self-reports and Finger Movements: Whatever Happened to Actual Behavior? *Perspectives on Psychological Science*, **2**, 396–403

Brink, M. S., Kuyvenhoven, J. P., Toering, T., Jordet, G., & Frencken, W. G. P. (2018) What Do Football Coaches Want from Sport Science? *Kinesiology*, **50**, 150–154

Bronfenbrenner, U. (1979). *The Ecology of Human Development: Experiments by Design and Nature.* Cambridge, MA: Harvard University Press

Collins, D., & Hansen, M. (2011). *Great by Choice: Uncertainty, Chaos, and Luck – Why Some Thrive Despite Them All.* New York, NY: HarperBusiness

Corlett, J. (1996). Sophistry, Socrates, and Sport Psychology, *The Sport Psychologist*, **10**, 84–94

Duarte, N. (2010). *Resonate: Present Visual Stories that Transform Audiences.* New York, NY: John Wiley and Sons

Gibson, J. J. (1979). *The Ecological Approach to Visual Perception.* Boston, MA: Hougthon Mifflin

Greatbatch, D., & Clark, T. (2005). *Management Speak: Why we Listen to What Management Gurus Tell Us.* London: Routledge

Heath, C., & Heath, D. (2007). *Made to Stick: Why Some Ideas Survive and Others Die.* New York, NY: Random House

Jordet, G. (2016). Psychology and Elite Soccer Performance. In Strudwick, T. (Ed.), *Soccer Science: Using Science to Develop Players and Teams* (pp. 367–388). Champaign, IL: Human Kinetics

Jordet, G., & Moe, V. F. (2002). Philosophical Consultancy with Professional Athletes. In Herrestad, H., Holt, A., & Svare, H. (Eds.), *Philosophy in Society* (pp. 25–34), Oslo, Norway: Unipub

Jordet, G., & Pepping, G. J. (2019). Flipping Sport Psychology Theory Into Practice: A Context- and Behaviour-centered Approach. In Cappuccio, M. L. (Ed.), *Handbook of Embodied Cognition and Sport Psychology.* Boston, MA: MIT Press

Kahneman, D. (2011). *Thinking, Fast and Slow.* New York, NY: Farrar, Straus and Giroux

Reynolds, G. (2010). *The Naked Presenter: Delivering Powerful Presentations With or Without Slides.* Berkeley, CA: New Riders

13

Keeping them on the pitch

Andy Barr with Geir Jordet

Introduction

Injuries in professional sports cost organisations billions of US dollars every year. In addition, comes the personal traumas for the players affected by the injuries where they miss games and critical periods in their careers. Accordingly, appropriate systems and regimens for injury rehabilitation is a natural part of elite sport, and all teams have this in place. However, arguably, a smarter approach to deal with sport injuries is to try to avoid them in the first place. In this chapter, we build on over two decades of experience working in professional sports to look at how to reduce the risk of injury incidence, and to outline a proper philosophy, where it is a science and where it is an art, and to emphasise the importance of communication, among other things.

My path

I started my career as a professional football player in England, back in 1995. I did not quite make the grade, mainly due to injuries. So I decided to take an alternate route within sports, through the medical environment. I took a physiotherapy degree, and I was fortunate that from participating on that course I met a lot of contacts who were working in professional football at that time, as physios (but not yet chartered). I got a job straight out of university with Bolton Wanderers. Here I had the role as first team physio. I worked in the academy a little bit, then fast-tracked to first team physio because they wanted somebody who understood the football culture. The fact that I had played at a decent level was a massive help for me and probably outweighed my physiotherapy skills to some extent.

At that time, I was just trying to learn as much as I possibly could within the area of sports medicine. I was very fortunate that the philosophy of the people I was working with there was very proactive, and I really got an interest in trying to reduce risk of injuries. Because we did not quite have the talent or the finances to have a large squad, we had to invest in health and wellness of these players through the staff being high level. That is where I learned a lot on injury-risk reduction and working and integrating into a team. My role was first team physio, but I linked well with the strength coaches, sports scientists, and the massage therapists and the various other practitioners employed to help keep the players healthy. I got a really good foundation of how to work with an interdisciplinary approach from an early stage, which really molded my philosophy on athlete care and management. I did six years with Bolton, the first team, and learned so much in a team that overachieved to say the least. We had good systems in place, and really saw the benefits of having a forward thinking and proactive culture.

I took this experience and went to Southampton Football Club to be their head of sports medicine. I did that for a couple of years, and I tried to set up the same systems that we had in place at Bolton. Proactive approaches to athlete screening, integrative approaches, working closely with the strength coaches and sports scientists so everyone was at the same page. But then I got an opportunity to go back to Bolton and I worked there for a year before Manchester City asked me to work with them in an integrated role where I was linking the medical department and the strength and conditioning apartment, in the role of injury-risk reduction specialist.

During my time at Bolton, I did a master's in sport science, and I also got my strength and conditioning certifications. I studied Pilates and movement analysis, and my area of expertise focused on biomechanical testing to identify reduced movement control which I linked to injury risk and performance deficit. I created programmes that were guided by these test results and integrated my findings into strength and conditioning and player development plans. So, when I went to Manchester City, one of the key things I focused on was looking at player body awareness from a specific movement control perspective. The results gave guidance for individualised exercise programmes to support their general strength and conditioning work.

One off-season when I worked with Manchester City, I toured the USA and I visited the New York Knicks. While I was there, they showed interest in my skillset and offered me a job to do the same as I had done in football. I took the opportunity to work in the NBA, in which I looked at overall player development and used various assessments to capture basketball relevant data for baselines and programming. I integrated the training (physio /medical, strength and conditioning, sport scientists, psychology and coaching staff into the player development plans. I focused on integrating every area of my analysis to holistically develop players and used communication terms relating to basketball to optimise coach and player buy-in. It took a little bit of time to learn the basketball culture, but once I understood that, it started to become more effective as I was able to communicate more effectively. I did that for maybe four years, then I went into a more senior, performance director role. I had the same responsibilities but more influence and more interaction with the head coach and management.

From there I took a job with New York FC. This, again, was more of a managerial role, director of medicine and performance. I set up the practices and processes but then after 18 months I decided that I needed more diversity with my work. I wanted to help more athletes, different sports, and have more freedom, so I started to consult with the goal of great impact. I'm now based in an integrated high-performance facility in LA where I work with elite athletes from various sports. Our practices are guided by objective data from various tests that range from biomechanical analysis to biomarker analysis, providing athletes with insights and solutions that keep them as healthy as possible and performing optimally.

Since working in the US, I earned my doctorate in physical therapy also. Everything I have done education-wise has always been part-time, which has been really beneficial for me as I have always been able to really apply the stuff I was learning along the way. I always tried to focus my assignments on the things I was passionate about. This allowed me to maximise my studies and develop expertise in key areas of interest. It took me longer to do part-time education and there were times when the last thing I wanted to do was to prepare for an exam when I had a lot going on at work.

Philosophy/foundations

Every individual is different, so my starting point with an athlete is to first treat them as an individual and relate to them as a person. My philosophy is to build on that relationship and perform baseline assessments that start from the reference point of their sport and their positional demands. If you do it the other way around you risk not getting the complete buy-in. Having the reference of the athlete's sport-specific demands as a starting point is essential in my opinion.

First, it is crucial to have the training program periodised in a way that provides them with the best opportunity to stay fresh and avoid fatigue. This means enough recovery time and measured overload of their sports' specific actions. If you get that right, it is one factor that influences many others. This involves working with the coaches to devise a sports-specific training programme that incorporates incremental, gradual overload. Planning and monitoring the quantity and quality of the athlete's sports actions through a periodised plan and monitoring to ensure actual outcomes match expected outcomes is imperative.

Second it is important to understand and track the factors that influence the quality of those actions and their ability to cope with the demands of that programme consistently – specifically, their energy levels. Maximising their energy levels and understanding what influences this is vital. Reduced energy levels changes the quality of how they move and perform their actions and also reduces their ability to increase the quantity of those actions. Some of the energy factors that influence the quality of their actions are sleep, nutrition, hydration, and lifestyle. Stress levels (especially emotional stress) can really affect the quality of recovery which influences their ability to cope with the demands of the training programme. An athlete can have the same programme load outputs every week, but if they are under a lot of emotional stress, sleeping poorly and not recovering well, then their perception of that workload can change so it feels much harder to them.

Thirdly it is important to track how their bodily systems are responding to the many different stressors. Using modalities that track various responses such as cognitive (e.g. decision-making speed and quality), neuromuscular (e.g. force production/absorption), biochemical (e.g. hormonal and immune), tissue integrity (muscle, tendon, ligament, and bone quality) and physiological (heart rate variability) highlights the influence of the energy factors (sleep, nutrition, loading patterns, emotional stress etc.) and movement strategies used (for actions such as jumping and landing) on body status. Insight can then be gained in terms of how they are coping with everything on a whole and their readiness to perform optimally. Tracking these various system responses provides greater context, detects minor issues before they become problematic, and guides quick personalised interventions. For example, signs of fatigue can be detected by tracking changes in immune system or heart rate variability responses. This can help reduce the chances of an athlete moving with less efficiency (from being in a fatigued state) and increasing the stress and strain on the bones, joints, muscles, and tendons. Changes to these tissues can also be detected with scanners and other devices to provide a complete picture.

If you have a good periodised programme in place, then it is much easier to see if they have a response change that is more likely to be due to an energy factor as opposed to excessive overload from the programme. If you do not have a good programme in place, and you have a coach who constantly works on technical/tactical measures without focusing on understanding how to give them optimal overload and recovery within a technical/tactical framework, then their overload could be quite inconsistent. This could be what causes their responses to be different as opposed to just having a sleep, nutritional, or stress-related problem.

Having a long-term development focus is vital. Looking to improve the quality of their actions, for example, what are the key actions they do while playing? For a basketball player, we know that the jump shot is a key action, but if we break that down, the actual basic actions involved are jumping, shooting, and landing. So how do we improve the quality of those basic actions and monitor them? We can assess the various different elements necessary to perform that action with quality such as optimal mobility, strength, power, or movement coordination. This information can then be used to guide programmes led by strength coaches, or injury-risk reduction programmes led by athletic trainers or physios. We should all be working to improve the quality of the action.

One of my first lessons at Bolton was that to be effective, you have to understand that everybody has value and everybody working together is more powerful than an individual working alone. When you are working within an interdisciplinary approach with other practitioners and have the goal to maximise player development it becomes about the player, and we as practitioners don't work on the player in isolation. Ultimately the context should be in reference to what they are trying to do, which is the sport. When you have an integrated approach, everyone understands what is going on and the player development is maximised. In the beginning, this is more of a challenge I think, because you are going to have more communication, more meetings, and it is about relinquishing your ego and accepting that everybody has value in what they have to offer. It is not about you, but it is about the athlete.

This is being proactive and not waiting for a player to have an issue or a symptom. This way, you are predicting potential issues and planning in a way that removes potential risks. There are so many variables that influence injury risk that sometimes you cannot account for all of them. But what are the main factors within that sport, and which of these factors really are impactful for them? Being proactive is having a programme in place. We know that excessive overload is going to cause injury, so we do not want to excessively overload them, but rather incrementally overload them to avoid injury. Then we plan to allow for full recovery and freshness. Fresh players stay healthy. When you react to the effects of a programme or a coach's actions and try to buffer those effects by doing something to respond to players being sore, tired, or having other symptoms – it's too late. That is not proactive. Avoiding fatigue is being proactive and you do that by having a good programme and monitoring the responses to that programme. If you monitor the responses then you can see any fluctuations and you can put an intervention in place before it becomes an issue. This relates to all areas, like nutrition, sleep, or anything that is going to impact their energy or their ability to cope. By consistently monitoring and tracking things that are relevant to the sport and to the athlete you provide an individualised way to reduce risk.

The more individualised you can be, the more proactive you are. Rather than waiting for somebody to complain about a tight calf or groin pain, you can profile athletes at the start of the season by screening for any deficits in strength, power, movement control, coordination, force absorption, and how they utilise their elasticity potential. This is always in relation to the game, and then, you can assess what needs to be addressed. For example, we know if they have a blocked or stiff ankle, it can affect their ability to control hip movement such as internal rotation or adduction which increase the stress on the ACL, at the knee. So we can track the ACL stiffness, improve the gluteus medius control and improve the ankle range of motion. With this we are being proactive because we know that all those things are injury-risk predictors, so to avoid that risk, working on these things is part of the development programme. We also may know that a player has an asymmetry left/right in his ground contact time, so we have to address that. We know that he has reduced ability to absorb force or he has strength issues. So rather than just doing a generic programme we can individualise the programming, and that is being proactive to identifying factors that might relate to injury risk. And, then providing the tools so that he can develop what he needs to do to jump and land effectively, so he has a better-quality action which will then take the stress off his ACL ligament. Consequently, the chances of injuring the ACL or meniscus are reduced as the shear forces at the knee are less and the tendons are not overloaded excessively in one direction. The forces are more evenly distributed through the ankle, knee and, hip with more control.

Science or art

Where is this work a science, and where is it an art? I think I had to learn through science. You have to be guided by science and evidence; evidence-based practice is the best way. Science and evidence help guide practice. Innovation comes in the application and use of science in your processes. Your understanding of the culture; your sense of the environment and of someone's personality; and your ability to communicate and to build relationships combined with the best way to apply the relevant science for a given situation is the art. The science is like your database and your knowledge, while your application is really the art of it.

From an injury-risk perspective, you have to look at the key evidence about injury-risk reduction. There is evidence surrounding excessive overload and also specific movement strategies in relation to increased injury risks in certain actions. Previous injury history is the best injury-risk predictor, so addressing things that make players more robust related to their previous injury history is important. Then there is ample biomechanical evidence that relates to certain tasks and actions performed in certain sports. The questions then are, again, what is the sport, what is the task, what is the action that they do, and then what is the evidence linking this from a movement perspective?

Obviously, ACL injuries cause players to lose a lot of time. There is much evidence out there in terms of the movements specifically within an action that is higher risk for ACL injury. So being able to improve the control of those movements within the action is part of using the research and evidence to guide your programme. For instance, jump/landing is again something that you see in basketball or in football. Within those actions, there are certain movement strategies that have higher risk of injury than others. For example, when cutting or jumping/landing you want to control your centre of mass – the position of the trunk when doing those movements. Excessive lateral sway or lateral trunk motion during these actions has increased risk of knee injury. Therefore, creating a programme that helps maximise the control of the centre of mass when performing these actions will reduce risk of knee injury. Applying exercises to improve the efficient control of lateral motion within those actions is effective practice. This is identifying the risk factors from the literature, and then applying an intervention linked into what is important in that sport.

Testing

When doing biomechanical testing, I look at specific risk movements during key actions that a player does. When explaining the test, I give conscious queues so the athlete knows what I am trying to get them to achieve. Then if the test is understood I then look at their specific movement control. For instance, when they jump and land, can they keep their knees straight, can they land with their feet straight and keep their body upright? If they cannot do this, the test will identify the specific direction they cannot control the motion which helps to guide programming and the specific exercises required to improve the quality of the landing action.

I use a specific biomechanics technology called QuantumperformX.com which is a sensor system that allows me to also collect objective metrics such as ground contact time, ground reaction forces, velocities, and joint angles as this helps capture more than the naked eye and also provides greater insights into specific performance deficits. I try not to do too much fitness testing anymore. My philosophy is to use the coaches' eyes to identify when the players start to show signs of reduced performance quality within the game. When the quality starts to reduce you know what the baseline is. Also, we know agility testing does not transfer into playing sport. Within the context of a game, players are recognising different things to react to and I think the way you can develop and test those things is by just playing modified versions of the game. Most of the testing that I do just focuses on the actual quality of the basic action, and how we can improve that in itself. Then we look at the fitness by playing the game. Where did we lose the quality? Okay stop, let's build the training programme around that.

Psychology

What goes on in the brain of an athlete really influences their physiological responses. The psychology, the cognitive function, and the overall player well-being stems from what goes on inside the brain. Without the brain or understanding what is going on inside the brain there is no performance. Obviously, physical training is psychological training too, because when you are training the body you are training the brain and the mind. So when you are training an athlete, you are overloading everything, including everything in the brain.

Knowing the psychology of the athlete involves how you communicate with them: it's about building relationships. This is a huge part of being an effective practitioner (and it will be covered in a separate section later in this chapter). I have worked closely with lots of psychologists within an integrated interdisciplinary setting. When you have got a good periodised programme in place, and when you see how players have issues around their energy, often there is something psychological that needs addressing. Having a good psychologist that you are working with can help improve a player's ability to recover and perform again.

In general, well-being is a reflection of an athlete's overall psychological state. I think there are ways to measure that. There is some great technology coming out that looks at facial recognition and emotional responses, which can give you an indication of someone's psychological status. There are also questionnaires, but daily face to face interaction tells a lot when trying to gauge an athlete's psychological well-being. Much is related to energy. An athlete that has good energy is usually in a good psychological state of mind. Psychology impacts levels of fatigue and influences energy. Factors such as sleep, nutritional habits, and how training is perceived gives an indication of the athlete's psychological status. Excessive sympathetic nervous-system responses are often a fear-driven or anxiety-driven issue, impacting recovery. Monitoring changes in physiological and biomarker responses can also provide objective insight into an athlete's psychological well-being.

Interacting and observing how athletes are communicating is of great value. If they trust the process, insight from well-being questionnaires can be gained, but often athletes don't answer honestly. Using questionnaires in addition to personal interaction and monitoring some of the other system responses mentioned previously can help give a clearer picture of where they are at or whether they are dealing with some kind of personal issue that is impacting their recovery. Having awareness of the impact of psychology and how that influences internal responses and recovery is extremely important.

Adapting to different sports

I was very lucky that I got to work quite a bit with Raymond Verheijen, and I use a lot of his methodology in what I do, which helps shape my practice. The way that I break it down in football, is similar to how I also break it down in basketball, starting with understanding the game demands and what is involved. With football and basketball, you have attacking, defending, and transitioning. Then from within that you have the actions – the football actions or the basketball actions. In football, you have closing down, creating space, attacking, heading, jumping, striking, passing, and shooting. And in basketball, there are specific actions in addition to rebounding, jump shots, and changing. Then, when we break them down again into another layer you get more basic actions. Understanding what these basic actions are and how they relate specifically to the game, allows for better communication and increased trust and buy-in from coaches and players.

Let's say we are trying to improve a basic action, such as the jump shot. The basic actions in a jump shot are jumping and landing. What is required to perform those actions effectively? Do we need to improve the ability to get into position? Do we need to improve the ability to react and respond? Do we need to improve the ability to coordinate the direction of the body motion? Or, do we need to improve the ability to make it more of an explosive action? If you look at the game and you are speaking to a coach, what are you trying to work on, what do we need to do? Is there a decision-making issue or is it about the ability to process information quickly and then have the ability to react quickly, which is different from making the right decision? So do we need to work on the execution of the basic action or does the coach need to work on the athlete's decision-making or his understanding of the direction he needs to run in? We also need to look at how quickly he is moving into that area or how quickly is he performing that task, because obviously we want it to be as explosive as possible and for him to perform the task quickly and execute the task well. Is it his actual ability to understand and make the right decision or is it that he is just a slow player who needs to work more on power and strength in his programme? If you understand the game components and the factors that decide if it is more decision-making or more execution of those actions, then you can create a programme that helps improve the execution. When it is broken down, what can the physical therapist, trainer, or strength coach do? If it is a decision-making issue, is it an issue of coaching and understanding the concepts from a technical/tactical perspective?

I took a lot of that from Raymond Verheijen. What I learned is that it is possible to take similar concepts and apply them in a different sport. I think the bottom line is understanding the game requirements, what players need to do in their positions and then how you break that down to develop it and be more specific. By doing this you get the buy-in from the coach, because they now understand why you do what you do and at the same time you're being more proactive with injury-risk reduction.

Typical mistakes

One of the typical errors people make is thinking that doing a lot of work in pre-season is going to make athletes fitter in the season. The error is to think that short-term overload is going to give long-term gain. Long-term overload gives you long-term gain. The key is to induce progressive overload. Looking for instant gratification is a major error and a massive problem. Long-term success comes from gradually implementing change, and we see that in all successful organisations and environments. When you go for short-term change, short-term overload, there is a big chance you usually get a short-term response often followed immediately by a negative response.

A key example is pre-season training. Historically, coaches do not get to work with the players as much as they want in the off-season. So when pre-season arrives, they want to work with them more, thinking that doing more is better. Overloading athletes is important, but it is imperative to measure and gradually apply overload to allow a player to avoid injury risk and fatigue, and keep his freshness while maximising performance. Another mistake occurs when teams lose, thinking that working harder the next week or doing more overload is going to result in winning. An incremental conditioning plan should not be changed based on game outcomes, but maybe what should change is the tactical strategy being applied. Working athletes harder as a consequence to bad results is an extreme emotional response. Emotional decisions are often what cause problems as opposed to a strategic objective decision where you can be more impactful. If you change the periodised programme, then all of a sudden you do not know the reason for torn hamstrings. Is it because of sleeping issues, stress, or because of a sudden change in the training programme? If you keep the training programme the same and you have a clean approach to monitoring that, the rest are just things you have to focus on and manage. But when everything is all over the place you never know what to address or maybe you are addressing too many things and it just becomes a reactive approach.

I often see teams tired at the end of the season. You want to be at your best and fittest at the end of the season, but teams go for short-term gain, rather not long-term gain. Teams in the NBA should be peaking when they get to the play-offs, not dying. Most of them at this point are tired and done. Yes, the season is a grind, but it has always been a grind. What are teams doing between each game to make it less of a grind? This is about planning, being smart with the training, and making sure players are doing all they can to stay fresh. Teams typically do not do that and they blame the schedule for fatigue. It is the same in the premier league and in football in general.

Another big mistake is when all players are treated the same. For instance, unfit players do the same or more as fit players, which is just wrong. Unfit players should do less and be allowed to gradually improve their fitness. A similar mistake is when young players do the same as established players. Young players are still building their tolerance to the sport, and the demands of it, mentally and physically. There are so many more demands as they get to a higher level. They need more time to adapt, so they should not be treated the same as an established player. Likewise, if you want to get the most out of an older player, they can often perform the same if they are given more time to recover. We know as you get older you recover more slowly. Similarly, more explosive players should not be treated the same as less explosive players. More explosive players create more muscle damage. If they have more muscle damage, they need more time to recover. You often see players that are more explosive get more muscle injuries and reoccurrences of these issues, and that is because they are not treated as individuals or there is a lack of knowledge that they need more time to recover.

Generally, too often there is a fear of not getting the work in. People sacrifice freshness to say that they actually worked. Unfortunately, you cannot cheat physiology. It takes time to adapt, so you can only do an optimal amount, and if you go past that, you are going to induce fatigue or create injury. Being smart with what each individual needs based on where they are currently at, and having a tailored programme for each individual, is definitely best practice.

Finally, I think another error is not accounting for travel and the impact travel (including time zones, sleep deprivation, and other circumstances) has on the body. That is why you monitor, so you can modify your programme slightly when external factors come to play like emotional load, stressful events, or sleep deprivation from travel. Having a plan that allows for this is rare. Players should have less physical load before and after to allow for the fact that they are not getting their usual recovery, because of a time zone change, sleep deprivation and travel fatigue. So, if you plan for that, then you are being proactive. If you don't plan for that, you are being reactive. In general, I think it is a lot easier to manage football schedules and planning than it is for basketball because there are fewer games and less travel. Usually teams travel on a Friday if they play Saturday. Friday is generally an underload day anyway, so that isn't really an issue. Thursday is as well if you are smart, and Wednesday is your overload. But if you, for instance, have a mid-week game or you have a European game where you have to travel, you need to change the load and players who are not playing need to maintain their programme. It is often a mistake when players who are not playing are not getting enough exposure to game-related fitness work. Then later down the road when they are called upon, they break down because they are not continually developing. This is about managing the squad differently, about planning, taking time, and communicating. Often because these things take effort, unfortunately they are overlooked.

Communication

Out of everything addressed in this chapter, I believe that communication is most important. On every level, if you cannot communicate well you will never, ever be effective in anything you do. This refers to all types of communication – verbal, body language, indirect communication, communication via email or text. Your ability to communicate really allows you to be effective and build relationships most effectively. With poor communication, people make assumptions, they take things personally, and when things are not clear, confusion arises and poor decisions are made. But if you can communicate well, the language that you use is something that everyone can understand, and you can be more effective. Poor communication is one of the biggest stumbling blocks between sport science and medical community and coaching staff. A lack of integration or interdisciplinary action, it is a result of a communication break-down, because the language that is used is foreign. If you are speaking to a coach using sports science or medical language, he is not trained in that jargon, so to him you might as well be speaking a different language. You need to speak in the football language or the basketball language; that should be your starting point. That comes from having the reference of basketball, having the reference of football, and then being clear with what you are trying to do. By doing this, you get better buy-in with the coach, because you are speaking the same language and you communicate at the same level. However, if you start coming at coaches and players with data and numbers, things that are going to confuse them, you set yourself up for failure. You need science to support your actions, but you do not want to come at coaches with the numbers first.

Listening is key to communication. By listening you gain trust and respect, and then you can really start to solve a problem. Listening helps you to be able to relate and find common ground, which lays the foundation for conversations that build relationships and trust. I believe doing something away from the team setting, outside the team, helps you to understand the athlete as a person or the coach as a person, which is the most important thing you can do. Don't see them as a coach, don't see them as a player. See them as a person first and then think about how can you help them become a better coach or player. If your approach is, how can I help you?, you are going to be more effective. I think understanding them as people makes it more of a purposeful event. You also get more fulfilment with your job when you start to help people as people. They can be more impactful with what they do and you can be more impactful too.

That is one of the things I learned from my first experience with Bolton. I was able to get to know the other staff outside the team environment on a consistent basis; we just became very close as friends, and we wanted to help each other improve our lives. We genuinely cared about each other and as a result we functioned better as a cohesive unit.

I think understanding people's background and culture – really getting to know people on a deeper level – allows you to better navigate the way you communicate. What I try to communicate with my athletes is that I am doing this for them, not the team, not the coach, I am trying to help them. Everything I am doing is to help them. When they realise you have their best interests at heart you are going to get more buy-in, more trust, and a better relationship with them. Your communication drives the core of your relationship.

Conclusions

Develop your communication skills because they build relationships. Understand the sport-specific culture, the environment, and the language that is required. Specialise in one area while appreciating all areas.

14

Medical practice with elite athletes

Bruce Hamilton

Editors' introduction

Bruce Hamilton completed studies in physical education and medicine at Otago University in New Zealand, prior to completing the Australasian College of Sports Medicine Fellowship in 2001. He has postgraduate qualifications in tropical medicine and sports law, has published over 90 peer reviewed manuscripts or book chapters, and in 2017 he was awarded a medical doctorate (MD) from the University of Otago for his research involving hamstring muscle injury.

Bruce previously worked at the Australian Institute of Sport, and was chief medical officer for Athletics Australia for 2001–02 prior to moving to the United Kingdom as the West Midlands regional lead physician for the English Institute of Sport. In 2005 he was appointed chief medical officer to UK Athletics before moving to Qatar in 2008, where he worked as a sports medicine physician and ultimately as chief of sports medicine from 2010–12 in Aspetar (Qatar Orthopaedic and Sports Medicine Hospital). In 2013 Dr Hamilton returned to New Zealand after being appointed medical lead for High Performance Sport NZ (HPSNZ) and the NZ Olympic Committee (NZOC). In his current role as director of performance health (HPSNZ/NZOC) Bruce is responsible for ensuring NZ has a world-class health service supporting elite NZ Olympic Athletes. Dr Hamilton has attended four World Track and Field Championships, two World Triathlon Championships, four Commonwealth, and three Olympic Games in a team medical capacity.

Introduction

Medical practitioners treated athletes in the ancient Olympic and combat events (Masterton, 1976, Bartels et al., 2006) and were again involved since the evolution of modern sport in the early nineteenth century. By the early twentieth century, doctors were increasingly visible in elite sports, being involved in both 'screening' for medical conditions and providing reactive care to athletes at the 1912 Olympics (Bergvall, 1913) and being recruited by universities and national teams. Internationally, medicine in sport evolved relatively independently with variations in approach to sport medicine resulting from differences in sporting, educational and medical norms, and societal expectations across nations. For example, distinct interpretations and influences of amateurism and social class between the USA and Britain in the early-twentieth century influenced the disparate development of sports medicine in both countries. The USA recognised the importance of medicine in sport relatively early, appointing doctors in sport education roles as early as the mid-nineteenth century, but the UK was later in achieving similar appointments. By comparison, Germany was the first country to establish a sports medicine representative body and the earliest to publish comprehensive texts on the topic of sports medicine (Weissbein, 1910, Hoberman, 1992). By the mid-twentieth century when the polymath sport physician Ernest Jokl asked the question, "What is Sports Medicine?" (Jokl, 1964), the international variation in approach was such that he was unable to find a uniform description (Shephard, 1974b). As medicine in sport evolved in the latter twentieth century, international differences in its organisation and culture remained, and sports medicine as a role descriptor now includes a broad range of disciplines and approaches (Boggess and Bytomski, 2013). This chapter will focus specifically on the role of the medical practitioner in the elite sport environment.

As a result of the organic growth of the sports medicine doctor role, there is neither a single international approach to training doctors for working in sport, nor a single model for doctors to operate within the elite sports environment. For example, professional teams in USA differ in both their approach to the engagement of medicine within teams/clubs and their expectations of practitioner education compared to similarly resourced clubs in Europe. Those expectations will differ again from British and Commonwealth approaches, which will differ again from less well-resourced sports codes. As a result, any detailed discussion of the role and approach to medicine in elite sport is challenged by underlying international differences in organisational style. Hence, the line taken in the following chapter will be to address broad principles and concepts which should underpin approaches to the application of medicine in elite sport, irrespective of setting.

The role of medicine in elite sport

Traditionally, the domain of medical practitioners in elite sport was largely one of injury diagnosis and treatment (Stevens and Phelps, 1933, Shephard, 1974a). However, by the 1960s it was recognised that the role of the doctor also encompassed the non-injury related health concerns of athletes (Williams, 1965). In modern high-performance sports, the role of medicine may be considered the "maintenance and optimisation of health" of elite athletes in the demanding sports environment (Speed and Jaques, 2011). This broad remit includes both 'proactive' health promotion and 'reactive' diagnosis and management of acute and subacute injuries and illnesses experienced by athletes. Since illness may include a broad spectrum of physical, psychological and social conditions, a great breadth of knowledge and experience is required by doctors working within elite sport. This required breadth of knowledge has been met by a range of different means around the world. In some countries, a range of hyper-specialised practitioners are recruited to form part of a large multi-disciplinary health team, while in others, the specialist 'sports physician' will be expected to be able to manage the full range of (non-surgical) conditions. In my experience both of these extremes have challenges. For example, in a large team it can be unclear who is responsible and accountable for making decisions and, as such, issues can fall between areas of expertise. By contrast, in the 'sports physician' generalist type approach, individuals may be required to make decisions which lie outside of their area of competence. Subsequently, a mixed model, with clear leadership but the ability to easily call upon appropriate expertise, is my preferred approach to ensuring the best care of athletes.

Health promotion strategies relate to both injury and illness prevention and optimising health status. The former requires being able to translate epidemiological and aetiological evidence of injury and illness risk in specific sporting codes, into practical, effective strategies for risk mitigation. Furthermore, optimising health requires a clear understanding of the demands of individual sports, and an equally comprehensive understanding of individual athlete needs (Dijkstra et al., 2014) Hence, while doctors who are 'fans' or have a history of participation in a given sport may have an intimate understanding of the sport, if they are not well-read from the medical literature, they will be providing an incomplete perspective on athlete care. Sports-specific knowledge, combined with an evidence-based approach to care, is what delineates the best approach.

Unfortunately, over the last 60 years in elite sport, medical practitioners have also played a role in the doping of athletes (Hoberman, 2002). In conflict with both medical and sporting ethics, doctors have figured in almost every elite level doping scandal over this period. The paradox of having those charged with athlete's health and well-being facilitating doping processes in elite athletes, illustrates one of the key challenges faced by practitioners working in elite sport – that of promoting health in a potentially unhealthy high-performance environment. This latter issue is one of the great challenges facing modern elite sport. How do doctors and sports organisations balance the long-term welfare of athletes against the short-term requirements of elite sport? For example, should athletes with an Anterior Cruciate Ligament (ACL) rupture be expedited back into sport quickly for the benefit of the team (and perhaps financially for the athlete), when we know that the risk of injury is higher in those returning to play earlier, and more injuries means greater morbidity (eg. osteoarthritis) in the years that follow? If not the doctor, who should be advocating for looking after the long-term well-being of the athlete? In the highly conflicted world of elite sport, this is consideration is often overlooked. The high-performance arena can place exceptional demands on medical practitioners, with a range of conflicting imperatives imposing challenges on the provision of optimal care. Fiscal, team, selection, aspirations, and coaching factors can all impose relatively (but not entirely) unique challenges on doctors operating in the high-performance sporting world. Hence, in order for a medical team to appropriately manage the broad range of medical and musculoskeletal issues experienced by athletes, the structural, organisational, and ethical considerations for medical support must be clear within any given team environment.

Organisation of sports medicine within elite sport

Given the impact that injuries and illnesses have been shown to have on sports performance, there has been relatively little documentation in the sports medicine literature of how to establish an appropriate medical presence in elite sport (Eirale et al., 2013, Dijkstra et al., 2014) By contrast, sociological literature in recent years has highlighted numerous challenges confronting the operation of medicine in the elite sporting environment. For example, until very recently, the recruitment of doctors in the UK for professional football has followed a distinctly unprofessional approach (Waddington et al., 2001) Partly as a result of this unprofessional engagement model, doctors working within professional sport have been shown to have their autonomy compromised, have motivation other than the primary care of patients, work in less than optimal physical environments, lack clinical authority, and have varying levels of training in the challenges faced in practising medicine in elite level sport (Malcolm, 2006, Anderson and Jackson, 2012, Bal and Brenner, 2013). In reality, this has in the past translated into doctors who may lack appropriate experience or training, working in heavily compromised situations, supporting the most high-profile of athletes, in the most pressured situations.

Subsequently, it may be interpreted that the organisational structure of medical support within elite sport, impacts upon the medical supports' effectiveness in supporting the well-being of athletes, and the risk of exposure to unethical or borderline practices. An interesting framework for considering the organisation of medicine within elite sport, is to conceptualise the delivery of medicine within any organisation as being on a spectrum of sport integration. At one end, medical support may be fully integrated into the sporting environment, with clinicians totally embedded in the sport, a so-called 'sportised' approach. At the polar extreme, medical support may be totally separated from sport, with practitioners working in a clinical environment distinct from the club or sport – the 'medicalised' approach. Any given approach may have a mix of both models, sitting somewhere within these extreme situations.

A 'sportised' medical service has practitioners highly immersed within sport, integrated into the sports performance (success) model, and relatively isolated from the broader medical world. In the 'sportised' approach, the medical role may be poorly remunerated, isolated from the broader medical community, have a low professional status within the sports environment in which it operates, and the practitioner may be heavily influenced by (and dependent on) the coach and club hierarchy, thereby by default exhibiting a high level of conformity to the sport or club goals (Freidson, 1960, Malcolm, 2006). Consequently, the fully integrated approach to the delivery of medicine, risks placing a doctor in challenging ethical conflicts with little support, which may thereby impede the delivery of optimal athlete support (Bal and Brenner, 2013, Poma et al., 2016) As one example of the unintended conundrum the 'sportised' approach to medical support may endear, consider the perception of injury risk. Injury is an inherent risk within all sport, but how much risk is acceptable varies between athletes and situations. It has been shown that a culture of risk acceptance potentially places athletes at an unacceptable or unknowing risk (Walk, 1997, Safai, 2003) and that social networks surrounding athletes have the potential to reinforce the risk acceptance. In the sportised model, it is argued that medical practitioners fully immersed within the sport environment may form part of a subculture that provides implicit and explicit messages minimising interpretations of risk, pain, and injury (Nixon, 1992) – potentially to the detriment of athletes well-being (Safai 2003). Take the post-ACL reconstruction return to play scenario described above. It is extremely challenging for the fully immersed practitioner, isolated from the broader medical environment, focussed on winning the impending championship, and constantly hearing the needs of the team, to step outside of the 'team' environment, and focus solely on what is best for the individual player – particularly if the doctor is employed by the team, to help the team win the championship.

By contrast, in the 'medicalised' approach to the delivery of care to the professional athlete the practitioner may work entirely outside of the team environment, act as a practitioner independent of the sport or club and consult from a separate medical facility (Bal and Brenner, 2013, Poma et al., 2016) In this model, the medical practitioner may be well remunerated, maintain a high professional status among non-sport colleagues, work from a clinical environment, and be less influenced by the sports goals. Clinical approaches may be more conservative, and evidence-based in approach (Freidson, 1960, Malcolm, 2006). This approach may prioritise the clinical needs of the individual athlete, but pose challenges to communication and impact within the sport performance environment. Utilising the ACL injury analogy further, the surgeon sitting in his hospital office, surrounded by colleagues, with no coach 'in his ear' and no emotional or financial engagement in winning the championship, is theoretically able to provide a more balanced clinical opinion – on the real risk to the knee. However, the flip side of this approach is that there may be conflict and uncertainty created within the team environment, if there is any difference in opinion between the external opinion, and the opinion of embedded clinical staff.

Awareness of the 'sportised' and 'medicalised' framework for engaging medical support in elite sport facilitates the recognition and mitigation of medical risks within any organisation. Professional approaches to the recruitment, ongoing education, oversight, and organisation of medical services can ensure the negative aspects of either polarised approach are mitigated.

Key considerations when establishing a medical team in elite sport

Based on the above discussion, establishing appropriate sports medicine support within the elite sports world is not as simple as just appointing a local doctor to a team. For medical personnel to be effective in the goals of 'maintaining and optimising' health of elite athletes, the following key factors should be considered.

Personnel

Given the large number of challenges posed by practising in the elite sport environment, engaged doctors should be appropriately qualified and experienced to manage the broad clinical and demanding interpersonal nature of the role. Until recently, many practitioners working in sports medicine, even at the elite level, have had no postgraduate training in sports medicine, inappropriately exposing practitioners and patient/athletes to risk (Malcolm, 2006). It is recommended that a transparent recruitment process is utilised, with a clear job description, reporting lines, accountabilities, and responsibilities. Minimum levels of medical experience and qualifications should be pre-determined. 'Shoulder tapping' practitioners based on word of mouth, informal, or casual contractual arrangements, and a lack of transparency in the approach to recruitment should be avoided when possible.

Internationally, academic training in sports medicine varies significantly, ranging from full specialist or subspecialty training, to no recognisable sports medicine training programme. Acknowledging the impact that having no available postgraduate training in sports medicine has on athlete care, organisations such as FIFA and the IOC now provide online diplomas in sports medicine, such that nearly every country can access learning resources. Given the complex medical and medico-legal environment in which elite sport medicine is practised, all doctors working in elite sport should have some formal postgraduate training qualification – in sports medicine! (Dijkstra et al., 2014).

Once recruitment is complete, sporting bodies should ensure that medical personnel establish a professional development plan with at least annual performance reviews by both sport and non-sport professionals. These plans ensure that doctors in sport keep up-to-date with the latest trends and management approaches to common problems, thereby optimising the care of athletes. Furthermore, regular and continuous external peer review is a critical element of practitioners' ongoing development, quality assurance, and ensuring appropriate care is being delivered; this should be mandated and audited by the sporting body. For example, the Australasian College of Sport and Exercise Medicine requires its Fellows to have at least ten hours of face to face peer review, complete an audit, and attend a National Sports Medicine conference on an annual basis. Without oversight, it should not be assumed that medical personnel will automatically maintain optimal professional development, particularly those working in a highly 'sportised' environment where collegial supervision is low.

Funding of doctors should be commensurate with the experience, qualifications, and responsibility of the role. Funding arrangements should be independent of performance outcomes, as this may deflect from the primary responsibility of advocacy for athlete health and well-being. In the modern world of elite sports medicine, doctors should neither be expected to work for free, nor participate in the exchange of 'envelopes with cash' as a result of successful team performances.

Physical environment

Establishing an appropriate environment for the practice of sports medicine is not always easy, but at the level of elite sport, an appropriate clinical setting is mandatory to ensure the appropriate care of athletes. Depending on the particular circumstances of a sport or medical practice, three distinct environments may be relevant. The area over which the medical team have least influence is typically the field of play, in which competitive events take place. Operation in this space is largely rule/regulation driven, and it is recommended that practitioners are familiar with resources, rules, and emergency procedures.

Often, the medical facility in the club setting is limited to communal changing areas or 'track/pitchside' care. Where possible, a private, clean medical area should be established to facilitate confidential discussions and interventions. The elite training facility is where the majority of health consultations typically take place and, as such, is a key environment for doctors working in professional sport. To ensure effective collaboration, the doctors workspace should be contiguous with physiotherapists and other health professionals. There should be an adequate space for confidential consultations, as well as a sterile area for any interventions. A meeting space for the health team, separate from the clinical work space, facilitates appropriate communication between disciplines. Trackside care, while valuable in enhancing engagement and sport specific knowledge for all involved, has significant limitations when attempting to provide world-class medical care – the latter requiring a work space not shrouded in sport pressures. Where possible, performing assessments or invasive procedures in non-hygienic, multi-use environments such as changing rooms or bathrooms should be avoided. The risks myself and colleagues have been exposed to in the past when performing intra-articular joint injections in stadium bathrooms due to a total lack of resources and facilities, should not have to be repeated in the modern era.

In addition to club-based facilities, doctors working with elite teams will often practice out of separate, 'medicalised' clinical settings, with athletes required to travel to a clinic for assessment (Dijkstra et al., 2014). While frequently perceived as problematic for athletes from a logistics and travel perspective, consultations external to the training environment have many advantages, including the ease of access to quality diagnostic imaging and laboratory investigations, and access to multiple specialties. Furthermore, this environment often may provide clinical oversight for practitioners, often isolated if working entirely in a sport setting.

The reality is that a balanced combination of these environments will provide the optimal support for the majority of athletes. When establishing a medical process, this should form part of the planning.

Organisational processes

The effectiveness of the medical practitioner within the professional team environment will be influenced by their training and experience, the physical environment in which they operate, and the organisational processes established around them. Many of the ethical challenges implicit in the practising of medicine in elite sport can either be mitigated or exaggerated by the implementation of effective or ineffective operational processes respectively.

For example and as alluded to above, while team environments tend to consider the good of the team ahead of individual needs, the goal of the doctor is to ensure the wellbeing of each individual (Devitt, 2016). In order to effectively achieve this goal, the doctor's clinical function should be independent of the performance outcomes of the team. Immediately, this creates a challenging situation, whereby a doctor employed by a team, may have to balance the conflicting imperatives of team and individual. As the team doctor employed by the organisation to help the team be successful, how am I supposed to balance the desire of the team and coaches, against the wellbeing of the athlete? The reality is that the operational structure established within a team may determine how effective, or otherwise, a doctor is in managing this situation. One proposed operating model suggests that the 'Chief Medical Officer' (CMO) leads a team of doctors, therapists, and performance scientists (including physiology, nutrition, biomechanics, psychology, and podiatry) and that this role sits alongside the 'head coach' but does not report to the head coach; rather reporting lines are to the chief executive, or performance director (Dijkstra et al., 2014). The approach of team coaches and doctors having distinct line management has the advantage of allowing the medical practitioners to engage in the performance environment but not be behoved to performance outcomes, and therefore to prioritise individual athlete health. However, while well positioned to allow the doctor autonomy in decision-making, this arrangement is not the usual situation, as in many professional sporting environments, the doctor will report directly to the head coach, and subsequently will have the team values heavily imposed. A further challenge of this model, specifically the inclusion of the sport science team under the line management of the CMO, may be challenging given the performance (as opposed to health) focus of many of these roles (Dijkstra et al., 2014). In my experience, sport science teams will have a heavy performance focus, with health and well-being an element, but not the primary element of their function. The merits therefore of their line management being a medical doctor whose primary function should be well-being, is questionable.

Irrespective of the formal line management approaches, optimal clinical outcomes in elite sport require high quality communication between coaching and performance staff and the medical teams. Opportunities for regular, formal and informal communication should be mandated between key members of health and performance teams within any sporting organisation. A mutual understanding of the contrasting imperatives, and respect for individual's roles, forms the foundation for quality communication. In the author's experience, mutual respect, active communication, and shared beliefs are the most important elements of an effectively operating health team. When this type of relationship doesn't exist, athlete welfare can be heavily compromised and medical delivery may be non-sustainable.

Clinical considerations

When establishing a medical team within an elite sporting environment, a number of key clinical topics should have clearly articulated strategies. In addition to ensuring where ultimate clinical responsibility sits within an organisation, strategic approaches to topics as diverse as anti-doping, supplement utilisation, cardiac evaluations, pre-participation and pre-signing health evaluations, confidentiality, ongoing education, concussion, injury rehabilitation and clinical pathways, management of mental health issues, inter-disciplinary communication, return to play processes, emergency preparedness, and injury/illness monitoring should be clearly documented. These significant topics should not be allowed to evolve organically within the sports environment, but should be strategically implemented based on best practice approaches, by the medical team lead. Implementation of these strategies will often be the responsibility of the individual team doctors, upon which the remaining discussion will focus.

The role of the team doctor

As alluded to above, the role of the team doctor can vary immensely, depending on whether one is working for the local junior football team, an Olympic sport, or a professional code. However, while expectations and working models may vary significantly, some principles which form the basis of the team doctor role, remain consistent.

Key relationships

Doctor–athlete

In many elite sports the risk of injury and illness may be considered high. For the team doctor to be effective in preventing and managing injury and illness in elite sport, an appropriate doctor–athlete relationship is critical. Recent examples have illustrated how the clinical influence that a doctor may exert at the elite level of sport can be exploited leading to inappropriate relationships and abuse (for a recent example from USA Gymnastics, where the team doctor has recently been sentenced for sexual abuse of elite athletes, see https://en.wikipedia.org/wiki/USA_Gymnastics_sex_abuse_scandal).

As discussed above, the doctor may often be required to balance the conflicting priorities of the team (and often the individual) of winning and subsequent commercial interests, with the short- and long-term health of the athlete/patient (Anderson and Jackson, 2012). Within the sport environment, and where a culture of risk acceptance may predominate (Walk, 1997) a doctor who is experienced, trusted, and able to negotiate effectively with athletes, may have a significant influence on health outcomes (Safai, 2003). In addition to time spent with athletes (which may be perceived by athletes as 'skin in the game'), education, peer review, supervision, and an appropriate environment will all facilitate the development and maintenance of appropriate professional doctor–athlete relationships. The value of time spent with athletes in the training and competition environment cannot be over-stated. In my experience, it is the time spent 'track-side' that facilitates both understanding and influence with both coaches and athletes. Where possible, these opportunities should be facilitated.

In the elite sport environment, it is often easy to become a 'fan' of athlete/patients/teams, which has the potential to bias decision-making away from pure athlete-centred priorities as laid out in the Olympic Medical Code (Committee, 2009). Similarly, social media may further blur this relationship, with doctors potentially being social media 'friends' with their athlete/patients. Hence, maintaining a professional relationship, which may involve establishing clear and often artificial boundaries is a priority for the doctor working in a team environment.

Case study

When working with UK Athletics as a relatively junior Sports Physician, my initial goal was to be perceived as part of the team. To facilitate this, I wore team kit to work each day (even though I didn't have to) and the work environment meant significant casual interaction with athletes, which I took as a positive. However, as a result, I found myself practising more 'corridor consultations'. Athletes felt it unnecessary to book a time, but just 'caught me' in the corridor for 'confidential' and often significant conversations. It quickly became apparent that I was perceived as available 100% of the time, and that I could do good medicine wherever. As a result, the quality of the work I was doing, and the care provided to the athletes was, in my view, declining. Subsequently, I changed my clothing, starting to wear a business shirt and jacket. I established a formal working routine, which, while still accessible, meant that athletes knew that they were being consulted, not having an informal chat. Finally, we separated the staff and athlete environment, recognising that there are differences in needs and expectations from both parties. These changes, required as a result of my initial naivety, enhanced the care to athletes, and meant that the role was effective and sustainable.

Ultimately, a positive, engaged, and professional relationship, with appropriate boundaries between the team doctor and athletes that facilitates the sharing of information, decision-making and informed well-being, is the goal (Elwyn et al., 2014).

Doctor–coach

An effective relationship between the team doctor and the coach is critical for the optimal management of athlete health and well-being. This is evidenced both in the frequency with which professional football (soccer) coaches forgo existing medical teams to embed their own trusted medical teams, and the examples of failed doctor–coach relationships on public record.[1]

As with many relationships, two elements may be key in the success of the coach–doctor relationship. The first element is role clarity. While the coach roles and responsibilities may be clearly defined, the off- and on-field responsibilities of the team doctor are often assumed, but less well articulated. As outlined above, consideration of athlete well-being can be in direct conflict with coaching performance imperatives, and with the team doctor position often reliant on the good will of the coach, a dysfunctional relationship can intensify a practitioner's ethical dilemmas. Clarity regarding responsibility on and off the field, decision-making regarding injury or illness availability, and shared awareness that athlete well-being is the primary concern of the team doctor, all facilitate an effective working relationship. In the examples alluded to above, had the respective roles and responsibilities been clear, many of the crises that occurred could have been avoided.

The second key element in the doctor–coach relationship is the ability to communicate in an open and trusting manner. Shared beliefs regarding the nature of the medical role, clear pathways of communication, transparent means of escalating concerns, combined with a mutual trust and understanding of the conflicting imperatives, facilitate a strong working relationship, which ultimately supports the welfare of the athlete – and team. In my experience, the ability to communicate effectively with the coach and to have an open approach to dialogue has been both the most rewarding and on occasion frustrating aspects of working in elite sport. Typically, the failings have resulted from both parties not understanding the respective responsibilities and pressures, and not taking the time to develop a strong effective working relationship. As with the doctor–athlete relationship, time spent with a coach can facilitate relationship building and communication.

Case study

In approximately 2003, as a relatively junior (but cocky) sports physician, I was fortunate to be appointed to work with UK Athletics (now British Athletics) in the West Midlands. It was clear from the very start *that my interpretation of 'an appropriate facility' and the 'role' of the doctor was quite distinct to that of the centre management and coaching team. The coaching team had been instrumental in establishing the role, and quite rightly felt frustration that I was not performing in the way that they wanted – that being standing trackside with the athletes and coaches, and providing constant immediate feedback. From my perspective, I felt the role was about developing a world-class medical approach, not about being a 'first aid' service. As a result, communication was never established, disagreements ensued, and it was generally pretty unpleasant and unsatisfying.*

However, both parties recognised the failing approach, and recognising that the environment wasn't sustainable and wasn't going to have an ongoing positive impact, the key coaches and I sat down to try and figure it out. The result was an awareness of each other's perspectives, an understanding of conflicting imperatives, but an understanding of the shared goal of having healthy, well-performing athletes. Subsequent to this 'enlightenment', regular semi-formalised meetings and appropriate balance of trackside and office-based workload were established. The positive outcome resulted from an ability to recognise shared motivations and a preparedness to learn and shift mindsets.

Doctor–paramedical and performance science

The only published work on the structure of the health team in elite sport suggests that the medical lead system is the most appropriate means of supporting athletes (Dijkstra et al., 2014). However, therapy, sport science, and other support staff may often operationally report to a range of clinical or non-clinical staff. As with the above relationships, communication, role, and responsibility clarity are key factors in establishing positive, productive working relationships.

Environment

Even in the elite team environment, many doctors function without a specific consultation room, without privacy, sterility, and without an effective means of keeping medical records, reports, or administrative support. In keeping with the primary focus on athlete well-being, it is critical that both an appropriate confidential space be available, and that administrative support be allocated to enhance the effectiveness of the medical support.

Key team doctor functions

The pre-signing medical and periodic health evaluation (PHE)

In many professional sports, the 'pre-signing medical' is a requirement prior to 'signing' an athlete to a team. In this role, the team doctor is working for the sport or team, in trying to understand the injury and illness history of a player, and translate that into future risk for the athlete and future team. It may include intensive investigation of areas of concern based on the individual history or the epidemiology of injury and illness within a particular sport. In this role, the team doctor is acting as an independent assessor of risk, on behalf of the club, and this should be clear to both the athlete and the club.

By contrast, the PHE is athlete-focussed, with the goal of assisting the athlete and medical team optimise the individual's health and performance (Ljungqvist et al., 2009) The PHE may be performed on a regular basis, and provide direction for ongoing proactive support.

The cardiac evaluation

The sudden cardiac death (SCD) of an elite athlete, while rare, has a profound impact on a family, club, community, and sport. Most organisations internationally now recognise the role of regular cardiac evaluation in identifying and quantifying the risk of SCD in elite athletes (Steriotis and Sharma, 2015). Cardiac evaluations may involve a clear history, examination, ECG, or other assessments as indicated. When embarking on a cardiac evaluation process, it is important that the sport has the expertise and resources to complete the process.[2] The team doctor is responsible for ensuring the accurate completion of a regular cardiac evaluation, including the provision of feedback to athletes on their risk. In the modern world of elite sport, the consequences of failing to have and follow a clear approach to evaluating cardiac risk in the elite athlete can be significant for athletes, families, doctors, and organisations are significant and life changing. This is a critical aspect of any sport plan which cannot be overlooked.

Medication and supplement management

Within club and team environments, ensuring the appropriate prescription and monitoring of medication management is a critical function of the team doctor. Where supplies are stored on-site, control of access, stock ordering, and management of out-of-date products are key functions for effective functioning. In combination with nutrition and/or physiology support, the team doctor should have oversight on the use of supplements by athletes.

In many elite team environments, limited resources mean that physiotherapists may travel without the support of doctors, and therefore act as the primary point of contact for all health-related matters. In this situation, it is vital that a clear approach to the prescription and delivery of medications is documented and monitored. Most commonly, a 'standing order' approach is utilised with physiotherapists, with the support of doctors at a distance, able to deliver a limited range of medications.

Anti-doping education and support

Throughout modern sport, the doctor has been found to be either deliberately or inadvertently linked to doping offences. In a team environment, the team doctor should be both an active advocate for ethical approaches to sport, and an educator of all team members on anti-doping principles and practice. Failure to ensure an appropriate education approach can have devastating effects on athletes, staff, and sport organisations.

Emergency preparedness

Preparation and training of key support members in the management of critical incidents both in training and on the field of play remains one of the primary functions of the team doctor. Depending on the specifics of sport, this may include management of the collapsed athlete, head injury, spinal injury, acute contact trauma, or other significant life or limb threatening incident.

On-field management

The most visible element of any team doctor role, on-field management of injuries and illnesses, requires a comprehensive understanding of both the competitive rules of the sport and the physical/psychological demands of the sport. A medical kit (always including an automated external defibrillator (AED)) appropriate for the requirements of the sport is a requirement, as is a clear understanding of the sporting rules and principles.

Injury and illness management

Management of injury and illness in the elite athlete setting requires experience and time in order to ensure optimal outcomes. Even minor injuries and illnesses can have significant impact on performance, and requires careful attention to detail.

Infectious disease

Ensuring sport-specific team hygiene protocols are established that minimise the risk of transmission of all forms of infectious disease, including the completion of an appropriate immunisation strategy.

Maintenance of medical records

Accurate documentation of medical consultations and procedures is mandatory for team doctors. Failure to complete comprehensive records can have significant consequences for both athletes and medical staff (Commons, 2018).

Ethical challenges for sports medicine in elite sport

As a medical subspecialty, sports medicine practitioners in elite sport are required to practice within clearly articulated medical ethical standards. Basic ethical principles which must be applied consistently within elite sport include autonomy (confidentiality, informed consent), justice (respecting the individual needs), beneficence (focus on athlete well-being), and non-maleficence (do no harm) (Devitt, 2016). Many sports medicine organisations have articulated ethical guidelines for those caring for athletes, all of which place the well-being of the athlete/patient as the focus.[3] Notwithstanding these guidelines and as alluded to above, the elite sports environment has specific ethical challenges, particularly in relation to the presence of conflicting obligations and the sharing of information (Anderson and Gerrard, 2005, Anderson, 2009).

Being paid by a club or team to perform medical services has the potential to place a doctor in a dilemma of meeting the conflicting imperatives of both the club or team (i.e. to be successful) and the individual athlete (i.e. to be healthy and successful). However, while this approach to the provision of health care to athletes has challenges, the alternative option, that all medical services are provided by fully independent providers, has significant limitations. Specifically, the latter situation limits the responsibility that any practitioner has for the care of the athlete, and will challenge effective communication with the club or team, thereby potentially negatively impacting upon the well-being of the athlete. By contrast, while the club-employed doctor has ethical challenges, as described above, these can be overcome by appropriate role clarity, responsibility demarcation, and high levels of trust and understanding amongst all involved. Having doctors with 'skin in the game' can work to the benefit of athletes and teams, when appropriately applied.

Confidentiality of the medical consult is fundamental in allowing full disclosure and comprehensive management of patient/athletes. However, a wall of confidentiality often frustrates coaches and support staff, who feel they would benefit from being more fully involved. Once again, trust and high levels of communication are key in mitigating the challenges of confidentiality in the elite sports environment. Balancing the confidentiality of the athlete with the needs of the team is a challenging task in many elite sport situations. Ensuring an athlete consents (without coercion) to appropriate sharing of information, and with whom, is an important component of the consultation process with elite athletes. Failure to clarify this during each consultation, can result in loss of confidence in the medical support from both the athlete and the club/sport. The downstream impact of this is a failure of the medical system, and reduced quality of care to athletes.

Failure to set, clarify, and meet appropriate ethical standards has resulted in many cases in compromised care for athletes, and exposing medical staff to sanctions (Anderson, 2011, Commons, 2018). Meeting appropriate ethical standards within the elite sporting environment requires a high standard of role clarity, responsibility delineation, mutual trust, and communication. Achieving these goals requires education of coaching, medical, and other support staff (Borjesson and Karlsson, 2014). Only with these elements, which involve all members of the team environment, will athletes' medical support be optimised.

Conclusion

Working as medical practitioner with an elite team or sporting code can be a highly rewarding experience. However, it is not an easy option, and in many cases neither undergraduate or postgraduate training adequately prepares practitioners for the demands place upon them. While a love for sport is a great starting point, it will not necessarily translate into a high-functioning doctor. Role clarity, clear organisational structure, ongoing peer support, regular process audits, an awareness of the environmental constraints, and a high level of communication skill will assist in ensuring athletes get the medical support they require.

Notes

1 See for example https://en.wikipedia.org/wiki/Bloodgate; https://en.wikipedia.org/wiki/Essendon_Football_Club_supplements_saga; www.express.co.uk/sport/football/598018/Chelsea-crisis-Roman-Abramovich-Jose-Mourinho-doctor-Eva-Carneiro.
2 For an example from football of where this can go wrong when not accurately completed, see www.39essex.com/content/wp-content/uploads/2015/02/Final-Hamed-v-Mills.pdf.
3 See for example: Australian Institute of Sport Best Practice Principles (www.ausport.gov.au/__data/assets/pdf_file/0003/531498/AIS_Sports_Science_Sports_Medicine_Best_Practice_Principles_FA.PDF); FIMS Code of Ethics (www.fims.org/about/code-ethics/); IOC Olympic Movement Medical Code (https://stillmed.olympic.org/media/Document%20Library/OlympicOrg/IOC/Who-We-Are/Commissions/Medical-and-Scientific-Commission/Olympic-Movement-Medical-Code-31-03-2016.pdf); ACSEP Code of Ethics and Professional Behaviour (www.acsep.org.au/content/Document/P015%20Code%20of%20Ethics%20%26%20Professional%20Behaviour.pdf).

References

Anderson, L. (2009). Writing a New Code of Ethics for Sports Physicians: Principles and Challenges. *Br J Sports Med*, **43**(13), 1079–1082
Anderson, L. (2011). Bloodgate: Were the Punishments Fair? *Br J Sports Med*, **45**(12), 948–949

Anderson, L. & Jackson, S. (2012). Competing Loyalties in Sports Medicine: Threats to Medical Professionalism in Elite, Commercial Sport.*International Review for the Sociology of Sport*, **48**(2), 238–249

Anderson, L. C. & Gerrard, D. F. (2005). Ethical Issues Concerning New Zealand Sports Doctors. *J Med Ethics*, **31**(2), 88–92

Bal, B. S. & Brenner, L. H. (2013). Care of the Professional Athlete: What Standard of Care? *Clinical Orthopaedics and Related Research*, **471**, 2060–2064

Bartels, E. M., Swaddling, J. & Harrison, A. P. (2006). History of Pain: An Ancient Greek Pain Remedy for Athletes. *Pain Practice*, **6**(3), 212–218

Bergvall, E. (1913). *The Fifth Olympiad. The Official Report of the Olympic Games of Stockholm 1912.* Stockholm: Wahlstrom & Widstrand

Boggess, B. R. & Bytomski, J. R. (2013). Medicolegal Aspects of Sports Medicine. *Primary Care Clinical Office Practitioner*, **40**: 525–535

Borjesson, M. and Karlsson, J. (2014). Ethical Dilemmas Faced by the Team Physician: Overlooked in Sports Medicine Education? *Br J Sports Med*, **48**(19), 1398–1399

Committee, I. O. (2009). *Olympic Movement Medical Code.* Lausanne: IOC

Commons, H. o. (2018). *House of Commons Digital, Culture, Media and Sport Committee. Combatting Doping in Sport. Fourth Report of Session 2017–19.* London: House of Commons

Devitt, B. M. (2016). Fundamental Ethical Principles in Sports Medicine. *Clinics in Sports Medicine*, **35**, 195–204

Dijkstra, H. P., Pollock, N., Chakraverty, R. & Alonso, J. M. (2014). Managing the Health of the Elite Athlete: A New Integrated Performance Health Management and Coaching Model. *Br J Sports* Med, **48**(7), 523–531

Eirale, C., Tol, J. L., Farooq, A., Smiley, F. & Chalabi, H. (2013). Low Injury Rate Strongly Correlates with Team Success in Qatari Professional Football. *Br J Sports Med*, **47**(12), 807–808

Elwyn, G., Dehlendorf, C., Epstein, R. M., Marrin, K., White, J. & Frosch, D. L. (2014). Shared Decision Makinga nd Motivational Interviewing: Achieving Patient-Centred Care Across the Spectrum of Health Care Problems. *Annals of Family Medicine*, **12**(3), 270–275

Freidson, E. (1960). Client Con Control trol and Medical Practice. *Americal Journal of Sociology*, **65**(4), 374–382

Hoberman, J. (1992). The Early Development of Sports Medicine in Germany. In Berryman, J. W. & Park, R. J. (Eds.), *Sport and Exercise Science. Essays in the History of Sports Medicine.* Chicago, IL: University of Ilinois Press

Hoberman, J. (2002). Sports Physicians and the Doping Crisis in Elite Sport. *Clin J Sport Med*, **12**(4), 203–208

Jokl, E. (1964). *What is Sports Medicine?* Spingfield, IL: Charles C Thomas

Ljungqvist, A., Jenoure, P., Engebretsen, L., Alonso, J. M., Bahr, R, Clough, A., De Bondt, G., Dvorak, J., Maloley, R., Matheson, G., Meeuwisse, W., Meijboom, E., Mountjoy, M., Pelliccia, A., Schwellnus, M., Sprumont, D., Schamasch, P., Gauthier, J. B., Dubi, C., Stupp, H., & Thill, C. (2009). The International Olympic Committee (IOC) Consensus Statement on Periodic Health Evaluation of Elite Athletes March 2009. *Br J Sports Med*, **43**(9), 631–643

Malcolm, D. (2006). Unprofessional Practice? The Status and Power of Sport Physicians. *Sociology of Sport Journal*, **23**, 376–395

Masterton, D. W. (1976). The Ancient Greek Origins of Sports Medicine. *British Journal of Sports Medicine*, **10**, 196–202

Nixon, H. (1992). A Social Network Analysis of Influences on Athletes to Play with Pain and Injuries. *Journal of Sport and Social Issues*, **16**(2), 127–135

Poma, C., Sherman, S. L., Spence, B., Brenner, L. H. & Bal, B. S. (2016). Rethinking the Standard of Care in Treating Professional Athletes. *Clinics in Sports Medicine*, **35**, 269–274

Safai, P. (2003). Healing the Body in the "Culture of Risk": Examining the Negotiation of Treatment Between Sport Medicine Clinicians and Injured Athletes in Canadian Intercollegiate Sport. *Sociology of Sport Journal*, **20**, 127–146

Shephard, R. J. (1974a). The Dimensions of Sports Medicine. *Can Med Assoc J*, **110**(10), 1167–1168

Shephard, R. J. (1974b). New Perspectives in Sports Medicine. *Can Fam Physician*, **20**(4), 49–51

Speed, C. & Jaques, R. (2011). High-performance Sports Medicine: An Ancient but Evolving Field. *British Journal of Sports Medicine*, **45**(2), 81–83

Steriotis, A. K. & Sharma, S. (2015). Risk Stratification in Hypertrophic Cardiomyopathy. *European Cardiology Review*, **10**(1), 1–6

Stevens, M. A. & Phelps, W. M. (1933). *The Control of Football Injuries*. New York, NY: A. S. Barnes and Company Inc

Waddington, I., Roderick, M. & Naik, R. (2001). Methods of Appointment and Qualifications of Club Doctors and Physiotherapists in English Professional Football: Some Problems and Issues. *British Journal of Sports Medicine*, **35**, 48–53

Walk, S. R. (1997). Peers in Pain: The Experiences of Student Athletic Trainers. *Sociology of Sport Journal*, **14**, 22–56

Weissbein, S. (1910). *Hygiene des Sports*. Berlin: Grethlein & Co

Williams, J. G. P. (1965). *Medical Aspects of Sport and Physical Fitness*. Oxford: Pergamon Press

Part III
The appliance of science
Interdisciplinary perspectives

In the previous section, an overview was provided on the role of various disciplines across sport science and medicine in elite sport. As conveyed by our contributors, each of these disciplines represent a unique and significant part of the 'performance machine'. Of course, these disciplines will be either more or less important, or more or less emphasised parts in different machines. Indeed, the best 'blend' will depend on the performer, team, or organisation in question, as well as, for example, the targeted goals and available resources. In this sense, optimal success for an elite performer, team, or organisation does not operate as a function of the number of sport science and medicine practitioners they have in support; or by having 'the right' practitioners. While the 'right' people certainly help, *greatest* return arrives when these disciplines are integrated and combined as a 'complete package'; also known as 'interdisciplinary' support.

Somewhat reflecting the maxim that an effective team is much more than the sum of its' individual parts, those who can achieve an interdisciplinary approach to sport science and medicine can therefore gain a significant advantage of their competitors. More specifically, an interdisciplinary approach harnesses insights from a range of relevant disciplines, meshing these together to find multifaceted solutions to what, in elite sport, are usually multifaceted goals, challenges, or issues. Taking an interdisciplinary approach can also limit the chances of coaches and the sport science and medicine team from barking up the wrong tree when it comes to identifying and working on these goals, challenges, or issues. For example, what might seem to be a psychological issue (e.g. flatness on competition day) may in fact have a significant physiological (e.g. training load), analytical (e.g. lack of clarity on game plan), nutritional (e.g. pre-performance snacking), and interpersonal (e.g. perceived pressure from a coach) basis. In short, the vast majority of performance factors are 'biopsychosocial': they are grounded in the individual or team's BIOlogy, PSYCHOlogy, and SOCIAL perceptions and interactions. Consequently, the best solutions for improving, delivering, or sustaining the factors are also usually 'biopsychosocial'.

On this basis, the purpose of this section is to provide perspectives on the application of science, in a more holistic and integrated sense, within elite sport. In doing so, this section starts with Graeme Maw's views on interdisciplinary support and how the evolution of sport science is proceeding on a 'big picture' level. From here, Chapter 16 then sees Fergus Connolly provide some specific thoughts on the development of performance through an interdisciplinary approach. In this contribution, Fergus offers an account on performance consulting, the nature and role of sport science as a collective service, finding a balance between specialists and generalists, and, the integration of practitioners so that they can solve problems as efficiently and effectively as possible.

As another contrast, and to build the perspectives considered, the remaining chapters in this section then consider the contribution of interdisciplinary leaders in embedded roles within elite sport systems. First, Ian Graham describes the role of data in football, including progress in game data, event data, tracking data, and psychological data, before describing the role of the research department and its cross-domain role in scouting, technology, sport science, and video analysis. Building on the research theme, Peter Vint then concludes this section by presenting his experiences of innovation through sport science. More specifically, Peter considers the nature of innovations in sport, how these are best linked to actual performance and, on this basis, how research that includes different scientific elements can fit into this agenda and be best delivered; including what makes an attempt at innovation successful and what tends to make it fail.

When interpreting the messages throughout this section, we encourage the reader to again keep a number of 'up-front' points in mind. First, it is worthwhile considering how decisions are made on which aspects of sport science are more or less applicable in a given moment for a given a goal, challenge, or issue. Second, principles that support co-ordinated communication and effort, both within the sport science and medicine team and between this team and others in the environment, also merit attention; especially given how different some perspectives and practitioners can be across the sciences. In fact, significant differences in perspectives and practitioners also often exist *in* the same science! Indeed, in a world where many can be inclined, and often reinforced by their organisations and social media, to show their 'place in the performance pie', the *ways* in which leaders work to create and maintain a truly interdisciplinary approach – operationally and interpersonally – are crucial. Moreover, there is also a risk – as seems to be apparent in some systems already – that the (science) tail ends up wagging the (performance or coaching) dog. More specifically, elite sport systems seem to be particularly susceptible to this when high levels of 'trust' in science and scientists exist in the sporting or wider culture, when there is a high level of investment in the service (i.e. we need to show that sport science is impactful because of the money we're spending!), and when there are limits in 'science education' for coaches (e.g. on understanding how to interpret, use, and challenge science). Once again, therefore, emphasis within this section is placed on the *how* and *why* behind effective practice.

15

Effective performance support

An integrated view

Graeme Maw

Origins and explosion of the sport science industry

A highly-prominent Olympic-medal winning coach recently tweeted "so much data so little sense".[1] Another multi Olympian athlete and coach cynically summarised an international peer-reviewed training article as "so it's just training specifically in other words. . .".[2] And a further elite coach simply said, "sport science has lost its way".[3]

As a scientist, devoted to sport, former sport science practitioner, and inaugural Vice President for Sport Science with the then Australian Association for Exercise and Sports Science (now Exercise and Sport Science Australia), this emerging rejection of 'my industry' saddens and worries me. As a high performance director and sports administrator, operating in outcome-oriented and resource scarce environments, I understand its forthright sentience.

Around my first day as a practising sport scientist, armed with PhD and lactate kit, I was recoiled by a then head coach who answered my question of "what can I do for you" with "go away until you can say what you can do for me" (or words to that effect). I was soon to appreciate that I could either laboriously and therefore detrimentally take up performers' time and energy or make a genuine performance difference – there is no neutral ground. Clearly, while sport science has grown into a mainstream industry, there are now concerns with making a performance difference.

Historical context

While science – or critical method – has always been applied to enhance sport performance, to my thinking it was really in the 1960s and 70s with the Eastern European regimens that the systematic use of scientists really took hold in sport. Early Olympic reports include reference to potions, strychnine and alcohol for the glory of gold. In the modern Olympic era, Doc Councilman and Forbes Carlisle were famously methodical in their training approach, in swimming for example. Landmark performances such as Roger Bannister's sub four-minute mile and Dick Fosbury's high jump 'flop' owed their conception to scientific forethought to training and technique. And when Greg LeMond won the 1987 Tour de France by the narrowest of margins, blazing down the Champs Elysees on 'aerodynamic' handlebars (compared to Lauren Fignon's flailing pony tail), his technology heralded from the progressive world of triathlon.

What characterised all these approaches was a clear focus on unlocking the performance puzzle, and ingenuity from a tight group of people (often just coach and athlete) fascinated enough to experiment in the field. Current England rugby coach, Eddie Jones, describes it as "chronically restless" for performance.[4]

De facto, what also characterised these trailblazers was the absence of an institutionalised plethora of sport scientists. In contrast now, we have what in many cases appears to be an industry justifying its own existence – from multitudinous university courses, to hundreds of positions and multimillions of dollars and pounds to perform often routine and mundane tasks.

When I first studied sport science and management back in 1984, I enrolled in the only University in England that offered a course – Loughborough. Now, according to the Complete University Guide, there are at least 81![5] The Australian Institute of Sport – a legendary scientific hub, launched in 1981 and recently overhauled – has been mimicked in each of the eight states and territories. The more recent English Institute of Sport – providing science and medicine support to British High Performance Programmes – has grown to over 350 employees at a staff-cost of £16.4 million in a total budget of £24.2 million.[6] In similar fashion, High Performance Sport New Zealand reserves approaching $10 million for Athlete Performance Support, compared to a budget of $35.4 million spread across the actual sports.[7]

Our sports institutes certainly seem to be assured on the need for science divisions, even though coaches are questioning. This leaves risk of the tail wagging the dog, especially when you consider the aspersions cast by British Parliament towards British Cycling and Team Sky, and knowledge of their vaunted philosophy of "Marginal Gains".[8]

The sport science 'industry' – academic or effective?

Publish or perish?

To understand the journey of sport science to institutionalisation, we perhaps need to consider the growth of an industry: something proves successful, demand goes up, and training institutions gear up to provide the supply. In the case of sport science, the demand spawned an explosion of university sport science departments, which in turn – as an attractive subject – grew their own demand.

It is interesting to note that even in relatively recent times, many of the great sport scientists delivered their impact from origins far from the pathway of undergraduate sport: Bob Treffene, who transformed Australian and world distance swimming, was a retired biomedical engineer who turned his knowledge to swim training; and Steve Peters, who optimised British Cycling's mental performance, was a clinical psychiatrist in the penal system with a passion for veterans' running. Both also stayed largely to the periphery of institutional roles.

Notwithstanding, the journey from Alois Mader delivering sport science in East Germany in the 1970s to developing disciples like Jan Olbrecht at the German University of Sports Science in Cologne in the 1980s and 90s does not deviate very far from tertiary education. And one of the main criticisms to this day of applied sport science is the academic irrelevance in the field. How often do research studies conclude that more research is needed? Or, particularly over time, contradict each other?

While Karl Wasserman, rather than Mader, owns perhaps first credit for 'identifying' the anaerobic threshold in the 1960s at Stanford University, the panacea of the 4 mMol blood lactate level has been both universally championed, and then debunked – displaced by a multitude of methods for establishing the 'definitive' anaerobic threshold, which still vary between them. The championing of carbohydrate-rich diets for the last three decades is now being challenged not just in sport but in health.[9] And, as above, when a published training review can be summarised by a coach in just eight words,[10] we have to wonder what's the point.

To my own frustration, as part of the physiology team supporting very successful Australian swimmers in the 1990s, my colleagues David Pyne and Kim Swanwick published an excellent analysis of step tests showing that while various deduced variables changed with training, none were directly associated with competition performance.[11]

Practice-based evidence or evidence-based practice?

The avalanche of sport science from academic institutions then lends itself to the current clamour for evidence-based practice – particularly in government: science can lend both the prior rationale for and the post measurement accountability of investment. Tail wagging the dog?

However, the very requirements of the academic world can be constraining in a competitive world. The publication cycle is lengthy and getting longer, and the typical probability of proof required of 5% (p=0.05) to publish is largely irrelevant to sports performance. Contrast both of those to the performance advantage of finding solutions that have not yet been published, and seeking gains that on balance might benefit an n of one working close to the margin, and you may understand the recoil from my early-days head coach.

In a probing critique, applied sport scientist Martin Buchheit put it like this:

> One solution might be for us to start where the questions actually arise (i.e., in clubs or federations) and then develop the structures required to conduct applied research, through research & development departments. Such sport scientists . . . are more than capable of creating relevant knowledge and best practice guidance within only a few weeks . . . contrasts with academic research that takes years to reach publication, before remaining inaccessible to the majority of coaches, athletes and practitioners.[12]

Practice-based evidence!

In medicine – a la TV physician Gregory House – practice-based evidence is already seen as a way of disciplines working together to find feasible solutions to complex real-life issues.[13] In industry, it is akin to product innovation, most effectively with a rapid cycle from idea to prototype to test and review. In sport, it certainly characterised those performance breakthroughs of Bannister, Fosbury, LeMond et al.

For my own part, my physiology degrees morphed in to competition analysis and modelling, movement dynamics coupling technique with energy cost, video capture, and all sorts, pulling in experts as needed to unpick the performance puzzle, glued together with the skill of critical analysis in the field. Along with the early years of Tim Kerrison's career (now Head of Athlete Performance at Team Sky) – where he coined "reverse periodisation" for sprinters[14] – we felt pioneering in 'performance science'.

Reductionism in a complex world

This integrated approach of the performance lens was not a module taught in my degrees, which rather took the reductionist approach of segregating rather than integrating subjects. This is the norm in sport science degrees and then in our institutes, where you will universally find departments of physiology, biomechanics, nutrition, performance analysis, psychology, and possibly others. Often these are competing for budget, prestige and coaches' time.

163

In contrast, human performance is inherently complex – complexity defined as any system of two or more distinct parts that are joined in such a way that it is difficult to separate them. It is well known, for example, that blood lactate levels are related not just to exercise intensity, but also nutritional status and technical efficiency. An inspirational colleague in Russia, Sergei Kolmogorov, showed that swimmers' drag is affected simultaneously by both form and fitness.[15] And physiological and perceived responses to exercise can be manipulated by sensory stimuli.[16] Performance-focused teams, rather than discipline departments, might be a better way to structure ourselves.

Thinking complex

Frequently we will hear of reductionism being countered through multidisciplinary teams. However, in my experience, these are different to performance-focused teams, typically functioning by sharing reports from individual discipline lenses, rather than re-integrating the whole. As Carlos Gershenson and Francis Heylighen explained in *How Can We Think Complex*,[17] once broken down in to its constituent parts, it is actually very difficult to re-envision the whole, especially for those trained in particular disciplines:

> through observation, an agent can in principle gather complete knowledge about any system, creating an internal representation whose components correspond to the components of the external system. This establishes a single, true, objective mapping from the realm of matter (the system) to the realm of mind (the representation).

Thus, until the 'representation' is itself seen as a complex, integrated system in the first place, it is difficult for the scientist to change their view: the physiologist champions physiology, the biomechanist favours biomechanics, etc., all competing for that scarce resource of funding and favour. Unless this paradigm is changed in learning, it perpetuates in practice. Yet a clear performance lens, rather than disciplines, was present for all the sporting and supporting greats.

Shortcomings of competency-based training

The challenge of reductionism is unfortunately further perpetuated in industry training and accreditation through the simplistic use of competency frameworks. Universities regularly now champion their vocational credentials, often taken as a needs-analysis generated tick list of tasks. Accrediting bodies do the same, with the British Association of Sport and Exercise Sciences listing 62 areas of competence for candidates to report to.[18] Included are only two references to multi-discipline and one to complex environments.

These approaches are plainly a mis-representation of the role of making a difference to elite sport performance. As coach educators once wrote to inspire creativity rather than rote-practice among England's elite cricket coaches: "Are you a cook or a chef?".

Constraints of institutionalisation

Of course, following reductionist recipes is much easier to organise and examine than original creation, whether in education or employment. The educational advocate, Sir Ken Robinson, attributes educational conformity to the industrial age, when organising production by time and classification was orderly, easily managed, and easily tested.[19] In his view, it has also led to a suppressed approach to creativity, which he champions as a fundamental characteristic of humanity.

Unsurprisingly, an industrial organisational model is also commonplace in predominantly government-funded systems, with discipline departments and a predilection with measurement and accountability. As discussed, these can foster competing discipline lenses rather than collaborative performance teams, and according to Jerry Muller at Princeton University, can lead to a Tyranny of Metrics that actually stifles performance through over measurement.[20]

Incorporating mavericks

Worst of all, as Muller eloquently says:

> Organizations in thrall to metrics end up motivating those members of staff with greater initiative to move out of the mainstream, where the culture of accountable performance prevails. Teachers move out of public schools to private and charter schools. Engineers move out of large corporations to boutique firms. Enterprising government employees become consultants. There is a healthy element to this, of course. But surely the large-scale organizations of our society are the poorer for driving out staff most likely to innovate and initiate. The more that work becomes a matter of filling in the boxes by which performance is to be measured and rewarded, the more it will repel those who think outside the box.

I had the privilege of leading sport at the renowned Somerset independent school, Millfield, founded by the incredible and eccentric Jack 'Boss' Meyer in 1935.[21] The school largely disdains the constraint of the English schools' academic league tables in favour of a commitment to holistic education, and in my time leveraged sport along the lines of Jean Cote's positive youth development.[22] Naturally, Millfield continually features among Britain's top sportsmen,[23] but less well known is consistently among the top two or three schools represented in UK Parliament.[24]

Training creativity

Models of training innovative and original thinking therefore do exist, and are perhaps increasing. Millfield fosters independent and holistic thinking through a platform of sport and music. Similarly, Bradford Primary School demonstrated improved academic results when including six hours of dance each week in to their curriculum.[25] In Canada and the USA, the benefits of visual and musical media are being recognised in training doctors.[26]

Situated learning

New Zealand secondary schools are effectively using Project-Based Learning to meld together knowledge and skills across curricula, to explore real-world, complex problems.[27] In junior sport, Teaching Games for Understanding has been a popular alternative to technique-based approaches for participant learning since the early 1980s. And all of these may be considered in or close to an umbrella of Situated Learning, to help the learner connect prior knowledge with new contexts.[28]

In a recent article for Statsbomb.com (available at https://statsbomb.com/author/tknutso/), renowned soccer analyst Ted Knutson championed that unlike almost every modern profession in the world, coaching is really an apprenticeship. Instead of learning via reading or attending lectures, the vast majority of knowledge you need to do the job comes via observing and doing. Theory is still important, but the practical element is dominant.

Ted's only error, in my opinion, was that such learning is not constrained to coaching, and often comes from situational contexts – including genuine performance-enhancing science – but it is rarely taught as such. According to the *Harvard Business Review*, we might all be better served as learners and experts spending more time "thinking about thinking" and "learning to reflect".[29]

The expert performance scientist

For our industry, any upsurge in situated learning and practice-based evidence is heartening in my opinion, with creative practitioners testing feasible concepts in the field. Of course, such concepts and ideas don't just appear from eureka moments, but from a strong basis of prior knowledge combined with a fascination and immersion in the puzzle.[30] The 'Performance Scientist' must therefore also have an expert grounding in basic knowledge.

This is different from considering the Performance Scientist as a generalist – rather an expert in performance enhancement unconstrained by disciplinary boundaries. Quintessentially, they bring analytical skill through a performance lens, rather than discipline competencies. As may be imagined from industrial conformity, they may be difficult to accommodate or manage in institutional systems and/or may be misrepresented as applied generalists. In reality, informing their performance lens, they are typically subject experts in one or more discipline, and moreover creative critical problem solvers; it is no surprise that many do not hail from undergraduate sport courses.

T-shaped expert

Perhaps a description of this practitioner can be drawn from the work of Kevin Bowring when head of elite coaching with the Rugby Football Union, in describing the T-shaped coach. At a time when discreet 'skills coaches' were proliferating arguably to the detriment of on-field decision-making, Bowring nurtured coaches to have a depth of expertise in one or more areas combined with a real breadth of appreciation of the game and player as a whole. In elite sport science, this would be akin to post-graduate expertise in one or more areas, allied with a genuine broad performance lens, integrated by critical problem-solving.

Tight teams

As already alluded to, many such colleagues have varied backgrounds, can be difficult to define and can prefer to work outside institutional systems. However, they forge tight relationships with coaches, in my experience primarily based on that deep fascination with the performance puzzle and an ability to make a difference. Bob Treffene in the 1990s was inseparable from Kieren Perkins' mentor John Carew. I reconciled my challenge with the Queensland Head Coaches. Tim Kerrison cut his teeth with the emerging coach Shannon Rollason and later right alongside Bradley Wiggins. And Daniel Plews is retained by Lisa Carrington's guide, Gordon Walker, despite leaving the New Zealand High Performance Sport institute.

These relationships are not surprising: expert coaches are notoriously time-poor, with a need to almost ruthlessly focus on performance. Yet, in contrast – allied to the training and proliferation of sport scientists – the apprentice coach is trained from foundation stages to expect to manage a plethora of practitioners, all requiring their place in the team. Sir Clive Woodward infamously led the 2005 British and Irish Lions tour to New Zealand with a backroom staff of 28 – up from ten for the previous 2003 Lions tour to Australia – to be white-washed in what became known as the Tour from Hell.[31]

It is a model that must and is being challenged. In New Zealand high performance sport at present, off the back of research into successful Olympic campaigns, it is apposite to talk of 'tight teams' wrapped around the athlete. This identifies those people most key to the athlete's performance, and typically numbers three to five; it is the inner sanctum of performance. The ability of the expert performance sport scientist to fit within this team is obvious – built on shared trust in the performance puzzle and the ability to make a difference.

Naturally, there is other knowledge and expertise outside this sanctum which can also make a difference, adding a key role of 'translator' to the effective sport scientist. As with many aspects of business and intelligence, it is necessary to take technical information into useable, under-standable form: the New Zealand Police specifically employ intelligence analysts as translators to "think analytically about a problem (of any kind), organise complex material clearly and logically, distinguish between fact and interpretation, and draw logical conclusions, and (convey it) clearly and succinctly" to the end user.[32] In sport science, this is often the distinction between academic and applied, with the added emphasis on problem-solving. It is then incumbent on coach educa-tors to develop coaches to be discerning users, rather than conformist consumers of sport science.

Conclusion

In short, effective sport science requires deep knowledge and advanced problem-solving through a performance lens, rather than a check-list of conformist competencies. While it may be convenient to position this at the advanced end of the scientists' development path, it can also be argued that unless the concept of complexity is accepted early, the reductionist approach may be difficult to put back together, and indeed hindered by institutional function. Institutes need to reorganise into genuine performance teams rather than discipline departments, and accommodate mavericks whose role may be difficult to define. The coach then is left to manage a tight-team inner sanctum, rather than a plethora of inputs whose performance return may be questionable. Yes, it is time for change – the sport science industry is burgeoning beyond gain.

Notes

1 https://twitter.com/joelfilliol/status/1006875330420858880.
2 https://twitter.com/jon_brown_/status/1041187683609960449.
3 https://trainingground.guru/articles/tony-strudwick-why-sport-science-has-lost-its-way.
4 www.eis2win.co.uk/2017/12/20/eddie-jones-on-being-chronically-restless-and-the-search-for-sustainable-success/.
5 www.thecompleteuniversityguide.co.uk/league-tables/rankings?s=sports%20science.
6 https://assets.publishing.service.gov.uk/government/uploads/system/uploads/attachment_data/file/627019/60229_HC_106_EIS_ARA_Accessible.pdf.
7 http://hpsnz.org.nz/content/uploads/2018/03/2018_Investment_Brochure_13.12.172.pdf.
8 https://publications.parliament.uk/pa/cm201719/cmselect/cmcumeds/366/366.pdf.
9 https://sportsscientists.com/2016/04/low-carbohydrate-diets-plea-balance-scientific-rigour-death-dogma/.
10 https://twitter.com/jon_brown_/status/1041187683609960449.

11 Pyne, D. B. 1., Lee, H., & Swanwick, K. M. (2001). Monitoring the Lactate Threshold in World-ranked Swimmers. *Med Sci Sports Exerc*, **33**(2), 291–297.

12 https://martin-buchheit.net/2017/07/03/houston-we-still-have-a-problem/.

13 Swisher, Anne K., PT, PhD, CCS, Editor in Chief. (2010) Practice-Based Evidence. *Cardiopulm Phys Ther J.*, **21**(2), 4.

14 www.ridemedia.com.au/interviews/tim-kerrison-coaching-sky/.

15 Kolmogorov, S. V. & Duplishcheva, O. A. (1992). Active Drag, Useful Mechanical Power Output and Hydrodynamic Force Coefficient in Different Swimming Strokes at Maximal Velocity. *Journal of Biomechanics*, **25**(3), 311–318.

16 Boutcher, S. H. & Trenske, M. (1990). The Effects of Sensory Deprivation and Music on Perceived Exertion and Affect During Exercise. *Journal of Sport and Exercise Psychology*, **12**, 167–176.

17 http://pespmc1.vub.ac.be/Papers/ThinkingComplex.pdf.

18 www.bases.org.uk/imgs/accreditation_competency_profile_feb_18504.pdf.

19 www.radionz.co.nz/national/programmes/sunday/audio/2018634594/sir-ken-robinson-why-schools-need-to-tap-into-kids-talents.

20 www.fastcompany.com/40577938/our-obsession-with-performance-data-is-killing-performance.

21 www.cricketcountry.com/articles/moments-in-history/jack-boss-meyer-eccentric-schoolmaster-somerset-cricketer-ranji-trophy-captain-738365.

22 Vierimaa, M., Erickson, K., Côté, J. et al. (2012). Positive Youth Development: A Measurement Framework for Sport. *International Journal of Sports Science & Coaching*, **7**(3), 601–614.

23 www.telegraph.co.uk/education/2016/08/04/talent-factory-how-millfield-produces-more-olympians-than-any-ot/.

24 www.suttontrust.com/wp-content/uploads/2010/05/1MPs_educational_backgrounds_2010_A.pdf.

25 www.theguardian.com/education/2017/oct/03/school-results-music-bradford.

26 https://files.eric.ed.gov/fulltext/EJ1094979.pdf; www.cbc.ca/news/canada/newfoundland-labrador/medicine-music-connection-1.4770372.

27 https://gazette.education.govt.nz/notices/1H9j1h-problem-based-learning-pbl-in-the-secondary-school/.

28 http://citeseerx.ist.psu.edu/viewdoc/download?doi=10.1.1.470.4539&rep=rep1&type=pdf; http://newlearningonline.com/new-learning/chapter-6/lave-and-wenger-on-situated-learning.

29 https://hbr.org/2018/05/learning-is-a-learned-behavior-heres-how-to-get-better-at-it.

30 www.ted.com/talks/steven_johnson_where_good_ideas_come_from?language=en.

31 www.lionsrugby.com/2004/10/21/woodward-unveils-lions-coaching-staff/; www.theguardian.com/sport/blog/2017/jun/04/2005-lions-tour-hell-new-zealand-alastair-campbell-clive-woodward.

32 www.police.govt.nz/sites/default/files/publications/intelligence-analyst-applicants-guide.pdf.

16

Interdisciplinary performance development in elite sport

Applied sport science

Fergus Connolly

Introduction

What are the essentials for providing effective performance development services in the applied setting? How do you use sport science effectively in practice? What is performance domain knowledge? What are the most crucial challenges and obstacles to effectively winning games and creating sustainable success? These are some of the questions we raise and answer in this chapter.

Performance consulting

My first goal when mentoring coaches or performance managers is always to help them identify their true personal purpose. For me, I'm a teacher by nature, I want to help people achieve the most they can. To that end consulting has always been my true passion, what I am best at, what I've always wanted to do. However, I knew from early on, in order to do that in elite sport I would have to gain experience and credibility in each of the different areas that I was going to support. Hence, over the last 20 years I have purposely worked in every major area of elite performance – soccer, international rugby, American football, Australian Rules, cricket, boxing, and with special forces groups – so that I could gain a breadth of experience and develop a skillset and experience unique to everybody else.

As I worked across sports I recognised that there were actually more principles in common across sports than were different. I saw the need to define these very principles that unify sports, unify the pure performance of teams. That is what I am most interested in. Yes, I have protocols, yes, I have techniques, yes, I have specific tactics. However, unless you have and understand the principles behind each element of performance to unify them, you cannot truly implement them.

The critical aspect is to be able to problem-solve, to identify limiting factors, i.e. what is most needed to improve the team at that time. For example, if you have correctly identified that speed is the factor that your team or player needs most to get better then you need to know how to improve it. Simply bringing in a speed coach to work on speed, or a nutrition coach to work on nutrition, is not enough. Unless you and they understand context, they are simply delivering drills, techniques, or recipes. That does not help in the long run.

It does not need lead to sustained success. You are then just giving someone an answer to a mathematical question, not giving them what they actually need. "Teach a man to fish, don't just give him fish".

My role is to help experts and organisations to identify where they need to improve, and to bring support for them to help them improve those areas themselves. It's not to simply deliver a training programme. To be truly successful, I have to support them, direct them, and help them identify what they need to improve, because sometimes they cannot see it themselves. Secondly, it's my role to help, source, or bring to them, the knowledge in a context they understand, what is needed for them to improve. Thirdly, and most important, I want to help them become more self-sustainable. Each one of these stages has specific principles behind them.

Interestingly, more recently much of my work has been on helping performance directors with the development of the 'soft skills' not taught in university, such as management, leadership, conflict resolution, and continuous professional development.

I do this work with the military (usually special forces and special operations), professional, and some collegiate coaches. There are one or two high school teams that I help because I want to give back to the grassroots. That is important to me. I have worked and done everything that I wanted to do in the professional area, and it's important to me to give something back to the kids and coaches at high school level because this is the last group that truly do it for the love of the game. Apart from kids and the military, most everyone else is doing it for financial gain exclusively and it's primarily a business first, entertainment second, and sport third.

Generally, I rarely work directly with players. I can, but I prefer to help the coaches to have a greater multiplying effect. I prefer middle or senior management, simply because it allows the development of a long-term programme of sustainable success and succession. If you only work with players directly and you leave, it's more difficult to develop a culture of sustained success or to establish a dominant system of play or coaching. But if you work from the top-down perspective and find out exactly what kind of issues they have, it is easier to propose solutions that will endure, not to mention you're addressing the root cause, not window dressing.

It is really a case of enabling and empowering. I want to empower and enable high performance staff to build a better environment and a better experience for the players, so they can solve their own problems. Good teachers make themselves irrelevant, ensuring the student becomes better than the teacher eventually. Insecure teachers want the student reliant on them. One of the biggest problems you have in this industry is that people tend to want to be in control and to be powerful. The goal is to develop people, not professionals only. The goal is not to give people solutions, but teach them how to find their own solutions, to become self-sustainable.

Really good high-performance leaders delegate responsibilities and support people. But they never quite abdicate their responsibilities to their players. They delegate to the people under them, and that is what I enjoy doing. I like to see people grow and develop, see them getting better. I get my personal joy from seeing other people be successful.

To what extent can consulting in this space be profitable? Let me answer that citing some facts. Turner Sport payed out ten billion dollars to show the national college basketball tournament for the next eight or ten years. The most recent NBA TV deal is on 26 billion dollars. The athletic programme at Texas brought in 161 million dollars last year. Manchester United spent more than 500 million in 2015. In the US alone, there are 128 Division 1 College football schools, 347 college Basketball teams, and 60 ice hockey teams. There is a huge number of teams, and they all need to improve and want to improve.

However, the biggest drawback that these organisations have is that these cultures have no time to improve because of short off-seasons and hectic game schedules. Seasons are very long and offer very little time off for learning or staying up to date. There are two further aspects to this. One is that the people hiring coaches, strength coaches, and athletic trainers, are not often educated in the areas they are hiring for. You may have a former retired player as general manager or athletic director, who is not a coach, who is just looking for the same kind of strength coach that he had ten years ago. Secondly, there is no international sport science organisation or accreditation. With this, there is a large room for improvement or professional development. There has also been an explosion in sport science and to be successful in a team setting, experience and knowledge in sports science are needed with the necessary 'soft skills' and honesty to implement it properly.

Sport science

Science is critical and has to be the foundation of any applied sports science programme, but in the applied setting, science alone is not a deliverable in itself; results are, hence the need for a balance – applied sports science encompasses more. I am interested in performance as the deliverable, with science as the foundation. Are you affecting the scoreboard or are you just moving chess pieces? Are you winning the game or just moving the pawns around? Those are the critical questions.

One could say that this is logical, but I would rather use the word honest, because I believe, fundamentally, there can be some dishonesty in the sport science industry. There is this claim that a complicated system or technology will bring you this result, when in fact it does not bring results. This becomes self-perpetuating. Make no mistake, there has always been sports science in sport, but there has never been a sports science industry like we have now, and this has clouded intentions and motivations.

One of the reasons that I wrote my book (*Game Changer: The Art of Sports Science*) was to create a foundational outline for the next generation of coaches based on deliverables. This next generation is currently misled by those who make things more complicated than they need to be. It is not an end, but a starting point to help those in team sports daily reach a holistic solution, that is yet out of reach. Winning is truly an art of science.

Like someone said once, the only fish who go with the flow are the dead ones. You must apply common sense to your specific situation, your team. Tell the truth as you know it, and if it happens to go against the grain, it goes against the grain. It is the search for the truth, and if that takes a different path than everyone else, it is just a road less travelled, not the wrong one. In the end, this is about constant questioning. I approach my book like this as well (and I refer to it because it is simply the most public example of my thoughts and ideas) – I will challenge the book in the next two to three years, when it has been edited and updated. I hope that the body of work helps people develop their own ideas. The goal of any great book is to inspire the reader to think and get better, not deliver a conclusion.

Getting results

The main question that guides me is, how do we get results? To get there, we have to ask – what is the objective? And, be brutally honest about the objective. What are we trying to do and where are we trying to get to? How do we do that in an ethical way?

Anybody can take over an organisation and break rules, or cheat. That is easy. But to do it ethically is a different question, and then to do it in a sustainable matter, to do it in a manner which is repeatable and consistent and protects player welfare especially. That is the most important aspect of our role.

As coaches we have to develop a breadth of skills too. Imagine you have an issue at your house, plumbing or the electrical system, and two different service men come to you. One has a small tool box with a limited number of tools and the other person is experienced, with many different experiences and tools. One of them is going to get the job done quicker and will have more options to deliver a sustainable solution, and not just a short-term solution, or fail to see the whole picture. That is what I do, help the client and team identify what the real problem is first, not what is assumed at a cursory glance, and fix it in a way that allows them to continue to be successful.

Again, I go back to purpose. What are your ethics, values, what is your purpose in life? What are we here to do? What are we trying to teach young men or young women through sport? What role models are we for the kids who watch us on ESPN on Sunday? It is not about win at all costs. The purpose of sport, whether it is amateur or professional, is to teach young people about life so they can have a wholesome life, contribute to society, and look out for each other. We have a duty to look after each other, no matter what race or background. That is what sport is! Sport is not life. Life is not sport. Sport exists within the realm of life and its duty, whether it is high school, professional team, or collegiate, is to raise young men and women to contribute to society. That is the fundamental basis for all sport.

An example of bad ethics would be if you choose to bribe or pay different people under the table, or if you decide you want to dope, or decide you want to break the NCCA rules when it comes to training, or regulations of the NFL about padded practices, or whatever that might be. So, you choose to work within the boundaries. Then, there is also the moral aspect of it. You have a moral obligation to look after everybody, whether they are the lowest ranked player on the team, the quarter-back, the running back, or whoever it is. Our duty is to look after people and develop people.

It is about people

All the issues that athletes face on the scene or off the scene, come from them as people. It rarely originates from the sport itself. So how do you develop these people to the degree that they can grow as people? For example, in the US, one of the most common profiles in college football is a 15-year-old kid from Florida or Georgia who is one of seven children with a single mother who struggles to keep things together. A college programme tries to recruit the player with the promise of a third level scholarship. They make a lot of promises, offers of a scholarship, and so forth. When the player ultimately arrives in the campus at 17–18 years of age, they are physically very well developed. But personality-wise and emotionally they are much younger. The biggest issues that this player will face as they journey through university and beyond will be personal issues, not sport issues or physical issues, because they can play the game, that is the reason why they were recruited. So, when a player fails on the field it will be because of the inability to manage life situations and challenges that they face in life. That is the biggest challenge. And that is why it is so important to look after the person first, not just the player.

The fundamental point is that you are looking after people, and they all come from different backgrounds. The older player has more experience, but an interesting observation in professional sport is that you are getting fewer and fewer older players. One reason for that is that fewer and fewer players have the life skills to survive the league, on and off the field.

If someone asked me, what is the most important thing for a young player who is in his first rookie year in the NFL, NBA or the Premier League, I would say, their first job is to survive. Because the longer you survive, the greater the skillset you develop as a person. Not as an athlete, but as a person. If you can survive, then you will learn the game. But your first job is to survive in the industry, and to learn. The older player who has survived has picked up habits, skills, tips, and hacks that enable him to survive in the industry, whether financial acumen, recovery, or lifestyle management skills. And that is why they are valuable. By surviving as people, they build up an experience, a toolbox of experiences that allow them to develop as players. They become more and more valuable because of that experience. But some teams fail to realise this, that by developing the person first, the foundation is laid for a longtime career in the league or competition.

What are the obstacles, internally, to such an approach? It really comes down to the ownership, to the people who own or run the organisation. Do they want instant success or sustainable success? Everybody wants everything instantly nowadays, so it is a case of whether they want it instantly as opposed to something that is going to survive and deliver a lasting legacy. So that is the question, do you want to build something that will last for a period of time, or not? That is a big question that the organisations need to answer.

Anybody can bring an organisation together and push them very hard, but the life cycle for that is only three years. You cannot bully a group for any longer than three years in my experience. The reason for this is that I can go to any team and promise them the world, and push them really hard, train really, really hard and get them through the season, and they will be very successful because we outwork teams. Just purely based on quantity, volume, the capacity that we have. But sustained success requires quality.

But there are three things that organisations needs to have in order to be really successful: one is capacity, which means, how much more can you do, and what is the limit? There is a limit, and many organisations do not realise that. The second is capability, quality. Do you have the quality, do you train for quality? This is something that often suffers or is absent. Quantity of practice is easy, but quality is harder to achieve. Quality is the perfection of basics, being tactical and technical under pressure, not magic.

The third aspect is character. A coach can take over any organisation and push them really hard and you can build capacity and outwork someone with false promises. Year two, if he doesn't have character, if he is not being honest with the team, not developing people first, the players will soon think to themselves: "Ok, things didn't quite go like he promised, but I'll give him the benefit of the doubt one more time". So, the second year, he works them even harder than the year before, because that was the recipe that worked last year. But again the coach is not improving capability, just capacity, work-rate, or effort. You only improve your capability by working on quality. So, if you do not improve the quality, your capabilities are not going to improve. Your capacities have developed, so your second year might be good, but you will get beaten by teams of better quality. And these teams are more efficient and more effective.

Like I said, if the coach is someone of low character by the third year players are thinking: "I don't trust this guy". Therefore, by year three, there is a choice. The coach changes personnel, changes coaches, quits or is fired. And that is the life cycle.

That is generally why there is a three-year itch, a three-year life cycle. To be successful in year three, where you build capacity, character, and capability all together, you have to do things the right way as a person, by building quality and developing capacity simultaneously, not isolating them.

Theory and research

I believe in pragmatism and action-based research. My research was an action-based PhD thesis on computer optimisation in manufacturing. That was my first introduction to action-based research, and the value of that in sport is that the results can be applied far quicker. Progress is faster. It is really important that you have the ability to constantly improve and develop. So, I read and study research, but there is a difference between information, knowledge, and wisdom. Research will supply information, and this comes from studies in a particular context, very often isolated, academic or in a laboratory-based situation. But the application is where knowledge comes, and the ability to apply it is where I have an edge. I respect research and there is value to it, but at the end of the day when you face the barrel of a gun, your theories kind of go out the window. So, it is about how you apply it. Finally, wisdom comes with success, and failure when trying systems, protocols, and interventions in the real world.

Dynamic system theory is one approach that I have come across that supports and helps me understand the reality of the situation best for what I do. I think we can argue that there are so many ways to do things, but this approach has helped me understand and create models that work. We operate in a chaotic environment and a chaotic world, so I am trying to find models that work.

The fundamental principles that govern the game are so important in team sports. A lot of this is developed from the military. If you go back, primarily to special operations and fundamental military theories, you will find that many of these ideas have been thought about and discussed through necessity. Going back beyond even World War I, generals tried to understand very chaotic environments. What I have done is perfect an approach that helps coaches and teams understand what is happening in their sport and provide a model that works. Think of it as a skeleton. All I try to do is to provide a skeleton and help the experts in-house develop their specific solutions.

For me, these types of principles have come from a necessity to try to understand what is happening. A lot of this comes from understanding situations and context. What I have learned the most from, actually, is watching kids play; watching my friend's son play basketball for example. Just sitting there watching. In a state of mindfulness, if you want to call it that, realising that the principles here are the very same principles that you are going to see in the NBA on ESPN later that evening. Having worked in these different sports, I realised all these environments are asking the same question, but they are using a different language.

Specialists and generalists

One of the biggest challenges that we have had, and this is not criticism per se, it is more an observation of the educational system that we have, is the belief in the power of specialists. Over the years we have revered specialists, in physiology and kinesiology, biomechanics, and psychology. The ability to apply or to use these resources properly however can only be done through generalists with a holistic perspective. Generalists, with the help of specialists, should be best placed to understand both the specific requirement and the dosage of medicine needed. You can kill anyone if you use the wrong medicine, but you can also kill if you use the wrong dosage. Generalists should understand the complete environment and effectively help administer different types of medicine. In team sport, the solution is almost always multi-faceted.

It is also important that specialists are managed so they can be most effective. The other thing is the prioritisation of the solution. One example is teams who seem to lose or concede goals late in the game. The obvious suggested solution is that they need to get fitter. That is what a fitness specialist would go in and do: improve fitness. The generalist, should it be the head coach, would look at it more holistically and say "You know what, because we weren't efficient in the first quarter, we started slow, and that led us to be fatigued late in the game". The real solution therefore is to improve efficacy, scoring or reduce turnovers, and it may not be a fitness issue at all. That is just one simple example. Again, teams that lose late in the game are often deemed not to be 'mentally tough' enough under pressure. It might not be that. It could be fitness, or it could be simply tactical – substitution strategies. Unless you have a generalist approach looking at all of these things as a whole, you are never going to come to the right conclusion.

Integrating staff

It's important to be aware of or recognise other people's strengths and your own vulnerabilities. This can only be done in a safe environment where people are prepared to have some conflict. They must be secure enough in their own ability to debate issues and talk things through. Unless you as the performance director can create that environment of trust it will be very difficult. This only comes from a foundation based on honesty. You need trust, honesty, and conflict to truly progress. I call it conflict, but it is really the ability to debate constructively and come to conclusions everyone agrees with. Unless you have the awareness of both your strengths and your weaknesses, then you are never going to progress, as a group or team. Finally, recognising that if we all take the credit, then we all need to accept responsibility as well.

How do you get this collaboration to happen? The very first thing, apart from stopping using email and instead talking in person, is that people need to spend time with each other, and be prepared to be vulnerable. If you cannot do this, you will never accept what the other person can contribute to help your limiting factors. A leader must be aware, open, and willing to have those conversations. If you're not prepared to accept your vulnerabilities and the areas where you are not strong and understand that this other person can help you, then progress will be limited.

Clarity of the objective is essential. What are we here to do? Are we here to build a sustainable programme? Do we want to dominate the opponent, not just win once or twice? How are we all going to contribute to that and how are we all going to share the benefits?

Testing

There is an over-reliance on testing in team sport. The real test is the game. That is a quantitative and qualitative assessment of your ability to perform under pressure. Testing, fitness testing, can be interesting. Some of it is useful. But, for the most part it is simply just interesting. The game is the ultimate test.

Testing is typically done in isolation. And it is taken out of context. True direction for improvement comes from the analysis of the game. Unless you analyse the game holistically, we just isolate one quality. The most common mistake is that we focus on the physical quality because it is the easiest one to measure. Working with truly elite organisations in high pressure environments, their goal is to try to select those who can produce extraordinary results in very extreme situations and develop these skills, because very often the qualities that they present are unique.

How then, do you get information from the game beyond that we won or we lost? That is the most brilliant question to ask. You must take the context and understand the inputs into that black box so to speak, and try to assess and come up with a model. This is why the model is so important. We all have intrinsic models by which we understand and interpret life. For example, a doll house is a young girl's model of how she interprets life, family life. As we grow older people develop models for managing stress, etc. So if something happens we interpret that in our model. The same with the game. You need to develop a game model. How do you look at the game? What are the qualities, what are the inputs that you see that you can understand? Not me or somebody else. What is your game model, what does it look like? The richer that the model can be, the better you understand the aspect of performance. The richer the model becomes, the better you can interpret the game, and the world for that matter. It goes to the athlete, to the person and how they interact with other people.

One mistake we see very often today are the fitness coaches who spend time warming up the players during the game, keeping them warm. They do not often get to watch the game properly. The following day, they have to take the players for recovery, so they do not have the chance to study and analyse the game. I know of some teams where the analysis department alone analyses the game and presents the results to the coach. Nothing could be more ridiculous. It is the coaches that need to drive this. They need to study the game and analyse it. One of the best coaches I came across is Tony Smith, the rugby league coach, and he always would insist that all his coaches and staff analyse the game with a solid understanding of the game model.

One of the biggest mistakes teams make today are simply building large staffs, and that is a big problem. The idea that more people solve problems faster or better is completely misguided. The programming industry has known this for many years and refer to it as the mythical man-month. Again, this all comes back to problem-solving – solve problems properly. Solve problems with quality, not quantity.

17

Using data in football

Ian Graham

Introduction

Football is not a data-friendly game. The reason for this is that goals are rare. The number of goals is the vital piece of data used to determine the winner of the game. The best team does not always win.

In the good old days, very little data apart from goals was available – if you were lucky you could find out the attendance at the game, and maybe which players played, and which ones scored. Today there is a deluge of data about all aspects of the game. The duty of the data analyst is to use this data to try to determine the processes by which goals are scored and conceded. They can then begin to offer recommendations about how to score more and concede fewer goals.

This is a big challenge for geeks with laptops (and some experience with mathematics). How can they compete with the subject-matter experts that are employed by football clubs – coaches, scouts, and sports scientists with decades of experience? The answer is that they do not compete, they pool their analysis with the experts' opinions: data analysis is not a substitute for football expertise. A cooperative approach will produce better decisions than experts or analysts can produce on their own.

In one sense the data analyst cannot compete – in any specific situation the expert can see things which are simply not contained in the data. But in another sense the geek has something the expert does not: breadth of data. Today, we have basic data on millions of games, event-by-event data on hundreds of thousands of games, and detailed information about the position and velocity of every player every 0.04 seconds in thousands of games. The richness of these data sets can tell you something experience cannot. Is it a good idea to shoot from 30 yards in general? How about in this specific instance? Is it a good idea to try a short corner? To buy this player? To sell that player? To sell him for a higher fee? To put out a weakened team the week before a big game?

The unique traits of any particular team means that experts are needed to help make these decisions, but general patterns are difficult to refute. A player may score a goal from 30 yards out in a specific game, but he will not score ten goals from ten shots from 30 yards out.

Other fields, such as medicine and finance, have already experienced a data analysis revolution. Sometimes, the use of data analysis was met with fierce resistance. Some doctors, for example, were outraged when it was suggested they use a checklist of symptoms to help produce a diagnosis: "This stupid list cannot compete with my nuanced experience". But the data did help, and the doctors who understood the *real* use of the checklist – as a tool to improve, rather than replace, their decisions – were the first to reap the rewards. The same will be true for football clubs.

Here is one anonymous example of the use of data analysis: a star player is misfiring – he has not scored in seven or eight games. If his performance really has dropped, then maybe it makes sense to drop, or even sell, the player. But if he is still a star, it would be a mistake to sell him. What do we do?

In this case, an analysis of the player's shots on goal showed that he was making the same number, of about the same quality, as he was before his barren run. The only difference was that the shots were not becoming goals. Players with similar poor runs of form had usually 'regressed to the mean' – that is they soon reverted to scoring at their usual rate. That was the case for this player - he quickly returned to his old scoring rate. A costly and unnecessary exercise to replace him was avoided.

The beauty of this analysis is that it's simple. Counting the number of shots per 90 minutes and using the location of the shots to determine their quality is easy. Because the analysis is so simple, it is easily understood in football terms – football experts get it.

It is rare to be able to use such a simple analysis to recommend a decision. But, however complicated the analysis, it is always vital to translate and interpret the results into the language of football.

Historical development

The raw material for analysis is data. The recent interest in football data analysis is the direct result of a dramatic increase in the availability of data. In the early days, data was very limited, and the task was to wring out every drop of predictiveness, so that it could say something relevant about the game.

Today data is abundant, and the main question is what to do with it. Data consists of 'signal', or useful information, and 'noise', or useless information. The key to data analysis is to separate the signal from the noise, and make recommendations based only on the useful signal that is contained in the data.

Early days

In the early days, up until the early 2000s, football data was not easy to find. In order to analyse anything beyond scores, lineups, and attendances, you had to collect it yourself. The early pioneer in data analysis was Charles Reep. He invented a shorthand notation for recording the sequence of events in a possession and recorded 578 games between 1953 and 1967 (Bray, 2006).

Although his work was misinterpreted by Charles Hughes at the English FA, and was seen as responsible for the development of the long-ball game in England, his collection and analysis of data was decades ahead of its time and deserves recognition.

Reep, together with statistician Bernard Benjamin (1968) observed that one shot in nine became a goal – a fraction that has remained remarkably consistent over the past 50 years. They also developed the first "Expected Goals" model in 1997 (see the section on "Event Data"), again a decade ahead of their time. Reep's work is also discussed by Egil Olsen in Chapter 4.

Game data

I started working with football data in 2005. The main public data source was www.football-data.co.uk, created and maintained by Joseph Buchdal. The site remains an excellent source of free data.

The basic unit of measurement in football is the game, and football-data.co.uk gives us one record per game. For each game we get the date, competition, teams and scores, shots, shots on target, fouls, corners, yellow and red cards, and bookmaker odds.

Even with such limited data, much analysis can be done. Team strength models can be developed using goal counts – the most famous of these models was developed by Dixon & Coles (1997). A goal scoring rate and a goal conceding rate is calculated for each team. These rates can be used to calculate the probability of a home win, a draw, or an away win in each game. Comparing their model's predictions to bookmaker odds, Dixon & Coles showed that inefficiencies existed in the bookmaker's odds, even after taking their 11% profit margin into account. For clubs, an objective method of rating a team can help understand whether a team's strength is really changing during a run of good or bad results.

Many other interesting questions can be answered using this 'basic' data – what is the effect of a red card? How big is home advantage in football and what might cause it? How are corners and shots related to goals scored?

The development of football data analysis was led by gambling syndicates and bookmakers – clubs have been slow to catch up. The first major impact for clubs of gambling-focused analysis has been in ownership: in 1996, Dixon & Coles were academics at Lancaster University. Dixon went on to found ATASS, a company that provides statistical analysis for betting consultancy Starlizard. Starlizard's owner, Tony Bloom, is chairman and majority shareholder of English Premier League club Brighton & Hove Albion. Coles works for Smartodds, owned by Mathew Benham – the owner of the football clubs Brentford and Midtjylland.

Event data

Understanding games at the team and result level is interesting, but teams are composed of players, and clubs are interested in player performance. After all, players' performances combine to produce team performance.

There are many challenges in analysing player performance – a player's performance is dependent on the performance of his teammates and of the opposition players. Player performance naturally changes with age and experience. A player's recorded 'events' in a game do not necessarily say anything about whether he made the correct decision in any particular situation. For example, scoring a goal might be the 'wrong' decision if an easy pass to a teammate for a tap-in was available. Despite these challenges, event data can tell us a lot about player performance.

The most basic level of player data is a count of the number of different types of action a player makes during a game – the number of goals, shots, passes, fouls, saves, tackles, interceptions etc. Early player ratings models used this kind of data because it was all that was available. A good example of a model using player counts data is the official Premier League ratings system – the ACTIM Index – developed by Ian McHale (McHale, Scarf & Folker, 2012). The ACTIM Index estimates the effect of player actions – passes, dribbles, interceptions, and bookings – on the quantity of shots and goals scored and conceded by their team. This approach related non-shot actions to shots. For example, a successful dribble was associated with 0.12 extra shots, and a yellow card was associated with 0.25 fewer shots.

The weakness of using counts of player actions is that it relies on correlations. For example, red cards are correlated with goals conceded, but the data alone does not reveal why they are correlated. Making inferences from correlations without using football knowledge is dangerous. The number of saves a goalkeeper makes is correlated with goals conceded by a team. The number of offside passes a team makes is correlated with the number of shots on goal they make. The football reasons for these correlations are clear: lots of saves mean a keeper's goal is under siege. Many offside passes suggest a team is playing well enough to attempt lots of dangerous passes. But it is ridiculous to suggest a save is a bad thing, and an offside pass is a good thing. In other words, "correlation does not imply causation". Offside passes do not cause goals, despite their correlation.

To improve on correlation-based performance ratings, it is necessary to analyse data event-by-event: where on the pitch did this event happen, and what happened next? By analysing the sequence of events, it is easy to see that saves are usually a good thing, and offside passes a bad thing. The spurious correlation between goals scored and offside passes can be ignored, because we can see that offside passes lead to a guaranteed loss of possession.

Event-by-event data was first widely collected and sold by Opta (now Perform) in 2006. Knowledge of the location of each event enabled better analysis and prediction of player performance. It clearly showed the shortcomings of 'traditional' football statistics such as pass completion percentage and shots on goal. I developed the Castrol Index in 2007, which improved on traditional statistics by using a location-specific passing rating, and an "Expected Goals" model.

The most 'successful' passers on a team are often central defenders. A high proportion of their passes are short, sideways, and in their own half. By analysing the location of the passes, it is easy to see that the lower pass completion rate of attacking midfielders is due to their attempts to thread difficult forward passes to strikers. Again, this is something that is intuitive and obvious to any club video analyst, but it took a long time for statistical analysis to catch up with football experts' intuitions.

Or consider shots: an attempt from 30 yards out results in a goal much less often than a shot from ten yards out. By controlling for the context of the shot – the location and situation – one can better analyse a player's shot selection and outcomes.

Weighting each shot by its probability of producing a goal, gives a value called "Expected Goals". Expected Goals is the success story of football data analysis in terms of public profile – Opta's Expected Goals numbers are shown after each game on the UK's Premier League highlights show, "Match of the Day".

Expected goals was first introduced in a paper by Pollard and Reep (1997). Their analysis is sophisticated: they account for the distance of the shot from goal, the angle of the shot from goal, whether it is a first-touch shot, defensive pressure, and whether the shot came from open play or set play. My 2007 version of Expected Goals took various elements directly from this seminal paper.

Expected Goals can describe the quality and quantity of shots but say nothing about how a team might create more high-quality shots. The next iteration of Expected Goals will concentrate on *how* good-quality shots are generated. In order to understand how the opportunity to create a high-quality shot arises, tracking data is needed.

Tracking data

Even detailed event data is not very good at describing football. Creating and exploiting space is an important part of the game and event data says nothing at all about it. A forward whose run drags opponents away, making space for a teammate to receive a pass, does not record an 'event'. To account for these facets of the game, it is necessary to know what every player is doing at every instant. 'Tracking data' uses video cameras to record the trajectories of all 22 players. It allows us to see what is happening off the ball as well as on it.

Tracking data was first collected in the Premier League by a company called Prozone. The initial application was summarising the physical performance of players. For the first time, it was possible to measure in every game the total distance players' covered, the amount of distance covered at high speed, and the number of sprints completed.

These summaries have been useful for sports science, where coaches could begin to tailor training to the requirements of the game. Physical preparation is important, but (in the Premier League at least) there is little correlation between physical statistics and game outcome. It is easy to lose games having outrun your opponent.

In 2013, the Premier League contracted ChyronHego to collect data for all 380 games each season. This increased availability of tracking data has led to an increase in its analysis. Over the past three years, the MIT Sloan Sports Analytics Conference has featured research papers using football tracking data. The 2018 conference featured four papers using football tracking data, from STATS.com, Hudl, and FC Barcelona.

The basic question that tracking data research asks is "how does space affect scoring opportunity?" The most promising method has been to define "pitch control". Pitch control assigns a value to each location on the pitch, based on the proximity of attacking and defending players. The idea is that a team controls an area of the pitch if their players are closer than the opposition. It is a natural framework for understanding why counter-attacks lead to more dangerous chances than playing against a deep defence.

The pitch control idea can be extended to analyse player skill and player decision-making. If a player can pass or receive into tightly guarded spaces, it is indicative of skill on the ball. If a player always chooses to pass to the receiver in the best combination of space and pitch location, it is indicative of good decision-making.

With the advent of tracking data, football data analysis is finally able to begin answering the questions of real interest to the coach.

Psychology

Psychology is clearly very important in football, but not easy to analyse. General patterns from behavioural economics (Kahneman, 2011) can certainly be observed in football. I believe that loss aversion is common in football, with teams becoming too defensive when leading in a game. The nature of a low-scoring game also leads to clustering illusions, where too much importance is given to a short winning or losing streak.

Palacios-Huerta (2014) discusses some psychological studies of football. In a penalty shootout, the team to take the first kick wins about 60% of the time, rather than the 50% that would be expected. The reason must be psychological, although the exact mechanism is unknown.[1] Referees also experience psychological pressure: they favour the home team, and award more injury time if the home team is behind by one goal.

My path

Any individual's career path can only be seen as a list of facts, rather than containing any general insight or advice for the success of others.

At school I liked science and maths, and really, really hated PE. In South Wales the main sport is rugby – a highly physical sport uniquely unsuited to those of a sensitive nature. Avoiding playing rugby as much as possible, I did a degree in physics and a PhD in biological physics.

Biological physics is a fascinating subject, where we try to apply the powerful mathematical techniques of physics to the messy and complicated world of biology. It was a relatively new field of research in 2001. The reaction of biologists was often "I don't understand these equations". A lot of time was spent trying to convince biologists that the physics approach was valid. Later, in football stats, there was a similar struggle to convince football experts that the data analysis approach was valid.

I left academia in 2005 to join a startup company called Decision Technology, simply because their job advert asked: "Would you like a career analysing football data?" It was pure luck that I saw the advert and decided to apply, since 'sports data' was not a career at the time.

My role was to develop mathematical models of football. Clubs were not interested in this for many years, and the main consumers of our analysis were bookmakers and the media.

I did research for a weekly column in the Times – "The Fink Tank", written by Daniel Finkelstein. This was a brilliant lesson in communicating the results of statistical analysis to a general audience. I also developed a player ranking model – the Castrol Index – that was used for the European Championships and World Cups between 2007 and 2014. Although it was a media application, these player rankings are what finally interested clubs in our work.

Decision Technology started working with Tottenham Hotspur while Damien Comolli was director of football. Our job there was to provide player recruitment advice and strategy consultancy.

In 2012, Liverpool FC offered me a job.

Role of the research department

The responsibility of the research department is to collect, organise, store, and analyse all data related to football operations. By making data easily available, and analysing that data, we help staff at the training ground make better-informed decisions.

The general questions that a data analysis approach can help answer are:

- What is our level of performance?
- Are our results in line with our performance?
- What is the benchmark for a league-average performance?
- What is the benchmark for a Premier League team?
- What can be done to improve our performance?

The 'performance' can be anything – the result in the next game, the league position next season, the impact of newly signed players, the physical performance and fitness of the squad, or the club's financial performance.

Introduction

Starting at a club, it is tempting to try to do as much as possible: how can we help sports science? How can we help the video analysts? The Academy? The medical department? A cost-benefit analysis showed that the greatest impact would be in squad management – buying and selling players. So we concentrated our efforts there: it was more important to make the best possible tools to help in one area rather than spread our efforts across many different projects. The project was successful, and we now had a case study of "why do I need this?" that we could show other departments.

Scouting

Transfer fees and player wages is where the bulk of most teams' money is spent. Clubs who sell well can also use recruitment as a source of income. One approach to transfers is this: for every transfer that another team makes, we ask "are we happy that we did not make that deal at that price?" For example, if a good 30-year-old defender who would improve our squad was sold to another team for £10 million, are we happy that we did not sign him instead? If he would improve our squad, maybe we should be unhappy. But if his age and price meant the player was poor value for money, then we should be happy that we didn't sign him, especially if better options were available.

To really gauge our happiness at making or not making a transfer, there needs to be a system to analyse players, to judge whether a potential transfer would improve our squad, or our first 11. There also needs to be a system to model squad depth, to forecast how many starts a potential transfer is likely to make. In addition, there needs to be a financial model in place to understand what the market would pay for a similar player.

These systems all have a statistical model behind them. The type of statistical model depends on the data available and what you are trying to measure.

Player performance is a difficult thing to measure, and the data typically used is not very eloquent in describing the player's impact on a game, as discussed above.

My approach for player performance analysis is to build a model that values each possession on an event-by-event basis. Assuming a pre-requisite for scoring a goal is to have the ball,[2] any event that moves the possession into a situation with a higher likelihood of scoring should be rewarded.

The challenge with a bespoke approach is that it requires a lot of reworking of data and specific mathematical models that are not available 'out of the box' using standard statistical packages. The benefit is that the football-based theory behind the bespoke model can better predict player and team performance.

The second challenge is to interpret player performance. The interpretation of model results for football experts is the critical component of doing data analysis at a club. If your results are not understood – or believed – by colleagues then the analysis, no matter how good it is, will not be acted upon.

When browsing player performance ratings, there will always be surprises. Why is this player that I dislike highly rated? Why is my favourite midfielder so badly rated? Many assumptions and calculations go into every statistical model, and making these clear is very important. For example, some players are set-piece specialists – they are good at taking free kicks and corners. An analysis might show that they create many dangerous goalscoring opportunities. But interpreting *why* they look good is important. If a team already has a good set-piece taker the marginal impact of anyone who rates well on set-pieces will be lower.

The third challenge is to convince decision-makers to act upon your results. In my case, I have been lucky to work with colleagues who genuinely bought into data analysis and accepted that it brought a new objective viewpoint, independent of the opinions of scouts and coaches.

Technology

Football data has become unwieldy. In 2005 it was possible to do a lot of work with text data files. Today we have hundreds of thousands of games containing thousands of events per game. We have thousands of games of tracking data – each game contains millions of records. It has become necessary to know about databases and cloud computing in order to analyse football data.

Six years ago, the typical workflow was to buy some data, convert it into text files, and run the data through our models. The model output was more text files, which could be visualised using a tool like Microsoft Excel. The workflow was fine for analysing a few games but maintenance was a chore. Every time a colleague wanted an updated analysis, the process had to be repeated, and the results mangled into a presentable form.

We wanted a more elegant solution. We set up a database, and wrote tools to automatically import data and run it through our various analyses. The results were published to an internal website. The power of this approach is that it put the analysis directly into the hands of the users and freed up time to develop better models.

The technology side of data analysis is not trivial and is often tedious. However, automation is increasingly necessary. Otherwise the scale of the work that can be done is fundamentally limited, as all the time is spent repeating the same analysis for next week's games.

Sports science

Sports science is an area of football that generates a lot of data. Physical performance data is collected for every player, in each game and each training session. The relationship between physical performance and the result of the game, or the results over a season, is complex. The correlation between team running statistics and results is weak, but a team that wasn't allowed to run during a game would almost certainly lose. The challenge for sports science is to use the many different variables of physical data to understand what effect it has on performance.

Our work with sports science has included projects to validate the different technologies that collect the physical data, and to derive novel statistics to better understand physical performance in a game.

Video analysis

Game data can be used to understand performance, and the performance of opponents. Post-match we can ask whether the result was in line with the underlying performance of the teams. For example, a 1-0 victory might have been an early goal followed by 80 minutes of last-ditch defending. If this game was played at home against a weak opponent then we might not be happy with the performance, even if we are happy with the result.

Data analysis that is produced post-match can also give context to the underlying performance. In each aspect we can compare how we did compared to expectation, and compared to a typical performance by a top-four team.

Opposition scouting can also benefit. Data analysis can provide information about the opponent's style and ability: are they a crossing team? A long-ball team? How effective is their crossing? If a team has new players, what might we expect from them? Do they change their style away from home, or against stronger opposition?

Academy

The same analysis that is used for the first team can also be useful for the academy, although the application is different. The academy is interested in player development more than results.

By analysing the performance of youth teams in the same way as the first team we can forecast how players might develop into members of the first team squad.

With many seasons of detailed data on academy players, we can begin to compare the youth performances of players now at top Premier League teams with those who play senior football at a lower level. This allows us to study which aspects of youth performance might translate to success in senior football.

Conclusion

Data analysis can help clubs win. Even basic analysis – creating and visualising a list of meaningful statistics – can steer clubs away from bad decisions.

The fundamental problem with data analysis in football is that it is a long-term investment producing long-term returns, whereas football is a short-term, results-driven business. The frequent turnover of managers and owners is testament to this short-termism.

The variance in game results is huge – the best team doesn't always win. A team employing the best data analysis practices may not see an immediate improvement in results over the course of a season, even if underlying performances improve significantly.

I have worked with clubs who experienced exactly this scenario. It was very difficult for decision-makers to stick with the process, even though everyone believed in it. The reward for perseverance with a data-driven process is that, in the long term, both performances *and* results improve.

Data analysis is still very new within football clubs, and there is still resistance to its use. This is not so surprising, given the poor historical track record of data analysis in English football. Convincing football people of the use of data is not easy. It is important to find open-minded coaches, scouts, and video analysts to work with and to be prepared for hostility from some colleagues.

Finally, the data analyst should always listen to sensible criticisms from football experts. The data cannot account for or predict everything that can happen on the pitch – the game is played by humans after all. Friendly coaches and video analysts have a wealth of experience and knowledge about the game – data analysts must take advantage of it.

Notes

1 This is the case in the traditional shoot-out when penalties are taken in turns, known as "ABAB". This analysis led to the suggestion that penalties should be taken in the order "ABBA", and is being trialled by FIFA.
2 This is not always true – for example own goals can be scored without a team possessing the ball.

References

Bray, K. (2006). *How to Score*. London: Granta Books
Dixon, M. & Coles, S. (1997). *Journal of the Royal Statistical Society: Series C (Applied Statistics)*, **46**(2), 265–280
Kahneman, D. (2011). *Thinking, Fast and Slow*. New York, NY: Farrar, Straus & Giroux
McHale, I., Scarf, P. & Folker, D. (2012). *Interfaces*, **42**(4), 339–351
Palacios-Huerta, I. (2014). *Beautiful Game Theory: How Soccer Can Help Economics*. Princeton, NJ: Princeton University Press
Pollard, R. & Reep, C. (1997). Measuring the Effectiveness of Playing Strategies at Soccer. *Journal of the Royal Statistical Society: Series D (The Statistician)*, **46**(4), 541–550

18

Research and innovation
Seeking and securing competitive advantage

Peter Vint

Introduction

Contests in elite sport are often decided by fractions of an inch and in fractions of a second. Sure, once-in-a-generation athletes like Usain Bolt, Michael Phelps, Serena Williams, and Katie Ledecky can make winning look easy. The reality, however, is anything but.

Across all pool- and open-water swimming events in the 2016 Summer Olympics in Rio de Janeiro, the *average* difference between gold and silver medalists was 0.72% while the average difference between the bronze medalists and fourth place finishers was 0.34%. In athletics running events, ranging from the 100 metres to the marathon, these differences were 0.66% and 0.40%, respectively. During the 2018 Winter Olympics in PyeongChang, the *average* margins of victory among all time-based events were even smaller with gold medalists beating out silver medalists by just 0.49% while fourth place finishers missed the podium by only 0.44%

With performance levels among the world's best athletes and teams tighter than ever, and with the financial incentives[1] and media recognition[2] associated with winning and losing growing larger, sporting organisations have been aggressively seeking, developing, and investing in tools, technologies, and methods to gain competitive advantages and sustain these over time.

This chapter is devoted to exploring the potential of research and innovation programs in elite sport. I have decided to discuss these ideas through the lens of my own experiences with the hope that a more personal rather than academic approach may resonate with readers who are interested in this topic.

My history

In 1997, I earned a doctoral degree in biomechanics and had, during the course of this work, spent a significant amount of time becoming familiar with personal computers and computer programming. In a strange way, I feel fortunate that I had started my training, years earlier, when human movement studies required cumbersome manual digitising of processed 35mm film. Had I not experienced the sheer drudgery associated with these early methods, I am not sure I could have fully appreciated the remarkable improvements that computerisation and digital technologies would later have in my work.

So, perhaps it comes as no surprise that my earliest connotations of the word, 'innovation', were most strongly associated with new technologies: gadgets, tools, and software applications. I think I largely held this notion for years, interchangeably using the word 'innovation' for the latest and greatest 'shiny thing'. It would be years later, during my work as senior sport technologist with the United States Olympic Committee, that I would learn a few important and, yes, painful lessons, that would forever change my understanding of what 'innovation' is and what it is not.

From 2005–09, I served the United States Olympic Committee in the capacity of biomechanist, sport technologist, motor learning/skill acquisition specialist, and analytics enthusiast. My primary responsibilities were to deliver innovative performance measurement and feedback tools in support of Olympic sport coaches and athletes. My team and I spent considerable time listening to coaches, athletes, and performance directors. We learned about the challenges they faced, ideas they had, and performance questions they needed to answer. To this end, I felt successful and was having a great time in the process. Among the 'innovations' I had conceptualised, developed and/or managed, and delivered included:

- Custom-fit, modified-stiffness, energy-preserving insoles designed to improve vertical jumping performance and lateral acceleration among indoor volleyball players.
- Modification of off-the-shelf sensors to measure and provide near real-time feedback of BMX, bobsled, and skeleton start performances.
- Modification of off-the-shelf force plate systems, coupled with digital video and graphical force overlays, to measure and provide instantaneous feedback during dryland ski-jump training and swim start performances.
- Custom, video-based match and race analysis systems for beach volleyball teams and bobsled and skeleton pilots, respectively.
- A digital video- and computer-based perceptual skill training system to measure and improve advanced cue utilisation and performance among indoor volleyball blockers.

At the time, the technical proficiencies required by me and my teammates to execute on these programs felt relatively advanced. With each new program came a new set of challenges and end user requirements and, with these, opportunities to explore the advanced sensor space. Some of these projects were successful. And, the work was fun. However, it was becoming clear to me and my team that our personal enjoyment and sense of satisfaction had exactly zero correlation to the actual performance impact of our deliverables.

That was a humbling realisation.

How could it be that these innovative projects failed to have an impact on performance? Each had used the latest technologies and had been specifically designed and delivered to meet the stated wants and needs of coaches and athletes. However, it was clear that in some cases, this was simply insufficient to bring about measurable change.

There were probably a number of reasons behind this insufficiency. Perhaps one was my own hubris. Just because I thought a project was well conceived, well designed, and delivered on time and under budget, did not actually mean that coaches and athletes would instantly love it, let alone use it. However, another was my lack of understanding about managing innovation and the underlying research programs that are often required to inform and support innovation. Others still included siloed approaches to performance interventions, issues related to the lack of utilisation on the part of coaches and athletes, and the absence of personal, professional, or organisational accountability to actually measure the impact of any program that was launched.

As a result, I sought to learn more about how my team and I could improve. I found a substantial body of literature devoted to innovation management and programmatic assessment. I encountered dozens of definitions of innovation until I found one that finally resonated with me: "Innovation is something different that has impact".[3]

To me, Anthony's definition helped distinguish between the purpose of innovation (to create impact) and the easier but less effective pursuit of shiny, new, technologically-oriented things. It connected my frustrations with failed or underwhelming project deliveries with an opportunity to look at these experiences through a different lens.

However, this definition also appealed to me because it allowed me and my teams to address innovation in a *relative sense*. For example, some sporting organisations were already quite advanced. Introducing something new that would have impact in those environments may require the latest technologies and advanced methods. However, for organisations, coaches, and athletes who were less advanced or perhaps more traditional in their approach to performance, innovations may have simply included the introduction and adoption of well-established best practices into their current training and competition environments. Simple examples of this included the effective implementation of strength and conditioning, nutrition, and recovery programmes and improvements in the design and delivery of practice and feedback.

With this in mind, it is easier to understand that innovations must ultimately serve a purpose beyond their mere introduction. 'Different' is insufficient when it comes to creating a sustainable competitive advantage. At some point, 'different' has to result in measurable and positive outcomes. See Figure 18.1, for a simple illustration of this idea. For organisations that are relatively advanced and already effectively using best practices, 'innovation' may require more advanced or cutting-edge interventions. For those who are less advanced, 'innovation' may simply require introducing well established, best practices to their environments.

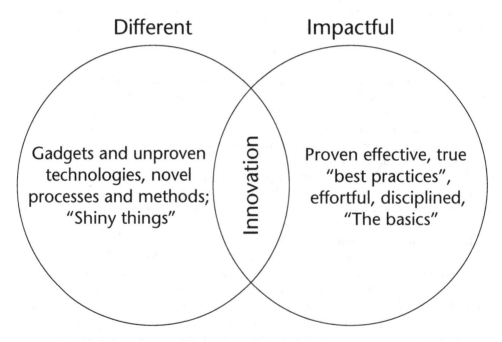

Figure 18.1 An illustration of Anthony's definition of innovation as the intersection of "something different with impact"

In the performance domain, these outcomes may include:

- Improved athlete, team, or organisational performance (sporting, financial, or otherwise);
- Increased athlete health, wellness, and career longevity;
- Improved return on investment of allocated resources (e.g. time, money, personnel) required to complete necessary tasks and/or perform at a particular level;
- Improving quality and/or quantity of actionable information.

Examples of innovations in sport

With Anthony's definition of innovation in mind, it is easy to find examples of things that were different and created impact in sport. Many of these have involved scientifically informed or research-guided modifications of existing equipment designs including the Klapskate[4] in speedskating, dimpled golf balls,[5] quick release ski bindings, aerobars, and bicycle derailer systems.

Some have emerged primarily from advances in materials, engineering, and manufacturing processes including the Fastskin LZR Racer[6] in swimming, cleated shoes, and any of the numerous improvements in the aero- or fluid-dynamic, strength, weight, resilience, and/or impact/vibration absorption characteristics of sporting equipment and environments (e.g. attire, bicycle, boat, brace, club, glove, helmet, pole, shoe, sled, ski, snowboard, racquet, and competition surface design).

Other innovations, however, have involved coach-guided or athlete-generated modifications in the techniques or sport specific movement patterns used during training and competition. Some of the most notable examples of innovations in this category include The Fosbury Flop,[7] V-style ski jumping,[8] non-linear sculling arm action in swimming, and the lesser known (and now illegal) somersault long jump[9] and Basque Style (spinning) javelin throw,[10,]

The growing ubiquity of wearable technologies and internet-connected devices, coupled with the dramatic rise in data analytics, has facilitated an improved access to individualised athlete data and the ability to make less biased and more informed decisions about nearly every facet of athlete and team performance. For some of these technologies, the potential to introduce something new and different to sport seems evident. The litmus test, however, will be whether they have created measurable impact in whatever they are designed to do.

Finding things that matter

The potential for any tool, technology, or process to create positive and measurable impact in sport is dependent upon a number of important factors. Successful innovations target things that actually matter to performance. They also target things that can sufficiently *change* within the rules of competition and within the timeframe available or being targeted (e.g. by the next competition, by the start of the playoffs, before the start of the next season, or by the next World Cup, Olympic Games, or World Championship). Fortunately, there are a number of systematic ways to identify the things that matter to performance outcomes. In my experience, the simplest and most effective of these is a process called deterministic modelling.[11]

In short, deterministic modelling provides a robust and reliable method to identify and measure the outcome of a performance and the factors contributing to it. The process of identifying factors and their relationship to the performance outcome is objective and unambiguous and strictly relies on physical, mechanical, and/or mathematical principles or on the rules and regulations of the sport itself.[12] They can be used to identify and evaluate critical factors in individual, head-to-head, and multi-competitor sports and can be effectively used with cgs sports,[13] judged sports,[14] and invasive combat and team sports. Deterministic models can be broad in scope or designed to focus on specific (bio-)mechanical, physiological, or even technical and tactical aspects of performance.

It is impossible within the scope of this chapter to provide a detailed list of known critical factors across every sport. It is possible, however, to describe some of these across broader categories of sports. Examples include:

- *Running and cycling sports*: Speed, distance, time, step/stroke frequency, distance per step/ stroke, forces/torques applied, duration of force/torque application, mass/moments of inertia, air, fluid, and rolling resistance, body position at pushoff and landing.
- *Jumping, throwing, and striking sports*: Velocity at takeoff/contact/release, relative height at takeoff/contact/release, air resistance, gravity, body position at takeoff, release, and landing, force/torque application, duration of force/torque application, mass/moments of inertia, coefficient of restitution (elasticity).
- *Sliding, skating, and rolling sports*: Speed, distance, time, stroke frequency, distance per stroke, forces/torques applied, duration of force/torque application, glide time, mass/moments of inertia, air and rolling resistance, cross-sectional area, air density, ice friction.
- *Swimming and boating sports*: Speed, distance, stroke time, glide time, stroke frequency, distance per stroke, forces/torques applied, duration of force/torque application, mass/ moments of inertia, buoyancy force, fluid resistance, cross-sectional area, fluid density, form, surface, and wave drag.
- *Judged sports*: execution score, difficulty score, speed, time, height, distance, rotation, forces/ torques applied, duration of force/torque application, mass/moments of inertia, body position at takeoff, at peak flight, and at landing.
- *Head-to-head sports*: points won, points conceded, scoring attempts, scoring efficiency, possessions gained, possessions lost.

Considering some of the major sport innovations mentioned earlier, each resulted in significant improvements in one or more of the factors listed above. For example:

- *Klapskate*: improved speedskating performance by increasing range of motion at the ankle thereby increasing the magnitude and duration over which propulsive forces could be applied during each stroke.
- *Fastskin LZR*: improved swimming performance by reducing surface and form drag and positively affecting buoyancy forces. These reductions in drag facilitated maintenance of higher average speeds during the glide and stroking phases of the race.
- *Fosbury Flop*: improved high jump performance by introducing a unique body configuration that allowed the body center of mass to pass underneath the bar during clearance.
- *V-style ski jump*: improved performance by introducing ski and body configurations that increased lift forces and allowed ski jumpers to remain airborne longer and therefore travel farther before landing.

When designed to a sufficient level of detail and applied to any single performance, deterministic models should capture every critical aspect of a performance outcome. Applied across multiple performances, however, the structure of deterministic models also provides an intuitive way to capture either within or between athlete and/or team performances and can be used for cross-sectional or longitudinal analyses. In this way, deterministic models that describe the results of multiple performances can be more appropriately considered *probabilistic* models and used as such.

Where and how does research fit in?

Recall that the ultimate goal of innovation is not simply to introduce something new or different. It is to create measurable impact. Therefore, regardless of the method(s) used to identify critical performance factors, whether through deterministic modelling, scientific literature, critical thinking,[15] brainstorming,[16] expert surveys,[17] 'gut instinct', or otherwise, we must commit ourselves to evaluating the effects of our interventions. Without this, we cannot really tell if our efforts have been successful. Without measurement, we'll never know if our 'something different' actually created impact.

Research should be considered a necessary element of any innovation program. It can help to identify what is already known, explore what is not known yet, describe how things work in isolation or as part of another system, and gather evidence to support, refute, or modify our current understanding. In the context of sport, research can improve both the efficiency and effectiveness of the work we do to improve performance by guiding us through the dizzying arrays of ideas and potential variables toward those that will most likely bear fruit.

In my experience, this is where innovation efforts can often fall down. We introduce something new. Ideally, we've done so after identifying and targeting critical aspects of performance that are changeable over time. We get excited, we launch, and we leave. In doing so, we've missed one of the most important aspects: measurement or validation. We need to demonstrate our intervention not only works, but that it creates measurable change that is not due to chance alone. This requires knowledge of how,[18] what, and when to measure and a genuine willingness to explore alternative or 'proxy' measurements, particularly if the intervention outcomes are traditionally believed to be 'intangible' or 'immeasurable'.[19]

Deep in the trenches of real-world sporting environments, research in and of itself, can be perceived to have marginal value. Time is short and pressure is high. Peer reviewed scientific literature can come across as esoteric and highly technical making it difficult to understand and apply. Criticisms regarding subject selection, sample size, and laboratory-based experimental designs have only served to further the divide between the theoretical and the practical.

This does not have to be. But, it is a valid and reasonable concern and points to an opportunity for forward-thinking organisations and individuals to address these problems differently. Among those, two approaches seem most common. In the first, organisations hire dedicated staff who have been formally trained and have specific domain expertise. In the second, organisations partner with university or industry experts to address performance issues on a project specific basis. There are advantages and disadvantages with either approach.

In the former, organisations can manage intellectual property issues directly and can manage priorities and project commitments internally. Drawbacks often come from organisational budget constraints that can limit the number, experience levels, expertise, management, and professional development opportunities of full-time staff. While some sporting organisations have significant player personnel budgets, operating budgets can be orders of magnitude smaller. As a result, sport science and medical staff members are sometimes asked to perform multiple roles, including some in which they have no significant experience or expertise.

In the latter, effective partnerships[20] can leverage exceptionally qualified personnel on a project by project basis. Experts are brought in and retained only as needed. While initial costs of acquiring such experts can be higher, these costs are often significantly lower than the overall expense of maintaining long-term, full-time staff. Challenges in partnership-based research and innovation efforts can arise in the form of finding the right experts, management of time and project priorities, and achieving mutual agreement regarding final work products and intellectual property. For many academics, this includes grant procurement and negotiating permissions to publish and/or present the results of their efforts in peer reviewed (public and therefore available to competitors for free!) formats. Further challenges can arise in assimilating outside experts with internal politics and cultural norms.

There are, however, alternatives to these approaches worth considering. The utility of these may depend on the ability of the sponsoring organisation to articulate specific needs or questions clearly and the internal capacity to manage, process, evaluate, and ultimately implement innovative ideas that result. But, for those organisations that are capable, crowd sourcing efforts like hackathons,[21] contest models,[22] and internal[23] or external[24] ideation platforms can effectively reduce costs, increase the number and diversity of ideas or solutions, and identify talented individuals that might have otherwise been difficult to find.

The (research and) innovation process

Launching a successful innovation program requires successful planning and execution. Politics, turf wars, siloes, and challenges associated with alignment, vision, strategy, budget, and organisational 'inertia' are all too common and can create significant challenges in moving programs forward.[25] While the business, behavioural, and management science literature can be helpful, it can also be daunting. Innovation processes like "Design Thinking",[26] "Agile",[27] and "Lean"[28] abound, as do approaches to effectively combine them.[29] And, while some approaches to innovation may be more appropriate than others, depending on circumstance, application, and desired outcome,[30] key steps in the innovation process that are most commonly cited are broadly summarised below in the context of sport performance environments.

Find inspiration, gather information, ideas, and data

Observing coaches, athletes, and staff during training, competition, and in preparation for these events, can yield considerable insights about their natural working environments. Notice how much time is taken to complete certain tasks, how communication and feedback flows; how engaged athletes are as coaches or performance staff speak; to what extent coaches and performance directors utilise the efforts of performance and analytics staff. Observe how coaches and athletes consume information. Are exchanges of information primarily verbal and face to face or remote and technology-based? Is one more effective than another?

Beyond observation, seeking to understand the perspectives of those closest to the sport can be facilitated by asking open ended questions. Examples might include: "What kinds of things tend to separate the top N athletes/teams in the world from the rest?"; "what do the top N do that the bottom N don't?"; "where, when, and how are seconds/inches/points most frequently won and lost?"; "what, in your mind, are the most important aspects of improving performance and how are you addressing these now?"; "who are the world leaders in doing these things?"; "what information would you love to have but struggle to get now?"; "what do you spend most of your time doing?"; "what do you find most time consuming or cumbersome, that if made easier, would have a positive impact on performance?"; "if we had one more dollar to spend, where would we put it to get the biggest bang for the buck?"

In addition to gathering insights directly from coaches, athletes, and performance directors within the immediate performance environment, a great deal can be learned by listening, observing, and becoming familiar with others that may work around the periphery, in other sports, or in other high-intensity, performance-centric industries like performing arts, military, aerospace, business, investment banking, or medicine. High-level sport performance conferences like those sponsored by Leaders[31] and CONQA[32] exemplify the broad and comprehensive applications of other performance domains in sport.

In my own work, finding inspiration from other sports and other performance domains has been deeply satisfying and surprisingly effective. Some of my favourite examples have included:

- A 3-D Doppler Radar-based technology[33] originally developed for the golf industry was transformed to provide real-time measurement and feedback of key performance variables in athletics throwing events.
- Analytical methods used to evaluate skill among chess[34] and video game[35] players were adapted to estimate international competitiveness among head-to-head and multi-competitor Olympic sport athletes and teams, respectively.
- Data visualisation methods used to display stock market performance[36] were reimagined to provide United States Olympic Committee (USOC) executives with a way to see historical, current, and targeted medal performances across all Summer or Winter Olympic sports in a single dashboard.
- Checklist methods used in the aviation[37] and medical[38] industries were modified for use during Olympic Games and World Championships in an effort to reduce unnecessary mistakes that had been previously observed in these high stakes, high pressure competitions.

Generate, refine, and prioritize ideas

Synthesising input from a variety of sources and industries, contextualised for sport- or environment-specific constraints, can consolidate insights about both general and specific types of challenges that exist and might be addressed. Frame challenges as opportunities and use active listening techniques to verify the intent and focus of new ideas. Define questions and refine the idea set as clearly and as concisely as is practical.

Maintain focus on opportunities that can create measurable impact. Ask questions like, "so what?"; "is *that* really important?"; "how important do we think this is and how do we know?"; "will this make us better and, if so, how and to what extent?"

Prioritisation is an important, and often overlooked, step in shaping an effective innovation strategy. Financial cost and performance impact are only two of the many aspects that should be considered. Others include development, implementation, testing, iteration time and complexity, end user interest and commitment, estimates regarding the frequency of use or application, and legality or probability of disqualification. Each of these considerations can be included in prioritisation assessments using qualitative or quantitative estimates, and, if desired, can be differentially weighted with respect to organisational priorities.

As important as the synthesis and prioritisation phase may be, it is important that the process is not so cumbersome that it impairs or inhibits progress. There will inevitably be high priority and high impact projects that are also big and complex and resource-intensive. There may also be projects that are somewhat lower priority that could be completed more quickly. If resources are available, moving forward with both types of projects – bigger, slower, more impactful projects with smaller, quicker, and perhaps somewhat less impactful projects – in parallel, rather than in series, can be productive and help build momentum to support a long-term innovation strategy.

Experiment, implement, and iterate

One of the most common recommendations regarding the innovation process is developing rapid prototypes that are directionally correct or offer some, but perhaps not all, of the solution features originally considered. Depending on the nature of the project, this may involve partnering with internal or external domain experts that have the skills and experiences to bring new ideas to fruition.

By definition, rapid prototypes are imperfect, but developing, launching, and testing new ideas allows feedback to be gathered quickly so that necessary changes can be made along the way. An idea considered to be a sure thing or failproof from a theoretical perspective may not actually work as intended in real-life performance environments. Or, even it does work as the innovation team intended, it may not be comfortable, suitable, or usable from the perspective of an athlete or coach.

The launch-test-feedback-improve cycle is an essential one. And it is also one that is sometimes neglected. It requires commitment, communication, time, and resources. It requires a clear and shared understanding between everyone involved about what is being done, what can be expected, and the conditions in which and/or timeframe over which a new program or idea might need to demonstrate measurable impact.

It can be easy for coaches, athletes, performance directors, and innovation personnel themselves, to get excited about the launch of a new product, program, or idea. This can be especially true if they have been actively involved in the concept and design requirements (which they should be) along the way. However, managing expectations regarding the necessity of iteration and communicating these expectations clearly and consistently can go a long way in helping everyone stay apprised of progress and stay focused on the end goal.

The willingness and ability of an innovation team and their targeted users to adequately iterate before launching a 'final version' often plays a critical role in whether a program is successful or not. For example, there were at least five major iterations in a program designed to improve US skeleton performance that was eventually associated with a 2014 Olympic bronze medal in Sochi.[39] And, it took more than 18 months and a number of athlete- and team-specific customisations, before a relatively simple video review and match analysis program would be used effectively by the 2008 US Men's and Women's gold medal beach volleyball teams in Beijing.

Why innovation efforts fail

There are a number of examples from high performance sport where innovation teams have implemented 'solutions' that, for any number of a reasons, have failed to create a positive impact on performance. In every case, these interventions have been well intentioned and adequately resourced. And, in almost every case, they have targeted critical performance variables that should have resulted in substantial performance gains. So, why have they failed? Unsurprisingly, there are a multitude of reasons, any of which may derail even the most well-designed project.

Resources, including money, expertise, and time, can present significant challenges to innovation efforts. As mentioned previously, successful launches require not only prototyping and testing, but iteration and modification as well. If an innovation strategy is to succeed, budgeting and managing resources must be included to see projects through.

Risks and rewards, whether real or perceived, are constantly being evaluated, challenged, and balanced by coaches and athletes. Considering the short duration of most elite athletes' careers[40] and the terrifyingly short average tenure of professional sport coaches and managers,[41] the very real pressures associated with staying in sport are often manifest by coaches and athletes working with people, processes, and technologies they know and trust best.

If there is a perception that the risk of adopting something new will be greater than the potential reward, innovation efforts can be doomed to failure. These issues can be magnified if the unveiling of an innovation coincides with a major competition like the Olympic Games or World Championships. Here, the pressure to perform is so high that interventions launched at or immediately before the competition, for the sake of maintaining competitive advantage, can sometimes backfire.[42] Timing matters. As it pertains to the ability of coaches and athletes to feel comfortable if not empowered, planning needs to account for such periods of adaptation.

However, perhaps the most straightforward reason that the introduction of new, different, and potentially impactful things fail is that they simply aren't used. While much has been made about making marginal gains or finding the next 1% of improvement, the fact is, there is significant evidence that a lot of what we already know to be effective simply fails to get used. And, while this is a prevalent issue in sport, it is an all too common occurrence in other professions as well.[43]

In *Better: A Surgeon's Notes on Performance*, Dr. Atul Gawande explains this notion as perfectly and as concisely as I've ever encountered: "we have not effectively utilized what science has already given us. And we have not made remotely adequate efforts to change that".[44]

In the context of elite sport, a great deal of what we know about the science of performance and training is not utilised as completely or as regularly as it could be. It's easy to associate innovation with bleeding edge technology. And, in some cases, that's not only appropriate, it is necessary.

However, in the context of sport, even at the highest levels of competition, there will always be opportunities to 'innovate' by introducing things that we know to be true and that have been proven to make a positive and sustainable difference in the health, wellbeing, and performance of athletes. Ironically, these things are often the least expensive and most readily available to implement.

Conclusion

This chapter will end the way it started. Outcomes in elite sport are decided by the smallest of margins. Within these margins, everything matters. Athletes, coaches, and performance directors should continue to explore everything possible, within their means and within legal limits, to tilt the odds in their favour. Finding the things that matter most is a great place to start and can improve the efficiency and effectiveness of any innovation program.

Innovation, itself, is described as "something different that has impact". It is not just about introducing something new. It is about creating meaningful and measurable changes in performance outcomes or in the behaviours or attributes of things that contribute to them. Opportunities to improve lie waiting at the most basic and the most advanced ends of the sport performance spectrum. They lie in things we already know to be true and in things we have yet to discover. And, as a result, it really doesn't matter where we start. It just matters that we do.

Notes

1 E.g. Rohde, M. & Breuer, C. (2016). Europe's Elite Football: Financial Growth, Sporting Success, Transfer Investment, and Private Majority Investors. *Int. J. Financial Stud.*, **4**, 12; Walker, A. G. (2015). Division I Intercollegiate Athletics Success and the Financial Impact on Universities. *SAGE Open*; https://edition.cnn.com/2016/08/19/sport/olympic-rewards-by-country/index.html.

2 E.g., www.forbes.com/sites/kurtbadenhausen/2015/06/10/cristiano-ronaldo-heads-the-most-popular-athletes-on-social-media/#582953e44c97.

3 Anthony, S. D. (2011). *The Little Black Book of Innovation: How It Works. How to Do It.* Cambridge, MA: Harvard Business Press Review. p. 16.

4 www.sportsci.org/news/news9703/slapxtra.htm

5 E.g., www.pgatour.com/equipmentreport/2014/12/30/dimples-golf-balls.html; http://assets.press.princeton.edu/chapters/s6-6_10592.pdf.

6 https://en.wikipedia.org/wiki/LZR_Racer.

7 https://en.wikipedia.org/wiki/Fosbury_Flop.

8 www.olympic.org/ski-jumping-equipment-and-history.

9 www.si.com/vault/1974/07/29/616167/the-flip-that-led-to-a-flap.

10 https://perryponders.com/2015/04/21/in-1956-a-man-broke-the-current-javelin-world-record-by-spinning-it-around-like-a-discus/.

11 Hay, G. J., & Reid, G. J. (1988). *Anatomy, Mechanics and Human Motion* (2nd edn.). Upper Saddle River, NJ: Prentice Hall; Hay, J. G. (1993). *The Biomechanics of Sports Techniques* (4th edn.). Redwood City, CA: Benjamin Cummings; Glazier, P., Wheat, J. S., Pease, D. & Bartlett, R. M. (2006). The Interface of Biomechanics and Motor Control: Dynamic Systems Theory and the Functional Role of Movement Variability. In Keith Davids, Simon Bennett, Karl Newell (Eds.). *Movement System Variability*. pp. 49–69. Champaign, IL: Human Kinetics.

12 E.g., see Chow, J. E. & Knudson, D. V. (2011). Use of Deterministic Models in Sports and Exercise Biomechanics Research. Sports Biomechanics, **10**:3, 219–233, doi: 10.1080/14763141.2011.592212; Mcdonnell, L., Hume, P. & Nolte, V. (2013). A Deterministic Model Based on Evidence for the Associations Between Kinematic Variables and Sprint Kayak Performance. Sports Biomech, **12**, 205–220. doi: 10.1080/14763141.2012.760106.

13 cgs (centimeters, grams, seconds) sports refer to those in which outcomes are described in terms of distance, weight, or time. Representative examples include high jump, weightlifting, and swimming, respectively.

14 Takei, Y. (1998). Three-dimensional Analysis of Handspring with Full Turn Vault: Deterministic Model, Coaches' Beliefs, and Judges' Scores. *Journal of Applied Biomechanics*, **14**, 190–210; Takei, Y. (2007). The Roche Vault Performed by Elite Gymnasts: Somersaulting Technique, Deterministic Model, and Judges' Scores, *Journal of Applied Biomechanics*, **23**, 1–11.

15 Paul, R. & Elder, L. (2014). Learning the Art of Critical Thinking. Harvard Business Review Case Study. Product ROT221-PDF-ENG.

16 Gregersen, H. (2018). Better Brainstorming. Harvard Business Review. Accessed online at https://hbr.org/2018/03/better-brainstorming.

17 While appealing, care must be taken when adopting expert survey and 'gut instinct' approaches. While beyond the scope of this work, excellent resources are available on the sources and consequences of 'expert' opinion and prediction. See Kahneman, D. (2011). *Thinking Fast and Slow*. New York, NY: Farrar, Straus, and Giroux; Tetlock, P. E. & Gardner, D. (2015). *Superforecasting: The Art and Science of Prediction*. New York, NY: Crown; and Tetlock, P. E. (2017). *Expert Political Judgement: How Good Is It? How Can We Know?* Princeton, NJ: Princeton University Press.

18 Important considerations include, but are not limited to, experimental design, calibration and testing, data reduction and statistical analysis, and the ability to interpret and report the results in the context of the experiment or application itself.

19 For excellent references on this topic, see Hubbard, D. W. (2014). *How to Measure Anything: Finding the Value of Intangibles in Business*. Oxford: Wiley; and Barr, S. (2016). *Prove It!: How to Create a High-Performance Culture and Measurable Success*. Oxford: Wiley.

20 www.uksport.gov.uk/news/2014/01/28/british-bobsleigh-use-bae-systems-wind-tunnel-technology-on-road-to-sochi, www.bmwusa.com/athletic-innovations.html, www.aerosportsresearch.com/ownthepodium.htm.

21 https://hackathon.nba.com, https://es.mancity.com/noticias/club%20news/club%20news/2016/august/hack%20mcfc.

22 www.kaggle.com/competitions, www.thehaguesecuritydelta.com/innovation/innovation-competitions.

23 https://hbr.org/2008/02/getting-the-best-employee-idea.

24 www.uksport.gov.uk/news/2009/01/28/uk-sport-announce-first-garage-innovators-award, www.innovationmanagement.se/2014/06/09/corporate-open-innovation-portals-an-active-part-of-an-open-innovation-strategy/, https://gwin.secure.force.com.

25 https://hbr.org/2018/07/the-biggest-obstacles-to-innovation-in-large-companies?autocomplete=true.

26 Brown, T., & Kātz, B. (2009). *Change by Design: How Design Thinking Transforms Organizations and Inspires Innovation*. New York, NY: Harper Business; https://designthinking.ideo.com; https://ssir.org/articles/entry/design_thinking_for_social_innovation; https://www.ideou.com/pages/design-thinking.

27 https://hbr.org/2016/04/the-secret-history-of-agile-innovation.

28 www.movestheneedle.com/all-blog/2018/8/14/what-is-lean-innovation-components-and-examples.

29 www.mindtheproduct.com/2017/09/understanding-design-thinking-lean-agile-work-together/.

30 https://hbr.org/2014/12/choose-the-right-innovation-method-at-the-right-time.

31 https://leadersinsport.com.

32 www.conqagroup.com.

33 https://trackmangolf.com.

34 https://en.wikipedia.org/wiki/Elo_rating_system.

35 https://en.wikipedia.org/wiki/TrueSkill.

36 www.facebook.com/cnbc/posts/have-you-checked-out-our-cnbc-real-time-exchange-heat-maps-on-air/199447060079077/.

37 www.boeing.com/features/innovation-quarterly/dec2016/feature-technology-checklist.page.

38 www.who.int/patientsafety/topics/safe-surgery/checklist/en/ and Gawande, A. (2011). *The Checklist Manifesto: How to Get Things Right*. New York, NY: Picador.

39 https://ceas.uc.edu/news-1314/skeleton-sled-designed-by-uc-professor-rides-to-an-olympic-medal.html.

40 www.wsj.com/articles/the-shrinking-shelf-life-of-nfl-players-1456694959; https://nfllabor.wordpress.com/2011/04/18/what-is-average-nfl-player's-career-length-longer-than-you-might-think-commissioner-goodell-says/.

41 Take your pick of the following: www.businessinsider.com/coaches-managers-tenure-nfl-mlb-nba-nhl-premier-league-2016-12, www.leaguemanagers.com/documents/55/LMA_End_of_Season_Report_and_Statistics_2016-17.pdf, www.theguardian.com/football/2016/may/26/sack-race-record-managerial-dismissals, www.wsj.com/articles/the-premier-league-cant-stop-firing-managers-1521213815.

42 A notable and recent example unfolded at the 2014 Winter Olympic Games in Sochi. See https://deadspin.com/ditching-the-new-under-armour-suit-didnt-help-speedska-1523482428 and www.wsj.com/articles/us-speedskating-asks-for-permission-to-change-suits-1392406996?tesla=y.

43 See Heath, D. & Heath, C. (2010). *Switch: How to Change When Change Is Hard*. New York, NY: Crown Business, in particular, the story regarding the 100,000 Lives Campaign led by Dr. Donald M. Berwick (www.ihi.org/Engage/Initiatives/Completed/5MillionLivesCampaign/Documents/Overview%20of%20the%20100K%20Campaign.pdf).

44 Gawande, A. (2007). *Better: A Surgeon's Notes on Performance*. New York, NY: Metropolitan Books. p. 232.

Part IV
Managing elite performance systems

In many respects, the first two sections of this book have, we hope, shed some light on the people and processes that elite performers usually interact with most often. Indeed, we have firstly considered how coaches are (or should be) essential ingredients for success across elite sport systems through their support of many of the 'day-to-day' or 'technical' activities that feed directly into 'on the day' performance. On a similar front, the role that formal science and scientists can play – both as a uni- and, much more so, an inter-disciplinary support package – has also been emphasised in the previous section. However, of course, for any elite system to be optimally effective, this more 'day-to-day' or 'technical' input needs to be locked to a broader, and long-term direction. Given the number and/or nature of coaches and support practitioners involved, these inputs also need to be optimally co-ordinated so that performers can develop, prepare, and perform as efficiently and effectively as possible. In short, a job that is overseen by the leader of the system in question.

Of course, the importance of leadership has long been recognised in a sporting sense, with a multitude of books, studies, blogs, and other media continuing to dedicate themselves to the topic. There are also a vast number of consultants who specialise in this area, offering services and guidance on what is an intriguing and hugely impactful aspect of team dynamics and social behaviour. Against this context, the purpose of this section is to provide a range of perspectives on the leadership process in elite sport systems. Recognising that these systems are highly variable, depending on each sport's demands, goals, resources, and culture (among other factors), these perspectives again cover a host of environments. Additionally, our focus remains on *how* and *why* these individuals work in the manner they do.

To kick things off, the first chapter from our group of leaders comes from Neil McCarthy, based on his experiences of managing academies and talent pathways in professional and Olympic sport. In this contribution, Neil describes the nature of professional sport academies, issues of coherence, the Olympic sport contrast, challenges for academies and talent pathways, and ideas on the nature of effective pathways and ways to optimise them. From this base, we then move to consider the co-ordination of a multidiscipline support service with elite sports in Ireland. In this chapter, Phil Moore describes leadership from a national institute perspective and covers aspects of vision and mission, the challenge of introducing a new system, the nature of this system's functioning and performance, the evolution of relationships, working in partnerships, and working with performers specifically.

Moving from support services to leadership in a national governing body, Chapter 22 sees Tim Jones reflect on his experiences as a performance director, namely with the UK's Olympic gymnastics and Paralympic athletics programmes. In this contribution, Tim offers an overview of the performance director role in a UK Olympic and Paralympic sport context, before considering the requirements of this role; including the ability to manage the early phases of your tenure, aligning the overall culture and philosophy of the programme, protecting and prioritising the programme in what is a contested and complex setting, and working against a long-term vision and plan. Finally, Tim offers his thoughts on the present and future of the PD role, including newly emerging challenges, its positioning in relation to other power structures, and learning how to lead.

Taking another step up the chain of influence, Chapter 23 then provides a perspective on the leadership of an entire national system, covering the co-ordination of elite performance programmes across multiple national governing bodies. In this chapter, Alex Baumann describes his approaches as CEO for both Canada's "Own the Podium" programme and High Performance Sport New Zealand. More specifically, Alex introduces the main responsibilities for CEOs of national systems before considering *what* to deliver in this role, covering strategic as well as 'people, culture, and environment' focused targets. From here, Alex then reflects on *how* he has worked to achieve these outcomes, including his approaches to developing a partnership approach, providing and promoting challenge, and embracing and enabling urgency.

Continuing with our pursuit of comparisons and contrasts, Chapter 24 is delivered by Frédéric Paquet and focuses on his leadership of professional sport organisations or, more precisely, professional football organisations. In this account, Frédéric reflects on his roles as CEO of AS Saint-Étienne FC and Lille Olympique Sporting Club in France and focuses in particular on the styles of leadership employed, why football is different to other sports and businesses, and obstacles faced in the job. Finally, and building on messages from Frédéric and others in this section, Kieran File then considers the importance of effectively managing and engaging with the media. In this contribution, Kieran takes an intentionally broad look at this feature in elite sport systems, considering how performers, coaches, and leaders can handle – and make the most of – their interactions. In doing so, Kieran discusses the role of impression management, the critical role of context, approaches to relationship management, and, finally, how the media are often used to achieve other interpersonal goals, such as positively impacting the perceptions of some and 'playing mind games' with others.

All in all, we hope that the variety in this section provides a useful comparison and contrast on the leadership challenge in elite sport – as well as, of course, highlighting some common themes. As a primer for these themes – and a backdrop to this section more broadly – the chapter that follows sees Andrew introduce some important considerations around the leadership role and process in contemporary elite sport. More specifically, Andrew discusses the overall goals of leadership in this domain, before exploring the value and nature of high performing cultures for achieving them. In particular, attention is given to the influence of the team, department, or organisation's purpose and identity, systems, structures, geography, and people. From here, some of the internal and external challenges faced by leaders when developing these pillars of culture are outlined, before considering some important processes, mechanisms, behavioural styles, and skills for succeeding in the job. Of note, these include a focus on the 'bright' *and* 'dark' sides of leadership behaviour, as well as the typically under-considered role of the leader's thinking skills.

19

Culture, leadership, and management with elites

Andrew Cruickshank

Introduction

As the formal organisation of elite sport continues to increase around the world, leadership is one of the most impactful factors for all of those operating across the domain. Indeed, the ways in which all groups function can be linked to the perceptions, intentions, and actions of those with responsibility for leading them (e.g., Sam, 2012). These leaders can be of both the *formal* variety (e.g. CEOs, performance directors, head coaches, academy managers, heads of sports science and medicine, team captains) and of the more *informal* variety (e.g. specialist coaches, expert practitioners, individuals who link different sub-groups together, influential parents). These leaders can also shape how their group operates through both the *presence* and *absence* of their perceptions, intentions, and actions (i.e. what is *not* said or done can be equally impactful as what *is* said and done). In short, what leaders feel, think, and do matters a lot for everyone!

Given the potential scale of their influence in elite sport systems, and to help set up the rest of this section, this chapter focuses on formal leaders; namely, those with ultimate responsibility for the performance of a whole team, department, or organisation (e.g. CEOs, performance directors, managers, heads of services, and head coaches). In many respects, the challenge facing these leaders has intensified in modern elite sport; or, at least, significantly evolved. More specifically, the pressure placed on formal leaders has become particularly intense and unforgiving in many settings, with the termination or discontinuation of contracts a common occurrence. This is particularly so in many professional sports; however, higher levels of turnover are now apparent in a number of domains (e.g. the performance director role within Olympic sports). Indeed, reflecting the fervent pursuit of success from boards of directors, funders, fans, the public and others – fuelled by a fast-paced and usually critical mainstream and social media – leader turnover is almost a 'standard operating procedure'. Of course, the turnover of leaders can sometimes have the desired effect; in fact, some teams, departments, and organisations have found that a regular change of leader is a viable strategy for long-term success (relative to their desired goals). On the flip side, and arguably in many more cases, elite teams, departments, or organisations often return to their previous levels of performance soon after a formal leader is replaced, or experience a continued downturn.

Against this general picture, the purpose of this chapter is to provide an overview of the leadership challenge in elite sport; reflecting both current contexts and trends on what the future seems to hold. More specifically, this chapter firstly considers the goals of leadership in elite sport to further establish a frame of reference. Secondly, attention turns to the role of culture in achieving these goals, with focus placed on some components that can optimise the functioning of a team, department, or organisation. As the implementation of these principles is often much easier said than done, however, the third section then outlines some of the key challenges in creating and sustaining high performing cultures from both 'inside and outside the tent'. On this basis, the final section then describes some particular processes, styles, and skills for leading effectively in the complex and contested world of elite sport.

The goals of leadership in elite sport

Of course, any consideration of what leaders need to do to be effective in elite sport has to be framed against the goals that they are ultimately responsible for achieving. In this respect, the most obvious answer to this is sporting success! Indeed, most if not all leaders in elite sport are tasked with delivering either *new* levels or types of success, a *return* to prior levels or types of success, or *sustained* levels or types of success. Significantly, such success is relative to the team, department, or organisation that the leader oversees. So, for example, this may equate to winning titles or reaching the 'next level' for leaders of senior elite teams, or to developing players who go on to establish themselves at senior level for leaders of elite sport pathways or academies. In sum, leaders in elite sport are tasked with constantly pushing the bar and delivering outcomes that surpass expectations and/or their competitors; especially those with whom they share a long competitive history.

That being said, the extent to which various stakeholders perceive the 'relativeness' of success (in what is a chiefly "here and now/we need success today" world) is a different question! Indeed, as well as different perceptions on what appropriate success is, boards of directors, fans, the public, the media, and, of course, those within the team, department, or organisation itself, can all have different opinions on whether they have been successful; or achieved this in the best *way* (e.g. the playing style of a football team). These points will be returned to later in the chapter as they are crucial in shaping the way in which leaders lead (and how they are perceived). For now, however, the key message at this stage is that leading in elite sport is focused on a pursuit for new, greater, or sustained sporting achievement.

On this basis, one clear implication for those leading in elite sport is the value of their team, department, or organisation's culture. Indeed, the chances of any type of success being achieved (i.e. of the 'new', 'greater', or 'sustained' variety) will be boosted by the presence of a strong, enduring, performance-supporting culture. Indeed, developing such a culture can help an incumbent or new leader to survive in their role; it can also give a newly appointed leader a better chance of survival when this culture is already in place. But what exactly are high performing cultures and what are they made from?

Achieving success: high performing cultures and their components

Despite being one of the most commonly referred to factors in elite sport, 'culture' is still often vaguely defined and deployed by those working within and commentating on the domain. Indeed, although it is often held up as one of the major reasons for achievements or under-achievements, culture is still often used as a catch-all for any behaviour within a group – positive and negative, or more socially desirable and less socially desirable. In this sense, and as obvious as it seems, it is important to remember that culture is a group-level factor: the practice and performance of individuals within the group *may* tell us a lot about the culture in which they operate; but they may also tell us little. Instead, when thinking and talking about culture, it is important to focus on how a whole *group* and its *sub-groups* operate; and even more specifically, how they operate *normally*.

Certainly, while many detailed and sometimes elaborate definitions of culture exist, perhaps one of the simplest and most useful is that culture is "what is *normal* for how *we* do things on our best days, on our worst days, and on our typical days". For a culture to be truly high per-forming, this 'normality' will encourage and reinforce individuals in (a) making day-to-day, moment-to-moment decisions that support their group's goals; and (b) regulating this focus and way of working both within and across generations of their group (i.e. as personnel change). It is important to note, however, that high performing cultures are not inherently 'nice' or 'com-fortable'; at least as defined by wider society. Indeed, as with any group who seek to truly push the boundaries of which they are capable, a degree of ruthlessness, conflict, and intense debate is often needed to catalyse *optimal* progress. In this respect, the reference to high performi*ng*, rather than high perform*ance*, cultures is intentional: even though all elite teams operate in high perfor-mance and may achieve notable success, this does not inevitably mean that they are making the most of their potential. As such, a high performi*ng* culture is shown when a group's *normal* ways of working: (a) optimises their short-term performance; (b) persists across time; and (c) leads to consistent long-term success relative to resources.

High performing cultures: some notable components

In the grand scheme of leading in elite sport, identifying what the goals are for a team, depart-ment, or organisation – and recognising how a strong culture will help to achieve these – is the relatively straightforward part. Far more difficult, of course, is actually making them happen. Clearly, what is normal for a specific team, department, or organisation is shaped by a large number of components. More specifically, establishing, evolving, or sustaining a high perform-ing culture is influenced, amongst other factors, by the group's *purpose and identity, systems, structures, geography*, and *people*.

With regards to *purpose and identity*, the normal workings of a group are of course shaped by the goals that they are ultimately striving for, the broader vision and mission that drives why they do what they do, plus a sense of "who we are" in relation to competitors. In terms of *systems*, these relate to the ways in which a group works on a more procedural level; which includes aspects such as funding, selection, and recruitment, reward and reinforcement, per-formance management, and internal/external reporting. As well as what the group does, the *structures* within which they work are also key in shaping normal practice. For example, this can include the extent to which organisation is hierarchical or flatter in nature, the levels or grouping of staff/performers, and use of decision-making bodies (e.g. senior leadership groups). *Geography* is of course another powerful influence on what is normal for a given team, depart-ment, or organisation; with the proximity or distance between members of the group – either on a local, national, or international scale – shaping what can and can't be done on a day-to-day basis. Finally, but arguably playing the greatest role, the *people* who make up the group are clearly fundamental in influencing how a group operates.

While an awareness of these components of culture can help leaders to channel their efforts, it is also important to recognise that no one purpose and identity, system, structure, geographi-cal spread, and type of person is innately 'right' or 'wrong' for building, evolving, or sustaining a high performing culture. As stressed throughout this book, the extent of one approach being 'right' or 'wrong' depends on the specific challenge and the specific context. In this sense, and as each group is characterised by its own history, goals, and resources, no one type of culture can deliver success for all, or arguably even most. Further complicating the challenge for leaders in the high exposure world of elite sport, the environments in which they work are also highly contested. Indeed, with a multidimensional focus on performance, entertainment, and financial security, what is 'right' or 'wrong' for a *group* is rarely aligned to the interests or opinions of *all*, or sometimes even *most* of its stakeholders.

Cultural challenges for leaders in elite sport

Building on this point of contest, the primary challenges facing leaders in elite sport can be broadly classified as relating to *internal interests and influence* and *external interests and influence*.

Internal interests and influence

In contrast to environments whereby power and control typically flow in a more top-down manner within a team, department, or organisation, power and control in elite sport can also flow, to a significant extent, from the bottom-up and laterally. For example, with the mix of high egos, high wages, the public nature of performance, and high exposure in the media, senior performers can often hold major authority when it comes to their team's functioning. Indeed, many performers in elite sport earn more than their coaches, support staff, or leaders, with major implications on team dynamics and management approaches. In fact, scenarios whereby individuals work against their group to pursue their own interests are commonplace; either by being actively-disruptive (e.g. player revolts) or passively-disruptive (e.g. refusing to follow a new training plan). Notably, this isn't just a strain for leaders of senior athletes; academies and talent development programmes are replete with equivalent challenges, if less extreme, from influential performers.

From a staffing perspective, leaders in elite sport also need to typically co-ordinate the work of a diverse range of staff; covering disciplines such as technical coaching, strength and conditioning, nutrition, physiotherapy, sport psychology, and scouting. However, as each of these disciplines is guided by their own distinct codes of practice and/or objectives, the risks for damaging conflict are often apparent. Add the ego element to this pot again – given that support staff have had to outperform their peers to acquire their roles and naturally aspire for their own progression – and the challenge becomes even more apparent. In sum, predictable social hierarchies seldom seem to prevail within the teams, departments, and organisations of elite sport.

External interests and influence

As well as the challenges brought by internal interests and influence, the organisation, funding, and public consumption of elite sport means that a host of external stakeholders also play a key role in shaping what is 'normal' in the domain. Based on their ultimate decision-making authority, boards of directors (or oligarch owners in the case of many professional teams) reflect one such source. Problematically, many owners and members of boards are rarely experts (and are sometimes even relative novices) when it comes to understanding and supporting *performance* sport. Indeed, compared to the complexity that they may see in their own professional domain, owners and directors can often see the challenges in sport to be easier; perhaps due to the product being on public display and open for comment from *anyone* – as fuelled by the regularity or scale of the fixtures/events, their coverage by the mainstream media, and the interest they stir on social media.

In some cases, the challenges facing leaders in elite sport are further complicated by the role of external funding agencies/sources and sponsors. Indeed, these groups can have a major stake in the performance of the team, department, or organisation that they support; and therefore a major say in how things operate through the conditions (both 'written' and 'unwritten') that they set for continued investment. Additionally, and as suggested above, the media can also play a significant role – sometimes *the* most significant role – in shaping the practices and performances of different cultures in elite sport. In this respect, a clear concern for any leader is when the media start leading the agenda for fans and/or the public, who already exert significant influence with regards to what is expected from the performers or team in question. Combined with the power exerted from other bodies and groups, such as national and international governing bodies, external service providers (e.g. institutes of sport, facility owners), the local community, an organisation's wider (i.e. non-performance) staffing and membership, and former performers, the picture is even more complicated!

In summary, elite sport is a socially complex and dynamic system that generates and extenuates challenges both continually and rapidly. More specifically, the involvement of a range of powerful stakeholders – with their own particular interests, agendas, and opinions – means that the elite sport domain is politically-charged and relatively unpredictable. As such, to build and sustain a high performing culture, leaders require a set of processes, behaviours, and skills that can help them to gain and stay in control as much as possible.

Processes, mechanisms, styles, and skills for leading and managing in elite sport

Processes and mechanisms for leading and managing

Based on goals of elite team leadership (i.e. to deliver 'new', 'greater', or 'sustained' success), alongside the internal and external challenges just described, one particularly key process for elite team leaders is that of *change management*. Indeed, whether trying to guide a group, department, or organisation towards new, greater, or sustained success, the ability to oversee change to catch up, match, or stay ahead of competitors is essential. Such work may equate to a change *in* culture (i.e. doing what's already happening but better), a change *of* culture (i.e. bringing in new principles or practices), or a change *for* culture (i.e. reorienting towards a new set of goals). In fact, the demands of elite sport often mean that a combination or all three of these are needed at the same time (e.g. in response to major funding changes). In this respect, our own research has highlighted a number of steps that support such change processes: including a detailed analysis of the challenge and current environment, managing internal and external stakeholder perceptions, delivering 'quick wins' as change is starting to be rolled out, holding back on other actions until the group is ready to evolve, and recruiting and harnessing cultural allies and change agents (Cruickshank, Collins, & Minten, 2014, 2015; or "cultural architects": Railo, 1986). Inherent across these steps is a focus on developing a view that: (a) the old culture or way of doings things is no longer functional, engaging, or rewarding; and (b) the new culture or way of doing things holds greater potential for individual and shared success.

As part of the change process – and leadership in more stable times – it is important that a leader adopts a 360-degree approach if they want to build and sustain the most robust culture. Indeed, rather than a one-way process, cultures are most robust when leaders work in a multi-directional way; as depicted in Figure 19.1.

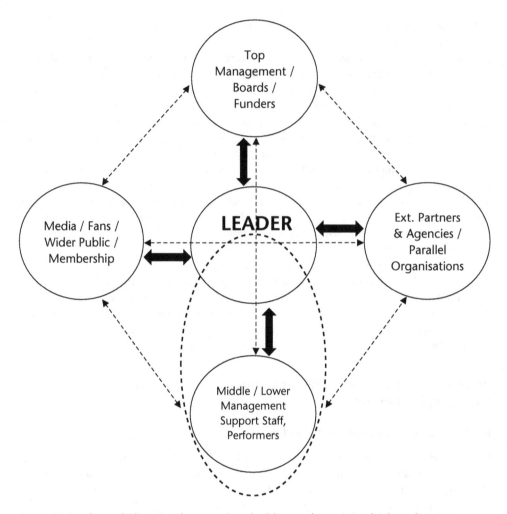

Figure 19.1 The multidirectional approach to building and sustaining high performing cultures

Source: Adapted from Collins & Cruickshank, 2012

In other words, if a leader tries to develop a 'cultural bubble' by working only with those that they are directly responsible for (see the dashed oval around the leader and middle/lower management, support staff, and performers), then the risk of this being 'popped' by those *above* (e.g. Boards of Directors, funders) or by those *laterally* (e.g. fans, media, the public, external partners, and agencies) is elevated. As such, a multidirectional view recognises the power, agency, and influence of *all* stakeholders in the wider environment; and that this power, agency, and influence opens and closes doors for a leader to lead in a certain way at a certain time (e.g. secure funding for a lengthy period of time can allow the leader to develop performers in a more long-term manner). A 360-degree view also works to help the leader to gather social and political information so that their team, department, or organisation adjusts to the evolving perceptions and demands of those around them. Moreover, this approach also allows the leader to have greater impact when consistent messages are sent through a variety of channels (e.g. upwards to the board, outwards to the media, downwards to performers). Such work is vital when recognising that it is often easier to revert to a previous or common perception or attitude than continue establishing a new one.

As suggested by this description, the relationships with stakeholders in elite sport can rarely be one-way if everyone is to get the *best* out of each other; whether that be in terms of the best support or the best performance (hence the solid, 'two-way arrows' emanating from and back to the leader with each key stakeholder group in Figure 19.1). In short, the power in these systems is usually "decentred" (Bevir & Richards, 2009): so it flows across the entire spectrum of stakeholders and can assist or restrict what everyone can do; especially the leader of the team, department, or organisation in question. As such, the implication is that a flow of information and power between leader, followers, and stakeholders is essential: when this is present, the chance for co-ordinated action is increased; when this is missing, the opposite occurs. Of course, this point may seem rather intuitive; however, given the challenge of just overseeing the team, department, or organisation for which the leader is responsible, finding the time, energy, and intent to engage in what often feels like more peripheral issues (e.g. how the media are reporting on current form; the board's concerns over the noise from other coaches in the system) is not straightforward. Indeed, building and sustaining a culture requires much plate-spinning!

Given the challenges of dealing with multiple interests and opinions, the need for a leader to operate both *overt* and *covert* agendas also becomes clear. More specifically, overt work relates to that which is 'visible' and clearly attributable to the leader (e.g. face-to-face interactions; introduction of new systems). In contrast, covert work relates to that which is much more indirect and subtle; important in the sense that it can help leaders to push things along without engaging in unfitting or unproductive levels of opinion-checking, debate, and negotiation across stakeholders.

In this sense, leaders often work to enable the emergence of desired perceptions and behaviours more 'naturally' from within the group; or at least with less obvious top-down direction. More specifically, and grounded in ideas from behavioural economics (Thaler and Sunstein, 2003), leadership effectiveness is often linked to the ability to shape the context in which stakeholders act and make decisions, rather than directly negotiating these actions and decisions; a feature that we have also found in our own research in elite sport, and one that is reflected in other chapters in this section of the book (Cruickshank, Collins, & Minten, 2013). As such, the challenge of agreeing what is 'right' or 'wrong' for everyone can be evaded or softened to some degree as stakeholders instead base their actions and decisions on what they feel to be *normal* or *desirable* (rather than overtly encouraged, requested, or demanded by the leader). In other words, leaders can create physical, structural, and psychosocial contexts that: a) encourage stakeholders to make their *own* decisions on adopting culture-supporting behaviours or not; but b) be *more likely* to adopt these than not (think about the reason why sweets and chocolate are placed near the conveyor belt in supermarkets!). Such shaping may involve things like a public presentation of performance data (to nudge players to outperform each other), building depth across positions in a squad (to elevate effort in training due to the increased level of competition), designing training sessions to expose the limitations of older players who have become negative influences (to adjust their standing in the team), bringing the media into a team environment when travelling to or at competitions (to encourage more favourable reporting), highlighting areas of wider challenge/less obvious progression to the media (to encourage a board to see the bigger picture), and working closely with less obvious cultural architects, such as those who glue different sub-groups in the team, department, or organisation together (to keep the *weight* of perceptions onside, not just those of the formal leadership group, such as captains or assistant coaches). Overall, effective leadership in elite sport is done as much in the background – sometimes even the shadows – as it is upfront.

Behavioural styles for leading and managing

One other key point to recognise from this picture is that leaders, to achieve sustained success in their domains, have to be dynamic and adaptive in their approach. Indeed, rather than finding a style that works and sticking to it resolutely, those who survive and thrive the best are usually those who are adept at sourcing feedback and new information, then using this to adapt (for a comparison, see Theodoridis & Bennison, 2009). Indeed, if leaders are to build and sustain a common and consistent approach in their complex and contested settings, the need to consciously switch between different styles of behaviour becomes apparent. Tying in with an earlier message in this chapter, it is also vital that these styles fit their team, department, or organisation's vision, mission, and goals. As an effective way to demonstrate this, consider the noticeably different styles of leadership that are successful across different sports, in the same sport, and even in the same team (e.g. when a new head coach with a different style gets more from the same group of players than the previous head coach did). As well as the success of different styles, these differences are also usually demanded by those responsible for appointing leaders (e.g. a board of directors identifying the need for a new style to take a sport onto 'the next level'). Finally, there might also be major costs when leaders persist with a style in the face of feedback that suggests that adaptation is needed (e.g. to respond to a series of poor results, negative perceptions of the team's performance from the media, or performers becoming bored with training methods).

Overall, therefore, one clear implication to emerge from this situation is that, to have the best chance of delivering sustained success, leaders need a broad behavioural repertoire; in other words, they need to be able to act in lots of different ways given that they face a lot of different situations and challenges (Cruickshank & Collins, 2016). In this respect, no *one* style of leadership can provide 'the answer' for leaders in elite sport; sometimes impact will come from a transformational approach, sometimes a transactional approach, sometimes an autocratic approach, sometimes even a 'dark' approach (i.e. using behaviours that most followers or observers would consider to be 'socially undesirable'). Indeed, although many autobiographies, textbooks, documentaries, studies, and commentators regularly point to the 'bright' (or socially desirable) parts of a successful leader's repertoire, much less reported are the actions taken to, either primarily or exclusively, further their own agenda and/or influence, exploit, block, or derail the agenda of others. In fact, acts of a Machiavellian, ruthless, socially dominant and cynical nature, for example, are common and – significantly – can be beneficial for most members of the team, department, or organisation in the long-term (e.g. engineering the exit of a senior performer who is suffocating the development of others: Cruickshank & Collins, 2015). In this way, socially undesirable behaviours can often serve socially desirable outcomes; just as much as socially desirable behaviours can often serve socially undesirable outcomes (e.g. lowering the social status of older performers by inspiring younger players to outperform them in new training drills). Again, the realm of leadership in elite sport is far from 'neat and tidy'!

Of course, leaders who consistently engage the dark side of leadership aren't likely to last long (or as long as they might) in their team, department, or organisation; we know that leaders who are successful in the long-run work towards more positive, inclusive, and shared aspirations overall. However, socially undesirable actions can and do play a role in enabling positive outcomes when they are used in an *intentional, intermittent,* and *appropriate* fashion. The 'dark side' of behaviour is, of course, a sensitive topic given that such behaviour is more commonly linked to negative outcomes. Nevertheless, the fact that socially undesirable acts are, in many respects, an entirely normal and predictable element of leadership means that it is naïve to overlook this area; it is also naïve to class any use of the dark side as automatically inappropriate. For example, a leader's self-serving agenda in the short term (e.g. securing one's job by exposing the frailties of other staff to central decision-makers) *might* open a path to deliver greatest benefit for most members of the team, department, or organisation in the long-term (e.g. via the recruitment of more talented staff). In this sense, using the dark side cannot be fully *justified* by a leader's motive or the outcome achieved, but it can be *qualified* by their motive to help us to consider how appropriate (or inappropriate) it was *in context*. In sum, leaders in elite sport are not (and are often not expected to be) 'nice' or 'inspirational' all of the time or with most people. The dark side of leadership is also not inherently 'wrong' and, in fact, failing to engage it can sometimes cost a team in their pursuit for success; albeit that particular care is needed given the potential for events to spiral if used inappropriately.

Cognitive skills for leading and managing

Tying this message together with the need for adaptation, it is clear that leadership in elite sport, as with most endeavours where people work with other people, operates on an 'it depends' and 'shades of grey' basis. In other words, few 'rights and wrongs' or 'definitive answers' exist when the challenge is so complex and evolving. Instead, leadership has to be viewed in context and so – if they are to perform *optimally* – leaders in elite sport also need to have excellent thinking skills: almost every action needs to be locked to a clear goal (in the short-, medium-, and long-term), weighed up against alternatives, assessed by their anticipated effects, and then monitored and modified (Collins & Cruickshank, 2015; Cruickshank & Collins, 2016). In this way, excellence requires leaders to think about what approach should (and shouldn't) be taken, with whom (and who not), where (and where not), when (and when not) and why (and why not) one way over others. Indeed, the professional judgement and decision-making (hereafter PJDM) skill of a leader is an often under-considered and under-celebrated but absolutely essential driver of success. In short, it provides a foundation for – and explanation of – *why* leaders actually do what they do.

As one particularly relevant feature of PJDM in leadership, *nested thinking* – as was introduced in Chapter 1 – provides a useful lens for understanding and informing a leader's actions. More specifically, it is a core way for leaders to perform effectively, flexibly, and innovatively in complex, dynamic, and contested environments. Figure 19.2 demonstrates how leaders can set themselves up to act in a coherent and consistent way across the micro- (e.g. day-to-day), meso- (e.g. month to month), and macro- (e.g. year to year) levels of their behaviour. Through an awareness of the 'bigger pictures', day-to-day decisions and actions can then be locked *simultaneously* into the goals for that week, which are locked into goals for that month, which are locked to the goals for that phase, year, and so on (as supported by the feedback and feedforward loops between within levels of the plan: see solid, two-way arrows in Figure 19.2).

Overall, the point is that decisions and actions taken in the 'here and now' will be most impactful when they are placed within a clear short-, medium-, and long-term agenda – and to do so, this requires a clear agenda in the first place! Attending to any of the agendas in isolation will also, more often than not, curtail the team's potential and performance; even though this might not be immediately clear (e.g. consider leaders who have achieved significant early success but then failed to anticipate and prepare for what was to come next). In this respect, a leader's

Timeline & Objectives/Activities

Level of Action	Example Leader Agenda	Year 1	Year 2	Year 3
Long-Term (3 years)	**Performance:** Establish team in European competition while sustaining level domestically **Strategic:** Build depth within the squad through targeted player development and recruitment; stagger rotation of players in key blocks of games **Socio-political:** Establish culture that encourages players to push collective standards; engage CEO / fans and use media to manage expectations	Build preparation around key domestic blocks to sustain level; find 'our way to prepare & play' in European games;	[Defined objectives]	[Defined objectives]

Quick Wins plus Setting the Tone & Direction

Level of Action	Example Leader Agenda	Pre-Season	August-December	January-April	[Following blocks]
Medium-Term (1st season)	**Strategic:** Recruitment of 'multi-position players' to support rotation; investment / extra allocation of resources into high potential younger players who can fill gaps in squad / perform domestically soon **Socio-political:** Sell 'squad depth' needs to Board; send messages and set challenges through media around longer-term goals, plans, and expectations; **Tactical/Motivational:** Work on 'shared mental models' for European comp prep and play, plus ability to switch styles; develop players' skills in performing within defined rotation policy	Regular contact with Board and Head of Recruitment; exploit opportunities to integrate high-potential youngsters; introduce long-term 'Euro-play' principles	Exploit home Euro games and gradually expose young players to domestic level; key players freshest and focused for key games	[Defined objectives]	[Defined objectives]

Gradually Introduce & Reinforce Refined Style & Values against Long-Term Agenda

Level of Action	Example Leader Agenda	Week 1	Week 2	Week 3	Week 4
Short-Term (4-week block)	**Tactical:** Focus on playing to current strengths and help key players to build early momentum **Interpersonal:** Keep senior and influential players on board; as well as players who aren't playing much but who are influential for squad dynamics and contributing to future objectives	[Defined objectives]	[Defined objectives]	[Defined objectives]	[Defined objectives]

Figure 19.2 An example of an elite team leader's nested planning

Source: Adapted from Collins & Cruickshank, 2015

thinking skills are not just evidenced by the positive outcomes that they deliver, but also, in large part, by the smoothness of the journey. In short, it is the thinking skills of leaders that help them to get – and then stay – one step ahead.

Concluding comments

To set up the rest of this section of the book, this chapter has provided an overview of the leadership challenge in elite sport; as based on current contexts and trends in the domain. More specifically, this chapter opened by clarifying the basic goals that the leader of a whole team, department, or organisation is responsible for achieving. From here, focus then turned to the role of culture in achieving these – including a description of some key components – before highlighting some challenges that leaders face in their work on this area. In light of the messages to this point, final coverage was given to some relevant processes, styles, and skills for leading in the complex and contested world of elite sport. With regard to processes, change management, a 360-degree approach, enabling a 'to and fro' of power, and shaping contexts were identified as particularly useful. Similarly, the need for a broad behavioural repertoire was also raised, as were strong skills in perhaps one of the most under-considered, under-supported, and under-celebrated aspects of leadership: PJDM. If we have planned this right, the chapters that follow should now bring many of these themes and ideas to life – plus a few extras!

References

Bevir, M., & Richards, D. (2009). Decentring Policy Networks: A Theoretical Agenda. *Public Administration*, **87**, 3–14

Collins, D., & Cruickshank, A. (2015). Take a Walk on the Wild Side: Exploring, Identifying, and Developing Consultancy Expertise with Elite Performance Team Leaders. *Psychology of Sport & Exercise*, **16**, 74–82

Collins, D. & Cruickshank, A. (2012). 'Multidirectional Management': Exploring the Challenges of Performance in the World Class Programme Environment. *Reflective Practice*, **13**, 455–469

Cruickshank, A., & Collins, D. (2016). Advancing Leadership in Sport: Time to Take Off the Blinkers? *Sports Medicine*, **46**, 1199–1204

Cruickshank, A., & Collins, D. (2015). Illuminating and Applying "the Dark Side": Insights from Elite Team Leaders. *Journal of Applied Sport Psychology*, **27**, 249–267

Cruickshank, A., Collins, D., & Minten, S. (2015). Driving and Sustaining Culture Change in Professional Sport Performance Teams: A Grounded Theory. *Psychology of Sport & Exercise*, **20**, 40–50

Cruickshank, A., Collins, D., & Minten, S. (2014). Driving and Sustaining Culture Change in Olympic Sport Performance Teams: A First Exploration and Grounded Theory. *Journal of Sport & Exercise Psychology*, **36**, 107–120

Cruickshank, A., Collins, D., & Minten, S. (2013). Culture Change in a Professional Sports Team: Shaping Environmental Contexts and Regulating Power. *International Journal of Sports Science and Coaching*, **8**, 271–290

Railo, W. (1986). *Willing to Win*. Utrecht: Amas

Sam, M. (2012). Targeted Investments in Elite Sport Funding: Wiser, More Innovative and Strategic? *Managing Leisure*, **17**, 207–220

Thaler, R. H., & Sunstein, C. (2003). Libertarian Paternalism. *The American Economic Review*, **93**(2), 175–179

Theodoridis, C., & Bennison, D. (2009). Complexity Theory and Retail Location Strategy. *The International Review of Retail, Distribution and Consumer Research*, **19**, 389–403.

20

Developing elites

Academy systems

Neil McCarthy

Introduction

Having spent 12 years as a player with reasonable success, during a period of immense change within the game of rugby union on a global scale, I often feel blessed that I was playing during the onset of the professional game. Having to manage an alternative career alongside being as professional as one could be with a small 'p' in terms of the amateur status of the game has certainly influenced me as a coach and practitioner. A significant shift moving from working full-time to being a professional athlete almost overnight was a challenge. On reflection, my epistemological 'view of the world' has inevitably been influenced by the players I had the pleasure of playing with and against during my career, the coaching experiences I received as a player and finally the environments in which this was situated.

As such, having experienced a diverse range of inputs during these formative times as a player, I have always sought and felt the need for a balanced and pragmatic approach to my coaching practice. This has inevitably, and in turn, influenced my approach to providing talent development environments that offer a broad range of experiences aimed at what happens next as opposed to solely the here and now.

Reflecting on these experiences as a player has enabled me to think forward in terms of some of the key aspects that are essential to negotiating a talent pathway as an athlete or player. For example, at times I felt ill-prepared for various transitions across my career as a player, be it age grade through to senior level, or transitioning into the national squad with little to no support to prepare, process, and manage these experiences. Accordingly, I have always felt a need to prepare (formerly rugby players now aspirational Olympians) appropriately for the challenge of these difficult transitions in a way that is realistic and representative of the actual challenges that they will encounter prior to going through the real thing for the first time.

Essential to being able to effectively equip players or athletes with the skills to be able to progress to the top and stay at the top has been a focus for most talent development environments (TDEs) I have worked within. Mental skills have been highlighted extensively for many years as being essential to being an elite sport person and yet much of the provision, certainly from my experiences as a player, has been isolated intervention-focused transactional mental skills. The represents a limited 'Sport Psychology' rather than the embedded and transformational systems of 'Performance Psychology' that encompass a range of both mental skills and behavioural aspects nested within the cultural foundations of the TDE (Martindale et al., 2005; Henrikksen et al. 2010). This has been a key focus for me as a coach, which primarily has been influenced by my own experiences and perception of successful performance environments. I have simply sought to underpin and challenge my thinking and perception in these areas through study to provide a more robust evidence-based foundation to guide my practice.

Professional sport academies

I was academy director at both Leicester Tigers and Gloucester Rugby, both with significantly different approaches to talent development.

Clearly, Leicester Tigers is one of the most successful clubs within the English game and Gloucester Rugby is constantly striving to break in to the top four of the Premiership. Against this back-drop I have tried to establish evidence-based models to support the player development objectives of both clubs which sit within the broader academy landscape; a landscape that has evolved significantly from its inception in 2001 to the current time. The agreements that have been brokered between the professional clubs (PRL) and the Rugby Football Union (RFU) dictate a specific geographical recruitment area for each programme with strictly managed movement of players' protocols as part of that agreement.

In short, players from each academy can only be identified and developed within the outlined service area or a graduated compensatory mechanism (financial transfer system) becomes active; making simple identification of talented players potentially expensive. Of course, talent development is also expensive (Abbott et al., 2002) and, as such, these programmes are seeking to innovate and develop identification and development strategies to maximise their output in respect of talented players. There is, of course, a cost-benefit balance to be maintained for academy directors in the sense that senior performance environments are focused solely on performance and, therefore, simply identifying talented players rather than developing those players 'in house' can be persuasive.

Typically then, the academy system is represented by a series of staged progressions, each stage represented by age with the Developing Player Programme (DPP) and Player Development Groups (PDGs) accounting for identification and development pre U16. Post PDGs comprises the junior academy or other iterations of the same concept, which typically provide development for post-16 players and are layered thereafter in age bands comprising senior academy players generally post-18 years of age through until senior transition. Augmenting this system are the national age grade teams, which sit alongside the broad stages of the pathway at U16, U18, and U20 levels and are managed centrally by the Rugby Football Union (RFU).

The issue of coherence across the academy process and network

One of the most important challenges throughout this process is one of coherence between stakeholders. Traditionally, the community game (RFU) meets the professional game (professional clubs) at these early stages of the pathway, which over a significant period of time has made it difficult to strike a balance between the altruistic motivations of the community game and the needs of the professional game to identify, select, and confirm those few players that will form the basis of the academy system. These divergent views on the mechanisms and delivery of this stage of the pathway have led often to a lack of coherence in preparing players for transition beyond this initial stage.

Given the complexity at these primary interfaces with the talent pool between stakeholders (schools, local clubs, RFU, professional clubs), coaches, and practitioners across the TD and participation agendas, it is understandable that a lack of coherence across the network may be observed as a consequence. Therefore one of the primary issues in identifying and developing talent during the initial stages of the pathway is the notion of a 'best in best out' process, an approach which, having been highlighted as inaccurate through TID evolutionary processes can, given the coherence issues identified at the bottom end, potentially lead to a lack of coherence within senior management of professional clubs and their understanding of TD processes. Common sense is persuasive to CEOs/Directors of Rugby (DORs) and, unfortunately, much of the dynamics of TD are inherently unstable and often counterintuitive which does lead to a break down in understanding across the TD continuum, particularly when ambiguity exists throughout the TD system and amongst practitioners themselves!

Professional sport to Olympic sport

Having spent the best part of ten years working within professional sport I have taken much of the learning from this time and tried to apply a principles-first framework to my thinking in respect of my role as performance pathway and talent manager for British Skeleton. British Skeleton is the most successful winter sport for Team GB and UK Sport having achieved Olympic medals at every Olympic Games since its reintroduction into the Olympics back in 2002. My role is primarily to identify, recruit, confirm, and develop athletes with the capacity and potential to relatively quickly be successful at world level as part of the world class performance programme.

Clearly there are some significant differences between professional team sport and an individual Olympic sport in terms of the why, what, and how across the triad of athlete, coaching, and environment (Rees et al., 2016) and further in respect of the processes involved in the development of a system to support the differing objectives between the two.

For example skeleton in contrast to rugby union as a sport has little to no participation base to support recruitment of athletes and so many of the interface participation coherence issues do not manifest, however this brings a different set of issues when looking to recruit athletes for the world class programme.

The programme is underpinned by a need to artificially source talent from other sporting backgrounds through a range of initiatives focused on factors that form a large piece of the performance jigsaw (physiological measures). This is reflected in the nature and manner in which the programme is firstly able to identify potential athletes and secondly the development process to support those that are selected into the programme. Clearly many potential athletes are screened at a basic level to establish suitability for the sport. Typically these involve physical performance measures, which are then coupled with anthropometric measures unique to the demands of the sport. This process is refined and additional layers to the performance jigsaw are layered in such as 'perceptual cognition' and 'performance robustness'.

Accordingly developing a system that can assess relatively quickly the series of factors that will impact on progression is key. These factors can be broadly categorised into three areas. The 'CAN' factors i.e. the physical capacity and potential measures that are essential to the sport; secondly the 'HAVE' factors which are the experiences each athlete brings to the sport from the environments and sports they have encountered prior to selection, which is essential in determining capacity, potential, and signposting to areas of their global development that may need to be targeted; finally the 'DO' factors which when coupled with the 'CAN' and 'HAVE' factors produce an exceptional athlete. These 'DO' factors primarily centre on the cognitive, emotional, and psychological parameters of performance.

Academy environments and talent pathways – the challenges

The systems, models, and programmes focused on the identification and development of talent continue to evolve in their complexity and comprehensiveness (Cooke et al. 2010). Talent development (TD) is a costly business therefore accurate identification is now a major focus for many sporting bodies (Abbott and Collins, 2002).

In this context (rugby union) and reflecting on my experience, given the managed movement processes of junior players within rugby union, simply *identifying* players at specific points is now arguably as equally expensive. Unfortunately however, the empirical observations now prevalent within literature in relation to athletes' struggles to bridge the gap between junior elite and senior elite status indicates there is no clear theoretical framework in which to operate a model of high predictability (Simonton, 2001; Abbott and Collins, 2002; 2004). In fact significant evidence suggests the opposite and high burn out rates are consistently observed within TD programmes built on early identification, which brings these programmes usefulness consistently into question (MacNamara, Button & Collins, 2010a; 2010b).

In contrast to my experiences within rugby academies, skeleton fortuitously select athletes that have passed through many of the selection gateways that are prominent in organised sport. Therefore, we potentially benefit from other sports selecting and de-selecting early in their pathways. That's not to say that these athletes do not enter the pathway complete but certainly many of the unstable factors around maturation are established even if the effects linger.

It appears therefore that much of the focus over time in this area has been tailored towards creating models of identification that primarily engage talent at the earliest opportunity, in the hope that selecting talented youngsters will automatically produce a talent pipeline of the best adults. Certainly, for decision-makers in relation to funding this appears to be a common sense approach to ensuring a senior programme is suitably stocked with sufficient quality of athlete to be called upon when required. Unfortunately, these models have generally sought to identify talent through a limited range of one-off proficiency focused measures such as current performance (generally national age grade selection, for example in rugby) and anthropometric/physical performance data (the big kids) that fails to acknowledge the evolving nature of talent (Abbott and Collins, 2002; 2004).

Therefore, predictive identification models that utilise static and isolated conceptions of talent (technical and tactical/physical/anthropometric) variables could be described as problematic at best and simply inaccurate at worst, as they do not account for the evolution and interaction of talent over time particularly if these selections are made pre or during maturational disturbances (Simonton, 2001).

The non-linear nature of the development journey has been highlighted through a substantial body of research (Simonton, 2001; Abbott et al., 2005) and is leading a shift away from one-dimensional identification models, to models that acknowledge the multidimensional non-linear framework in which talent evolves. Despite the increasingly robust evidence against mass early *identification* and mass early *de-selection* of athletes owing to this non-linear progression, many potential athletes/players that could have gone on to be successful have been deselected as a consequence of this notion of a '*best in best out*' philosophy. Typified by those players or athletes demonstrating at a specific point in time, qualities that may not transition into senior level through maturation over a period of time. As a consequence, perhaps we see some being completely dis-enchanted with the experience and thus exiting sport even at recreation and participation level (Abbott and Collins, 2002; Abbott et al., 2005; Güllich and Emrich, 2012).

Modelling the pathway

Conversations abound in this space that are focused on managing the conflicting dynamics within an academy or talent pathway in terms of 'performance' now versus 'performance' later. The reality is that it is very difficult to manage with stakeholders owing in the main to perceptions of ability linked to current performance. Even in the face of and irrespective of the theoretical underpinning and lack of evidence to support such perceptions, nonetheless one needs to maintain a level of pragmatism because of the potential impact on other areas of the development process such as recruitment and retention of players or athletes as well as funding streams.

Accordingly, clarity of purpose aimed at the long-term objectives, clearly articulated, AGREED, and finally disseminated throughout the pathway is of absolute importance. Gaining this clarity and acknowledging the associated dynamics with TD from boards and agencies is a significant piece of the planning process that is often forgotten when caught up in the day-to-day management of a pathway. Providing consistency in the narratives that form the basis of the pathway and the various levels within is essential to maintaining a level of coherence.

Developing sufficient organisational coherence within a pathway and maintaining clarity and consistency is essential but can be problematic, many facets of the talent development experience particularly for non-athlete stakeholders are somewhat counterintuitive in the sense that they can often seem to contradict the very essence of high performance. For example, there is a negative correlation with age grade or junior level competition success and eventual senior success (Martindale et al., 2005) and so winning at age grade level is of little importance in the long term, therefore shifting away from such a focus would seem a logical step in maintaining the efficacy of the development process.

Notwithstanding this, competition is an important feature of the development process and an opportunity to explore the boundaries of performance at a moment in time providing meaningful opportunities and experience for growth, however, over-preparing for competition with a narrow focus of 'win now approach' all the time at the expense of 'longer term' objectives can create fractures within the overall pathway strategy if this is not clearly articulated in advance with athletes, parents, and other stakeholders.

Of course there are other practical factors to consider in these scenarios, such as the broader organisational perceptions of success. Parents, players, and support staff are also integral to perpetuating beliefs albeit for some the 'here and now' can and often is the pinnacle of their careers, therefore a balanced and 'nested' approach coupled with the right blend and depth of experience on an individual basis throughout pathways should be a priority (Martindale et al. 2005; Henrikksen & Stambulova, 2017). This is an important factor in maintaining coherence in the sense that unless there is a connection through stakeholders and the notion of reward and/or assessment (i.e. winning and losing) is aligned to the overall objectives of long-term development and learning, people will seek and pursue what they perceive to be of importance leading to a breakdown in the of the system (Martindale et al., 2005; Henrikksen & Stambulova, 2017).

This level of 'nested' thinking blending strategic objectives/purpose of a pathway with the aggregated and progressive needs of the individual at different points in time or stages of a pathway are of importance in firstly establishing a system and secondly maintaining momentum of a system in the long term.

Creating unified models for developing players or athletes for senior elite environments is a much-debated subject. Within the rugby union landscape in England, all 14 licensed academies operate significantly diverse development models albeit in various pyramid frameworks, that appear to promote a logical sequence of progression. However the notion that broad bases of participation and levels of participating numbers systematically reduce in a bottom-up hierarchal process, until the top tier of the pyramid is defined by elite athletes and elite competition, is now contested (Bailey et al., 2010). This traditional thinking in respect of the journey to senior elite level has been consistently popularised with many National Governing Body (NGB) policy-makers and despite its historical popularity with policy-makers a number of criticisms have been levelled at this approach (Bailey and Collins, 2013), notably the systematic exclusion of athletes, irrespective of how good they are or crucially how good they could become, as fewer and fewer are able to access the tiered process. Further consideration must be given towards the 'end game' in respect of this type of modelling as it is suggested the top tier can only be as strong as the influences and experiences offered through the lowest levels. The presumption of a linear progression through the system from one level to the next has now consistently been challenged as to its actual effectiveness (Abbott and Collins, 2002; Bailey and Collins, 2013). Various maturational, environmental, and psychosocial factors that also include the assumption that everyone selected for the next level has been selected on merit provide sufficient doubt as to the efficacy of such models as an effective TD aid (Martindale et al., 2005).

Given the issues associated with low predictability of developmental systems, national governing bodies and sports clubs continue to operate pyramid systems that by their very nature dictate a drop off as athletes' progress, or not, up the pyramid ladder (Abbott et al., 2005; Bailey & Collins, 2013). Pyramid models presume successful progression is a consequence of an emergent ability when in fact research undermines this notion of identifying talent during these early stages owing to a range of mediating factors that influence ability and thus the ability to progress. These psychosocial and environmental factors, such as simply accessing the bottom end of the pyramid through parental support and guidance (Rowley, 1993) and other factors such as coaching and facilities, all conspire to make progression increasingly difficult for young athletes through throwing the "necessary six to get started", especially those from stressed socio-economic situations (Bailey and Collins, 2013).

For some players and athletes who can demonstrate and express perceptions of ability early, progression through pathways is initiated quicker than others. However some evidence would suggest this is not always appropriate as other performance components are under-developed which leads to one-off performance assessments that can be affected by physical, emotional, and cognitive maturity; consequently some players are written off and de-selected (McCarthy & Collins, 2014).

A good example of this during my tenure at Leicester Tigers was that a number of players who were de-selected for various developmental and performance deficiencies during transition into the senior programme have gone on to achieve senior elite status in the game elsewhere.

Of course, consideration has to be given to context and clearly the quality and status of Leicester Tigers at the time was such that it was extremely difficult to break into the first team squad. Accordingly, there is an argument that it is potentially far harder to produce players for certain individual clubs based on their individual status and indeed investment, conversely owing to a lack of first team success at Gloucester Rugby players were consistently targeted and picked off by clubs who were perceived to be more progressive and successful which contrasted with the experience at Leicester Tigers.

Dynamics that conspire to trip you up within the pathway

One such dynamic that consistently plays out in all sports is the Relative Age Effect (RAE). Research linked to maturity has highlighted the impact on the performance and selection of children within sports and, more pertinently, inclusion within and negotiation of the development journey (Carling et al., 2009). An abundance of literature highlights the obvious physical advantages associated with being relatively old; further, it is a robust concept that this advantage manifests in identification processes. The RAE has been highlighted within literature pertaining to talent identification processes and is considered a consistent and influential factor in the disproportionate selection and identification of relatively older children within sports (for a review see Musch & Grondin, 2001).

The inevitable chronological grouping of children as they enter the education system has been shown to create significant cognitive, emotional, and physical differences in children who are born just before, or after, the academic cut-off date. This manner of grouping children continues as they enter organised sports as most employ the same criterion as the education system; grouping individuals aligned to an academic cut-off date (e.g. 1 September in England and Wales).

Being relatively older within sports allows the potential for a developing athlete to demonstrate a performance advantage at early identification points (Musch & Grondin, 2001). In the main it has been argued that this is owing to a physical advantage, thus demonstrating more desirable attributes, although these are generally senior level performance markers. Unsurprisingly during my time within the academy system this was an ever-present challenge in terms of looking beyond the obvious when attempting to identify and recruit players.

At both academy programmes we sought to explore this phenomenon in greater detail and depth to inform our development processes, in short what we found was somewhat counter to the much-publicised issues that are reported within the RAE literature. For example, whilst as with most sports we found a significant RAE present at the Leicester academy on initial selection (McCarthy & Collins, 2014) we were surprised and intrigued to understand why, in addition to these initial selection biases, we also saw greater conversion rates from the academy into senior programmes from players who were relatively young. Given the traditional notion that these players were at a significant disadvantage by virtue of birth-date we wanted to understand in greater detail why this might be happening. Our contention was that the attritional experiences that these players had when progressing through both educational and organised sport developed a climate of challenge that was conducive to the development of an ability to cope or a bounce-back ability. Unlike their relatively older peers who it appeared had a far easier journey through the systems by virtue of being ahead at that point in terms of maturation and as a consequence failed to develop the appropriate coping skills that would enable them once maturation levelled out to transition in the same manner as the relatively younger players (McCarthy et al., 2016).

This had considerable impact; both in terms of how we structured our identification and development processes but also in terms of educating those responsible for identification and recruitment, in many respects this was the biggest challenge in terms of how to structure a system that enabled athletes who were at a relative disadvantage or advantage to be challenged enough to begin the process of developing an ability to cope but conversely providing suitable space and flex to accommodate those players that couldn't demonstrate the obvious attributes early on owing to maturation.

Clearly, this had implications for how, as coaches, practitioners, and scouts, talent was perceived. Accordingly, there was a need to acknowledge talent as a biopsychosocial concept that would account for the many overlapping areas of development. At both academy programmes, we worked within a framework that considered talent in this respect. Figure 20.1 highlights the key aspects and the basis of the developmental processes clearly highlighting the interaction of components of performance and how they can overlap and indeed in respect of development grow at different stages over time (Abbott & Collins, 2004; Abbott et al., 2005).

Given the acknowledgment of talent as a multi-faceted and layered concept, a significant challenge was shifting our thinking as a coaching and performance team to an interdisciplinary development framework and a move forward from multidisciplinary, that is somewhat typified by working practice within discipline silos and a lack of coherence across performance components.

Therefore Figure 20.2 depicts an integrated characterisation of human development that also considers working context as a basis of talent development (Bailey et al., 2010). Within each academy programme in which I have worked, and now within the skeleton pathway, this shift in thinking to pull the coaching process and performance support together in an integrated performance/development team has been challenging but essential in providing an environment that is genuinely holistic in its aspirations.

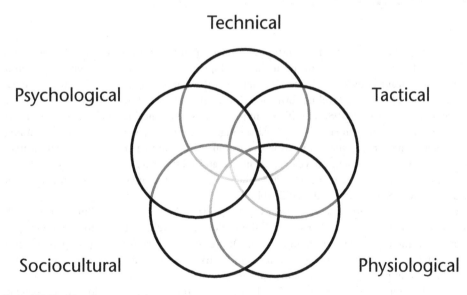

Figure 20.1 Five rings model
Source: Adapted from Abbott & Collins, 2002

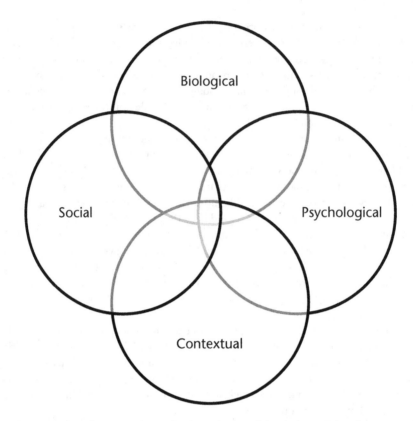

Figure 20.2 Interdisciplinary contextualisation of talent (biopsychosocial and contextual)
Source: Adapted from Bailey et al. (2010)

One of the key elements of a holistic interpretation and acknowledgement of talent is the role psychological factors have on both the development and transition of talent into senior level. A significant body of evidence now supports the role of psychological factors as determinants of successful elite level performance (MacNamara et al., 2010a, 2010b). For example, Orlick and Partington, (1998) identified a number of psychological strategies that contributed to success in elite performers such as goal setting, commitment, visualisation, and planning. Other key characteristics such as realistic evaluation of individual performance, commitment, engagement in quality practice have been identified and a distinction between elite level athletes and their less successful peers in regards to their engagement in mental preparation has been evidenced (MacNamara et al., 2010a; 2010b).

Research across performance domains (MacNamara, Holmes and Collins, 2006; 2008; MacNamara et al., 2010a) further supports the notion that psychological factors influence performance at the highest level of competition. Of greater relevance is the impact psychological factors have on facilitating the negotiation of, and entry into, talent development environments including the impact on the developmental capacity of an individual to then progress successfully. Furthermore, recent research has highlighted the importance of psychological competency as a key tenet in facilitating the route to elite level (MacNamara et al., 2010a; 2010b).

For example, constructs such as resilience (Sarkar & Fletcher, 2014), growth mindset (Dweck, 2006), grit (Duckworth et al., 2007) psychological characteristics of developing excellence (PCDEs) (MacNamara, Holmes & Collins, 2008; MacNamara et al., 2010a; 2010b) and 'mental' toughness' (Crust & Clough, 2011). This developing evidence appears to promote many of these constructs as determinants of successful transition to elite status, clearly motivation, commitment, and persistence are key factors in the ability to consistently keep moving forward in one's development. However, simply having the motivation, commitment, and persistence to commit is potentially not in its self sufficient to fully negotiate the journey. Athletes must also be resilient in the face of adversity (Sarkar & Fletcher, 2014). Resilience in a sporting context has been defined as having or developing the capacity to successfully adapt despite challenging circumstances (Sarkar & Fletcher, 2014).

As such within the various programmes I have worked I have utilised one such framework to form the basis of a curriculum focused on the elements that have been shown to play a key role in the realisation of potential. Psychological characteristics of developing excellence (PCDEs) (MacNamara et al., 2010a, 2010b) have formed the backbone of the pathways and environments I have managed. The PCDE framework incorporating a range of mental skills and behaviours allows young athletes or players to make the most of their development opportunities through targeted interventions to prepare them for the realities of life at the next level of the pathway. TDEs should not be comfortable places to be if we want to develop the capacity and competency to excel through and beyond the pathway (Sarkar and Fletcher, 2014; Rees et al., 2016; Collins et al., 2016).

Essential to this process is integrating the PCDE framework within our coaching practice and performance support to ensure a contextually defined and individually focused curriculum is suitably delivered in a systematic way. Bespoke interventions aimed at challenging and supporting athletes and players in various ways appropriate to their development needs and performance requirements can be initiated within the coaching process and broader TDE as and when required (Collins et al., 2016).

What is an effective talent development environment?

The primary objective of most talent development programmes in sport is to accurately identify, develop, and confirm the ability of an athlete with the aim of senior level success. This systematic approach to nurturing talent is thought to provide the most effective and efficient strategy to fulfil this primary objective (Martindale et al., 2005; Vaeyens, Lenoir, Williams, & Philippaerts, 2008). Talent development programmes therefore in recent times have generally been characterised and driven by a need to carefully nurture and protect significant investment in these athletes and the systems that support this process.

In short, the support systems that underpin the development process have sought to smooth the way and align athletes to a well-planned and often preordained development trajectory. The basis for this approach to TD is the perception that talent development is a relatively linear process with individuals once entering talent pathways progressing in a smooth and steady fashion with supporting structures and resource focused on eliminating challenging periods, experiences, and elements in their path as a way of protecting their investment in an individual (Abbott et al., 2005; Gullich, 2007).

However, evidence suggests that many of the problems athletes face when transitioning through a pathway are in fact a direct consequence of such challenge-free experiences during formative years of development and the over-emphasis from coaches and support staff to artificially smooth the experience (Gullich, 2007). Therefore recent work in this area has focused on the exploration of these challenge-filled experiences in more detail (Collins et al., 2016).

Optimising the pathway

Reflecting the need to prepare players or athletes for the realities of the next stage of the pathway and working towards developing the most appropriate attitudes likely to help through these transitions has been a key feature of all TDEs I have managed. Working within and through the PCDE curriculum and utilising a teach–test–tweak–repeat process grounded within Kolb's experiential learning theory (Kolb & Fry, 1975) we were able to plan, do, and review bespoke interventions centred on realistic challenges athletes and players are likely to encounter in a progressive manner. This was structured on an individual level and at team level to provide opportunities for developing the notion of "I have been here before and can deal with this" within the development process.

The mechanism for delivering this is through the individual athlete/development plan and the case conferencing of the individual player or athlete. Developing and facilitating a well planned, well managed integrated challenge strategy to develop a more psychologically robust player or athlete has strong merit (Collins et al., 2016). Key to the success of this process is pulling together the coaching and performance team in an integrated manner to ensure 'buy in' and coherence across the programme. With young athletes or players parental/guardian support becomes an ever-essential ingredient in managing the stress and potential fall-out from these challenging times, often well-intentioned parents/guardians striving to support their young offspring attempt to clear the path of obstacles, even when they have deliberately been put there! This is a crucial point which I can relate to and often in the past missed through focusing on the integration of the immediate TDE staff and the athlete/player, in reality particularly with young players or athletes contact time is limited and therefore to really gain the right traction educating the additional support mechanisms is of paramount importance to avoid disruptions and negative association with having to go backwards to propel themselves forward.

In that sense, periodising challenge in such a manner can be as simple or as complex as required dependent on the needs of the individual and the context in which they need to be delivered. Essential is the review and feedback processes that allow the learning experience to be reflected on and refined, as capacity develops and confidence is expressed through newly developed skills (Collins et al., 2016).

Next steps

This chapter has presented a personal perspective on what has proven useful in my years in academy programmes. I think the biggest next step is to ensure that future efforts are based on longitudinal tracking data rather than the retrospective work that has characterised the area so far. With this, we can pursue the agendas that are currently indicated with even more certainty. Exciting times!

References

Abbott, A., Button, C., Pepping, G.-J., & Collins, D. (2005). Unnatural Selection: Talent Identification and Development in Sport. *Nonlinear Dynamics, Psychology and Life Sciences*, 9(1), 61–88

Abbott, A. & Collins, D. (2004). Eliminating the Dichotomy Between Theory and Practice in Talent Identification and Development: Considering the Role of Psychology. *Journal of Sports Sciences*, 22(5), 395–408

Abbott, A., & Collins, D. (2002). A Theoretical and Empirical Analysis of a 'State of the Art' Talent Identification Model. *Journal of High Ability Studies*, **13**(2), 157–178

Abbott, A., Collins, D. J., Martindale, R., & Sowerby, K. (2002). *Talent Identification and Development: An Academic Review*. Edinburgh: Sportscotland

Bailey, R. & Collins, D. (2013). The Standard Model of Talent Development and Its Discontents. *Kinesiology Review*, **2**, 248–259

Bailey, R. P., Collins, D., Ford, P., MacNamara, Á., Toms, M. & Pearce, G. (2010) *Participant Development in Sport; An Academic Review*. Leeds: SportsCoach UK

Carling, C., Le Gall, F., Reilly, T. & Williams, A. M. (2009). Do Anthropometric and Fitness Characteristics Vary According to Birth Date Distribution? *Scandinavian Journal of Medicine & Science in Sports*, **19**(1), 3–9

Cooke, C., Cobley, S., Till, K. & Wattie, N. (2010). Searching for Sporting Excellence: Talent Identification and Development. *British Journal of Sports Medicine*, **44**(SUPP), i66–i66

Collins, D., MacNamara, Á. & McCarthy, N. (2016) Super Champions, Champions and Almosts: Important Differences and Commonalities on the Rocky Road. *Frontiers in Psychology*, 11 January, doi: 10.3389/fpsyg.2015.02009

Crust, L. and Clough, P. J. (2011). Developing Mental Toughness: From Research to Practice. *Journal of Sport Psychology in Action*, **2**(1), 21–32

Duckworth, A. L., Peterson, C., Matthews, M. D., & Kelly, D. R. (2007). Grit: Perseverance and Passion for Long-Term Goals. *Journal of Personality and Social Psychology*, **92**(6), 1087–1101. doi:10.1037/0022-3514.92.6.1087

Dweck, C. S. (2006). *Mindset: The New Psychology of Success*. New York, NY: Random House

Güllich, A. & Emrich, E. (2012). Individualistic and Collectivistic Approach in Athlete Support Programmes in the German High-Performance Sport System. *European Journal for Sport and Society*, **9** (4), 243–268

Henrikksen, K. & Stambulova, N. (2017). Creating Optimal Environments for Talent Development: A Holistic Ecological Approach. In Baker, J., Cobley, S., Schorer, J and Wattie, N. (Eds)., *Routledge Handbook of Talent Identification and Development in Sport*. pp. 271–284. London: Routledge

Henrikksen, K., Stamulova, N. & Roessler, K. (2010). Holistic Approach to Athletic Talent Development Environments: A Successful Sailing Milieu. *Psychology of Sport and Exercise*, **11**(3), 212–222

Kolb, D. A. & Fry, R. E. (1975). Toward an Applied Theory of Experiential Learning. In C. Cooper (Ed.), *Theories of Group Processes*. New York, NY: John Wiley & Sons

MacNamara, Á., Button, A. & Collins, D. (2010a). The Role of Psychological Characteristics in Facilitating the Pathway to Elite Performance. Part 1: Identifying Mental Skills and Behaviours. *The Sport Psychologist*, **24**, 52–73

MacNamara, Á., Button, A. & Collins, D. (2010b). The Role of Psychological Characteristics in Facilitating the Pathway to Elite Performance. Part 2: Examining Environmental and Stage Related Differences in Skills and Behaviours. *The Sport Psychologist*, **24**, 74–96

MacNamara, Á., Holmes, P. & Collins, D. (2012). The Pathway to Excellence: The Role of Psychological Characteristics in Negotiating the Challenges of Musical Development. In K. Swanwick (Ed.). *Music Education: Major Themes in Education*. London: Routledge

MacNamara, Á., Holmes, P. & Collins D. (2008) Negotiating Transitions in Musical Development: The Role of Psychological Characteristics of Developing Excellence'. *Psychology of Music*, **36**(3), 335–352

MacNamara, Á., Holmes, P. & Collins, D. (2006). The Pathway To Excellence: The Role Of Psychological Characteristics In Negotiating The Challenges Of Musical Development. *British Journal of Music Education*, **23**, 3

Martindale, R. J. J., Collins, D. & Daubney, J. (2005). A Critical Review of Talent Development and Implications for Sport. *Quest*, **57**, 353–377

McCarthy, N. & Collins, D. (2014): Initial Identification & Selection Bias Versus the Eventual Confirmation of Talent: Evidence for the Benefits of a Rocky Road? *Journal of Sports Sciences*, **32**, 1604–1610. doi: 10.1080/02640414.2014.908322

McCarthy, N., Collins, D. & Court, D. (2016). Start Hard, Finish Better: Further Evidence for the Reversal of RAE Advantage. *Journal of Sports Sciences*, **34**(15), 1461–1465, doi: 10.1080/02640414.2015.1119297

Musch, J. & Grondin, G. (2001). Unequal Competition as an Impediment to Personal Development: A Review of the Relative Age Effect in Sport. *Developmental Review*, **21**, 147–167

Orlick, T., & Partington, J. (1998). Mental Links to Excellence. *The Sport Psychologist*, **2**, 105–130

Rees, T., Hardy, L., Güllich, A. et al. (2016). The Great British Medalists Project: A Review of Current Knowledge on the Development of the World's Best Sporting Talent. *Sports Med*, **46**(8), 1041–1058. doi: 10.1007/s40279-016-0476-2

Rowley, S. (1993). Training of Young Athletes study (TOYA): Identification of Talent. London: The Sports Council

Sarkar, M. and Fletcher, D. (2014). Psychological Resilience in Sport Performers: A Review of Stressors and Protective Factors. *Journal of Sports Sciences*, **32**(15), 1419–1434

Simonton, D. K. (2001). Talent Development as a Multidimensional, Multiplicative, and Dynamic Process. *Current Directions in Psychological Science*, **10**(2), 39–43. doi: 10.1111/1467-8721.00110

Vaeyens, R., Lenoir, M., Williams, A. M., & Philippaerts, R. M. (2008). Talent Identification and Development Programmes in Sport: Current Models and Future Directions. *Sports Medicine*, **38**(9), 703–714

21

Supporting performance
A national institute perspective

Phil Moore

Introduction and context

Institutes of sport exist in various guises all around the world. Some have a long and storied history, others are relative upstarts. The concept of an Institute of Sport in Ireland was first mooted following the 2000 Sydney Olympics and it was established as an entity in 2006. Leadership roles began to be filled in the following year with an ambitious agenda, proposed facilities on the nascent National Sports Campus and a substantial and rising budget to implement programmes. The economic crash of 2008 severely impacted these plans (and all enterprises funded by the Irish state). Consequently, the development path of the Institute was adjusted to respond to the new reality. Throughout the recession Sport Ireland continued to invest in the Institute, despite a significant reduction it its own budget, and the Institute leadership team focused on using the available resources efficiently and building partnerships to help deliver its mission. In 2018, the Sport Ireland Institute (SII) has a team of around 30 staff (mix of full- and part-time) based in its purpose-built facilities on the bustling Sport Ireland National Sports Campus and is the primary agency for the delivery of support services to Irish Olympic and Paralympic sports.

I joined the Institute in 2007 as Athlete Services Director with a brief to establish a lifestyle support system for 'carded' athletes (athletes funded through Sport Ireland's carding scheme). In 2009 my brief expanded to include the science-based services and I was grandly titled Director of Performance Services. More recently, the 'services' tag was changed to 'support' to reflect an evolution in emphasis in the relationship that we wanted to have with our high-performance sports. So I am currently director of performance support which covers all science, medicine, and lifeskills supports to Olympic and Paralympic high performance programmes.

Vision and mission

Every organisation has a mission statement and naturally we do too. Typically, the finished product is pretty similar to every other vision and mission and ours probably fits neatly in that box as well as any other. However, the value is in the process of developing such statements of intent and there are usually some essential components that speak to that intent. In our case the two key words are 'partner' and 'impact'. As we have evolved as an organisation, we have focused our attention and our structure to make these central concepts in our thinking and action – hopefully this will be evident.

> *The vision of the Sport Ireland Institute is* "To be an essential partner in podium success for Irish High Performance Athletes and Sports".
> *The mission is to* "Drive excellence, create solutions, and impact performance".

The Institute's work is focused primarily on the senior elite athletes and teams and the NGBs provide most of the supports to the age-grade programmes. Other providers of support services include NGB employees, the University departments and private consultants. In addition, both the Olympic Federation of Ireland and Paralympics Ireland have provided a significant level of support over the past two decades. Thus the 'system' of support is quite complex – multiple agencies and individual providers are involved and most support teams comprise a mix of these providers. Moreover, each sport has its own structure, culture, established practices and history (as does the Institute) and of course there is a dynamic network of existing and evolving relationships between Institute and NGB personnel.

Consequently, a significant part of my role, is to build and navigate the relationships with the various stakeholders and consumers of our support services.

How did I get here?

My background as an athlete and coach was in lacrosse – I played for Scotland 48 times and was national coach for seven years (and have enjoyably revived my coaching career recently with the local U9 rugby team). I was a sport psychologist accredited by BASES and worked in a variety of sports but in an Olympic context was psychologist for GB and England Hockey men's and women's programmes from 1999 to 2005 during which time which I progressed to become their sport science and medicine team leader. Subsequently, I worked with Irish Hockey which led to the opportunity to work with Sport Ireland to help set up the Sport Ireland Institute.

I think it's been useful to have had a range of roles in sport as preparation for working in an institute of sport. I hope, having walked in the shoes, that I have some insight into the needs and wants of athletes, coaches, and managers. In particular, having managed support services in a sport when the English Institute of Sport was established I was aware of at least some of the challenges on both sides of the fence when a new agency is introduced into an existing system. It's a disruptive event, although 'event' suggests something that happens once and there's a clear before and after. The reality in my experience is it's a process that takes probably a minimum of roughly three years. Most of the 'before' stems from official papers that set out purpose, function, and structure of the new entity which generates lots of speculation and positioning. Typically this is followed by the recruitment of key personnel – both executive and oversight. These are the people that begin the process of bringing the concept to life, shaping the direction, rubbing up against the various pre-existing interests, and negotiating new relationships. Of course, this is a period of some friction which continues until the new organisation has carved out its space. The 'after' is a long tail of settling into new patterns of work and relationships. The notion that an Institute springs up fully formed and with a unity of purpose and vision is appealing but not reality. Although there may be a statement of purpose this is often modified in the early evolutionary process – shaped by the personnel recruited and other agents and agencies in the system and of course the broader national macro political-socio-economic context.

Emerging into an 'occupied' space

Most institutes of sport and certainly those established in the last 30 years emerge through a variety of lobbying interests into an already occupied space. In the absence of a centralised system, many university departments and individual practitioners have provided support services and NGBs have often developed their own network of support staff. So, the establishment of an institute is a disruptive event in the pre-existing complex high-performance sport system. This presents a number of challenges both for the nascent institute and the other stakeholders. I lived through this experience in the UK system whilst working for England Hockey as the English Institute of Sport came into being and was acutely aware of some of the potential difficulties (and opportunities) that a new institute would face in the Irish system. The most significant challenge I think was probably around the approach of the new institute to the extant individuals, teams, and organisations which could be could be crudely characterised as a choice of 'embrace or replace'. The message delivered early on in the relationship between England Hockey and the EIS was that it would be 'replaced' over time. In fact, the reality was much more of a partnership developed over time but the initial approach probably slowed the development of a trust-based relationship.

In my initial role with the Sport Ireland Institute, I was charged with developing an athlete lifeskills programme which actually was relatively uncontested – no NGB and very few providers were working in this area so typically, sports were generally happy that someone would provide this support. The science and medical services however were right in the middle of the contested zone. Many providers and interested parties had their own territory well established and were understandably reluctant to concede ground. Moreover, there was quite a range of different expectations or preferences for what the Institute would be and how it would work – from a network of (and for) sport science and medicine practitioners to a funder of support services to a research investor to a system leader. We were very clear in our own minds that our priorities were athlete and coach support and that other agendas would need to align with those priorities. In the main, our initial approach was to 'embrace' what was already in place and working, to contract the providers identified by the sports as their key personnel and, where we were able, to bring additional resource and expertise. We did make one significant structural change to the support system in 2009. This was to shift the access to support services from an athlete 'service credit'-based model (where athletes could use their credits to draw services from a list of approved providers) to a system where support was built into the performance plans and managed by the relevant Performance Director. The old system had been established in the early 1990s and worked well to provide athletes with access to science and medicine supports but by the late noughties, the high performance programmes had evolved and we thought the time was right to reshape the Institute provision to drive a more integrated and holistic athlete support within each programme.

Complex adaptive systems

It should be evident by now that I would view high performance sports (and their support) as complex adaptive systems. Of course, systems are dynamic and change is always happening – its just the speed and intensity that varies across time. Wishing for stability is fruitless and even problematic as it's likely to be unattainable – far better to embrace change as a natural part of a complex adaptive system that to try to stand Canute-like against the incoming tide. However, I would acknowledge that this is not a universally held view. I recall one senior swim coach who disputed my suggestion that he needed to be a change agent. His perspective was that he was actually trying to produce replicable, technically correct movement patterns and therefore stability and repeatability were his primary goals within his coaching and programmes. The flaw in this argument is that from a bio-psycho-social viewpoint change is continuous and even if his aim was to maintain stability, all the other changes have to be managed. In short, to stand still he would have to be in constant motion and consequently change-management and adaptability would still be of paramount importance.

The high-performance system as an ecology of ideas

Former Irish Hockey coach Gene Muller remarked once that he really felt he was coaching ideas as much as athletes. This led to a discussion around the notion that his function as a coach was to operate in an 'ecology of ideas' in which the best ideas thrived and killed off the weaker ones. In this picture, the arrival of a new coach into a programme was equivalent to an extinction event – many of the 'old' ideas would not survive the event and athletes and staff wedded to those ideas would leave the system unless able to adapt. Around the same time a conversation about complexity ideas in professional development with an old colleague, Mike Jess of Edinburgh University, sparked a different chain of thought. It was late 2012 and we were in the middle of a review of our high-performance coach support programme leading into the London Olympic Games. Feedback was very positive and several coaches cited examples of how they'd applied the support ideas and the network of relationships to positive effect at the Games. So we thought that we were getting something right but at the delivery end it felt a bit ad-hoc and that we were making it up as we went along. Mike pointed out that what we were doing was consistent with a complexity perspective of professional development and support (Jess et al., 2016). The programme embraced the need to build a network of relationships, it was driven bottom-up by the needs of the participants rather than a top-down ideal model of coaching, it emphasised adaptability skills by placing the participants in challenging situations and learning was identified in-action as well as after-action (cf. Carson & Collins, 2016), peer feedback played a significant role and the culture of trust was enhanced by disclosure of vulnerabilities. We recognised that we were orchestrating rather than leading and that much of the value was derived from the relationships built through the process. All of these factors contributed to the coaches' abilities to make good professional judgements (Martindale & Collins, 2012) and decisions under duress. At the core of both conversations is the proposition that relationships between ideas, activities, organisations and, of course, people are critical to the success of any high-performance sport system.

Why, you might wonder, am I taking you down this esoteric bywater? The reason is that these ideas began to permeate all of our work with sports including science and medicine support services.

Evolving relationships

As with our coach support work, we had generally very positive feedback on the science, medicine, and lifeskills services that we had been delivering to a range of sports. We had multidisciplinary teams working collaboratively with Performance Directors (PDs) and coaches, good collegial relationships between Institute staff and National Governing Body (NGB) staff and internally between the Institute team. And yet, at the same time we had that nagging feeling that we could be doing better, that we were too far removed from the performance. It certainly wasn't a lack of desire or intent but we knew that we weren't where we wanted to be with our essential relationships with the athletes, coaches, PDs and at an organisational level between the Institute and the NGBs. But why?

We needed to consider if in our own structure we were blocking a more multi-disciplinary, performance focused form of practice, and to consider how this was impacting on our essential relationships. So back to basics – using Mintzberg's (1983) organisational typology as a framework, we reviewed our structure and concluded that we were probably a hybrid professional bureaucracy – adhocracy organisation. In this type of organisational structure, practice standards and qualifications are typically set by the external professional bodies, and whilst internally, staff are grouped for administrative purposes by discipline, they are typically deployed as small multidisciplinary teams. Critically, these teams are led by expert project managers. When we looked at examples of other such organisations, there were numerous examples of consulting business that organise by disciplinary departments but that were agile in their deployment of dynamic mix of professionals to meet a particular client's needs. Our structure was departmental with lead consultants in each of the 'ologies and therapies although we had a lead or liaison consultant in each sport, their function was essentially coordinating the work of our staff in the sport. We recognised that our team were sitting in their discipline and working together but not stepping out of their own expertise to push into performance questions beyond their comfort boundaries. We needed to change.

We reorganised internally to move from a departmental hierarchy to a matrix (shown as Figure 21.1) which retained the department heads but introduced a role to lead focus on performance questions in each of the targeted sports – the head of performance support (HoPS).

Both roles are managers with equal weight. The heads of service are effectively the suppliers and the HoPS are the consumers of services. HoPS are responsible for getting close to performance – they are required to understand the drivers and limiters of performance in their sport from a coach/PD perspective. It's their job to work with the performance lead in the sport to get to the critical performance factors for their programme and then to challenge support staff across disciplines to work together to find solutions. We are in the process of rolling out this structure but already we have very positive responses from the coaches and PDs. Our own team are very energised by the change but also are experiencing significant stretch and discomfort. The energised response and part of the discomfort arises because they feel more immersed in the sport and closer to the outcomes – they now have more 'skin in the game' and an element of their accountability is about outcomes of the whole support programme and not

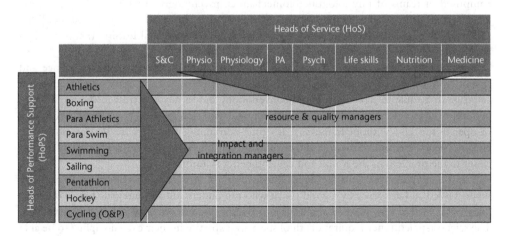

Figure 21.1   The refined matrix management model used by the Irish Institute. Cross disciplinary, sport-focused management replaces discipline-specific leadership

just their input from their own department. They have to come out of their disciplinary home territory and get inside the coach's perspective. The other part of both energy and discomfort is the negotiation for resources for their team. The HoPS described it as their "Hunger Games". They are in competition with each other for service time from the heads of service (HoS) of each discipline for their sport. The HoS have a limited staff capacity so bids for that resource are interrogated against a set of criteria:

- Medal potential of the sport/athletes.
- Impact potential of the service – will my support make a difference?
- Efficiencies and logistics – what will it cost in staff time and other resources?
- Health of the programme – clarity of purpose, communication, and leadership.

Ultimately, the outcomes of the robust negotiations arrive at my desk to arbitrate if needs be (rarely) but normally, to identify the human resource requirements to meet the needs of the sports. So our staff model is driven directly from sport needs. The ownership and leadership of our support work is vested in the people closest to the delivery and consequently, my role as director is more orchestration than direction. We have a distributed leadership model rather than command and control which we hope facilitates better performance support solutions by those best placed to find them.

Multidisciplinary support work

Finding best solutions requires our specialist support staff to work together in multidisciplinary teams. However, doing multidisciplinary or interdisciplinary work is challenging. It's a quarter-century since we outlined some of the challenges (Burwitz et al., 1994) and the reality is that in many ways little progress has been achieved in the intervening years. Recently, Wayne Goldsmith (2018) published a highly critical admonition to sport science that pretty much summed up the same key failings identified in our own work: in essence, too many silos of disciplinary focus that are too removed from performance questions. One of the drivers of this situation is that sport sciences are generally taught in their disciplinary streams by academics who have specialised in that discipline. University and college departments are often comprised of teams of physiologists, biomechanists, psychologists etc. Moreover, academic journals tend to be single-disciplinary and even those that are broader in scope still publish a vast majority of single-discipline studies. In short, there are structural features that maintain a largely silo-ed world in sport science.

However, I would readily acknowledge that doing multi or interdisciplinary science and support is not easy. It requires specialists to learn sufficiently of each other's perspective and language to be able to have meaningful conversations and to develop trust in the professional opinion of those specialists who may see things that you don't or can't see. A bit like trying to operate the UN without translators! It's time-consuming and as more staff are involved, becomes very expensive. However, the benefits are (or should be) that the support team can get closer to the problem in the round and develop better solutions.

The other challenge is that of depth versus breadth. Arguably, the best multidisciplinary support is led and delivered by a good coach who can understand and integrate lots of different 'ologies but with a very focused application to the specific performance needs of their athlete. The scientist-practitioner requires depth of specialist expertise in their own discipline to be able to bring something of value to the table. The application of that knowledge might well be of use to a broad range of athletes (i.e. the application of physiology expertise to understanding of performance in endurance sports). Both need the other AND the ability to talk to each other. Too often, the science is pitched for the scientist and is not useable for the coach. For example, a young intern came to me aghast at his perception that we weren't doing high-level science (certainly compared to what was going on back at the university labs). He had, on his own initiative, developed analyses of data to a level that we did not routinely provide and was keen to bring this to the coach. The coach was mildly interested in this work but couldn't see any practical use for it with the athletes at their stage of development. He was also mildly irritated that the intern hadn't provided the summary of results that the coach had requested in the format that he wanted. Frustration on both sides and no effective relationship between the two. The focus of the debrief with the intern was on the need to build a working relationship with the coach. He needed to listen, above all else, to the needs of the coach and deliver what was requested. Build the first steps in the relationship so that in time he could have meaningful engagement. If he didn't attend to this first and foremost, his scientific expertise was worthless. We are about support through the application of science not support as a vehicle for your science.

On the other hand, coaches can sometimes be defensive about their territory and occasionally don't let the scientist in. Of course, the stronger coaches tend to be very open and inquisistive and are often pretty good at working out who can help them and who will be too much trouble. Time is short and at the high end of performance you'll be quickly appraised for your usefulness (not your expertise necessarily) and discarded pretty quickly if you don't meet the mark. However, our own team have often found it difficult to get a coach or PD to articulate their performance questions. Often, the coach will direct the conversation back to a need for service (i.e. physiology lab testing or more S&C support) rather than engage in a conversation around the performance. Possibly, we haven't asked often enough for this to be normal. Possibly it feels like an encroachment on their territory (uncomfortable for both coach and support staff). However, by starting with a focus on building a trust-based relationship we are more frequently getting much closer to the performance questions.

Do you want to dance?

So, I've talked quite a lot about how we see ourselves as an organisation, my underpinning philosophy of practice, how this manifests itself in an organisational structure, and ultimately how we would like our relationships with sports to be. We want to be a partner rather than a provider, but what if you just want to buy a service? Sometimes we just get friend-zoned. In these cases, I do think it's important to be aware that, of course, my approach is one of many and in keeping with a complexity perspective, there are many different approaches that may all be effective to a greater or lesser extent. One of our aims is to try to meet sports, PDs, and coaches where they are rather than where we think they should be (which would be terribly arrogant).

So there is no one-size-fits-all model of engagement between the SII and each of the partner sports. In this situation, a command and control management model would be unlikely to work effectively. Equally, to have no operational consistency could result in such diversity that the Institute team would become entirely fragmented and our ability to deliver coherent support significantly compromised. We try to balance these tensions through our matrix structure (which I've outlined) and through our in-house professional development programmes. Whilst we provide support for conference and workshop attendance in disciplinary specialist areas, the main emphasis in our internal staff development work is around the challenges in the 'doing' of good multidisciplinary teamwork in real-life settings. To achieve this we use case-study scenarios, role play, show-and-tell presentations, as well as workshops around self-management and self-care. Interestingly, I think the show-and-tell sessions and case-study scenarios have generated the greatest responses from the team. The show-and-tell have been led off initially by senior staff and have involved disclosure around a particularly difficult or challenging professional experience. I delivered one of these sessions early on and found it very uncomfortable to publicly (within the team) expose some vulnerabilities in my own competence and practice. It was an emotionally draining experience and took much more out of me than I'd anticipated beforehand. However, feedback from the session suggested that it was important model from the outset the candour required if we as a team really aspired to be excellent at what we do and in our work with our stakeholders.

Relationship with athletes

So far, I've focused on the workings of the Institute and its relationship with sports at an organisational level and on the relationships between our team and the coaches and PDs. We of course work on a daily basis with athletes and their support is our primary objective. That said, we rarely have a relationship with an athlete in the absence of a coach, and when that is the case we are generally much less effective. However, the relationship between support staff and athletes is obviously important and there are some key considerations that need to be borne in mind when engaging in this relationship.

Firstly, the basics are the same as with the coach and PD – listen and try to understand where the athlete sees themselves, what they're trying to achieve and how you may be able to help. I encourage our support staff to engage in 'contracting' from the outset – setting of clear expectations and commitments on both sides. Sometimes, support staff can be too eager to please and set up an unbalanced relationship with the athlete. This is not healthy for either party – the athlete can develop a sense of entitlement or worse dependency. The provider becomes a resentful martyr. I recall a conversation with one of our relatively inexperienced psychologists who was complaining about what she perceived to be a lack of commitment and respect from an athlete (repeatedly missed or late for appointments, not delivering on agreed homework). We discussed the basis of the support relationship and it was clear that the psychologist had not established with the athlete their respective commitments and expectations. There were no consequences to being late or not completing work so this was normalised by the support provider.

Secondly, understanding your orbit is critical – by this I mean that as you enter into a sport, you are typically in an outer orbit around the coach-athlete relationship which is at the centre of this system. If you're good at what you do then your orbit moves closer to the 'sun'. Ideally, you position yourself so that you have sufficient influence and gravity in the system to create impact but without getting so close to the centre that you become part of the 'star' at the centre of the system. So it's a good idea to be intentional in positioning oneself within the complex social structure around an athlete and coach. Sometimes moving closer or being further out can be beneficial but too often I've seen support providers who have drifted unintentionally into ineffective relationships which end up with a lack of engagement on both sides (orbit too distant) or over-involvement, dependency – particularly problematic where a provider makes themselves indispensable (or perceived so by the athlete). The ideal that we're aiming for is a relationship built on mutual respect, with clarity of expectations that helps to foster the athlete's sense of autonomy and competence. This must always be a primary aim in the support relationship.

I try to ensure that, in every sport we support, we have redundancy built into the team – there's never one single provider in any discipline and although there may clearly be a primary provider, there's always a back-up. I do this for two reasons; one, it's better for the athlete not to be dependent on one person (what happens if for a multitude of possible reasons they're not available at a critical time). Two, as an organisation we want to ensure we're not 'held to ransom' by a service provider.

Related to this is the need for support staff to sometimes do nothing. Providers often feel a need to be seen to be busy all the time to justify their inclusion in a team – particularly around camps and competition. This is especially the case if you find yourself surrounded by others doing the same and you potentially have a PD looking at value for money. Of course, there are always small jobs to be done to help out, but on occasion I have seen providers compromise their effectiveness in their primary function by becoming a dogsbody. There is huge value in spending time with athletes (and coaches and other staff) to learn more about how things work and to build relationships. And as I've argued earlier, as relationships are the undervalued currency in effective support work, building them is a great investment in future impact.

Finally, psychological self-care is essential for the provider of support services. It's too easy to say yes to every request for help and end up feeling stretched and stressed. This path leads to burnout. I think in the most effective support relationships there is an engaged, emotional commitment – it's intense and shared with the athletes and other staff. Recognising the need to decompress after competition is critical as is an investment in 'normal' relationships. My own experience of about a decade of being heavily involved in direct support work was that over time my social network outside of the applied work dwindled – when you're away at camp and competition for extended periods, it takes effort to maintain relationships outside of the work and a healthy balance and lifestyle. Debriefing with colleagues can help to unpack, learn and close off episodes of high investment in support work and should be built into work programmes. From an organisational perspective this is a smart move as it protects our investment in our staff as we want to retain accumulated wisdom rather than replace burnt-out practitioners.

Summary

In this chapter I've tried to provide a viewpoint based on my own experience of both doing and managing support work within an Institute of Sport. I will readily acknowledge that this is not the only or 'correct' perspective and that other Institutes will operate on a different basis. I hope that I've provided an insight into the complex, dynamic, non-linear world of support work. If you take nothing else from my world-view, I would re-emphasise the centrality of the inter-related nature of the work and consequently the need to embrace more holistic and integrated approaches to doing applied support work with a clear focus on performance questions. Underpinning this approach is a need to invest in relationships between people, ideas, disciplines and organisations as a primary objective rather than as a by-product of doing 'proper' work.

References

Burwitz, L., Moore, P. M. & Wilkinson, D. M. (1994). Future Directions for Performance-related Sports Science Research: An Interdisciplinary Approach. *Journal of Sports Sciences*, **12**, 93–109

Carson, H. J., & Collins, D. (2016). Implementing the Five-A Model of Technical Change: Key Roles for the Sport Psychologist. *Journal of Applied Sport Psychology*, **28**(4), 392–409

Goldsmith, W. (2018) Sport Science You've Still Got it Wrong. Retrieved from: http://newsportfuture. com/sports-science/

Jess, M., Carse, N., & Keay, J. (2016). The Primary Physical Education Curriculum Process: More Complex than you Might Think!! *International Journal of Primary, Elementary and Early Years Education*, **44**, 502–512. doi: 10.1080/03004279.2016.1169482

Martindale, A., & Collins, D. (2012). A Professional Judgment and Decision Making Case Study: Reflection-in-Action Research. *The Sport Psychologist*, **26**, 500–518

Mintzberg, H. (1983). Power In and Around Organizations. Theory of Management Policy Series. Upper Saddle River, NJ: Prentice-Hall

22

The performance director's role

Tim Jones with Andrew Cruickshank

Introduction

Amplified by the levels of investment and interest in elite sport around the world, leading the 'performance department' or 'arm' of a sports organisation is an increasingly complex and dynamic role. In this sense, the *performance director* (hereafter PD) has become a key figure in elite sport systems; a figure who, in broad terms, is responsible for leading, co-ordinating, and managing the systems, structures, and processes that are intended to drive performers, managers, coaches, support staff, and other specialists to develop, prepare, and perform at the highest level. In this chapter, my aim is to offer a perspective on the PD's role in an Olympic and Paralympic sport context, as supported by reflections on my experience as PD for the UK's Paralympic athletics (2006–08) and Olympic gymnastics (2008–13) programmes. More specifically, I present my views in two parts: in the first I will outline some useful approaches and skills that are required of the PD; in the second, I will offer a perspective on some current trends and future needs for the PD. Before presenting my ideas, however, it is important to clarify that these views and messages are clearly shaped by my experiences in UK-based roles. However, as elite sport systems around the world share a number of similarities, in terms of their *general* focus and nature, my hope is that they can offer a useful comparison or stimulus for those in other countries and cultures. To frame this, I will now provide a brief overview of the PD's role in a UK Olympic and Paralympic sport context, before then moving to consider some key approaches and skills that can benefit a PD.

Contextualising the PD role in UK Olympic and Paralympic sport

Although the recent success of the Olympic and Paralympic systems in the UK cannot be attributed to a single event, one particularly notable moment was the nation's performance at the 1996 Olympic Games in Atlanta. At these Games, the British team won one gold medal and finished in their lowest position in the medal table in almost a century. In response to the high levels of internal and external criticism that followed, the UK reformed its elite sport system in terms of funding, organisation, and leadership, with 'UK Sport' established in 1997 to improve and sustain success in future Olympic and Paralympic Games. More specifically, UK Sport was – and still is – responsible for overseeing the strategic distribution of financial investment, primarily derived from the National Lottery and government sources, across a range of national sport organisations (hereafter NSOs). Over the last two decades, UK Sport's role has continued to evolve, with this agency also now directing and supporting NSOs with regard to their hosting of events, international influence and development, governance, leadership, accounting, and science, medicine and technology (www.uksport.gov.uk).

Tied to these changes, many NSOs in the UK have also focused on evolving the leadership and organisation of their high-performance arm (with their other main arms usually focused on participation and talent development). This evolution has occurred to a greater extent in some more than others; and more independently in some more than others. Indeed, it is fair to say that changes in some NSO's leadership and organisation have been driven primarily by UK Sport's desire for greater accountability in the system. As part of this evolution, funded sports are now commonly led by a dedicated PD.

Considering the evolution of the PD role itself, it is important to recognise that the original wave or 'first version' of the PD (in a UK Olympic and Paralympic context) tended to be one of the sport's 'master coaches'; and, significantly, a master coach who had worked in the sport for a long time, achieved credible results with their athlete(s) or team(s), and developed a depth of technical understanding (e.g. the technical attributes and skills that athletes or teams needed to perform at medal-winning level, or in current jargon, an individual version of a 'What It Takes To Win' model). At the time, this approach seemed logical to many – including on a political level. However, since this original wave, notable changes have occurred with regard to the 'type' of PD who NSOs and UK Sport have desired and appointed.

Broadly speaking, this evolution has reflected a growing understanding of (a) the actual demands of the PD role; and (b) where the PD has greatest impact. Regarding the former, PDs are usually responsible for notable or, in some cases, major funds. In my own case with British Gymnastics, our plan for the London cycle was built around £11 million of funding, with the plan for Rio built on £15 million. In sum, a PD is usually responsible for a significant budget which requires skills that typically aren't acquired through coaching alone (as per the typical 'master coach's' background). In terms of the understanding of where a PD has greatest impact, it is also important to note that a PD is invariably 'one step removed' from athletes, most of their staff, and actual 'on the day' performance; in other words, they are usually not directly involved in the day-to-day work of those in the 'training or competition environment'. Instead, a PD's efforts are typically focused on designing, leading, and evolving their sport's overall systems, structures, and processes. But, and turning to the first main section of this chapter, what specific approaches and skills can help PDs to fulfil this role effectively?

So, what do you have to be able to do as a PD?

Against this portrayal of the PD role, some clear implications arise for what PDs have to be able to do in order to be effective in their work. Importantly, however, these *general* implications are not, based on my awareness of other systems, just UK-specific. Certainly, similarities in other countries and cultures suggest that these implications are relevant to many operating in the PD role; albeit with country/system-specific emphases or slants. Of course, there isn't enough space in this chapter to cover most, let alone all of these implications. As such, I have decided to focus on what I feel are a particularly key set; as based on my experiences and reflections on those of my peers. Specifically, these implications are: *managing the early phase well; building and promoting culture and philosophical alignment; protecting and prioritising the performance programme;* and *working against a long-term vision and a 'nested plan'.*

Managing the early phase well

When first starting a PD role, it's obviously important to have ideas on what you want to do in the opening phases of your tenure, such as your first 30 days, six months, or year, and I have been pretty clear on these in my roles to date – particularly in relation to my time with British Gymnastics. However, as much as these ideas might relate to the systems, structures, and processes of performance, arguably one of the most significant goals is to position and establish yourself on an *interpersonal* level; in other words, 'how people see you'. In the case of my time with British Gymnastics, I was acutely aware of the challenge of not having competed, coached, or worked in the sport beforehand (I had instead competed, coached, and worked in swimming). As such, a pressing concern for me was the possibility that I would be viewed as almost a 'mouthpiece' for UK Sport: a 'UK Sport agent' or 'pick' who had been tasked to critique and completely change what British Gymnastics was doing, first and foremost, for the interests of UK Sport. Indeed, while a small number of other NSOs had appointed 'outsiders' as their PD, my sense at the time was that the role was almost imposed upon the sport. In this vein, it is fair to say that many in the sport didn't buy into the idea of 'the PD' as a way forward, especially a PD who was unknown to the sport and a potential 'UK Sport insider' (even though I'd never worked for UK Sport and had been employed by other NSOs directly in the past). In short, I recognised that my lack of history and connections in gymnastics would shape others' views on who I was, what I was in it for, and how I would work; views that I needed to manage quickly.

As a result, one major goal during the initial phase of my tenure was to establish where my credibility in the role sat: I couldn't (and wouldn't) come in to the sport and tell coaches how to develop their discipline or athletes technically. Instead, I identified that my credibility would come from my skills in building the broader system, cutting to the main issues, and bringing people together to work for a common objective. For this credibility to come across, it was vital to therefore position myself as someone who had the interests of the sport at heart; and an enthusiasm to work alongside those already in the system. Indeed, despite the 'cons' of being an 'outsider', there were 'pros' to this as well. More specifically, I worked hard to establish myself as a 'neutral' figure; someone who wasn't engrained in the sport's history, politics, and personalities, or biased along the 'tribal' lines that a multi-discipline sport can easily foster. As such, I was proactive in making sure that I committed time to meeting and listening to a range of individuals and groups after my appointment. This was particularly helpful for my future work with the trampoline discipline, who had come under the NSO's jurisdiction relatively late on (having been governed by a separate federation previously) and often felt that they were treated less favourably than the other disciplines. In sum, and even though it presented a challenge, my profile and background was arguably one of my biggest strengths coming into this PD role. Albeit with some careful work, it meant that I could assume a largely impartial position, see the system for what it was, and evaluate my findings with a clear 'performance view'.

Of course, this opening period of 'perception building' wasn't just important in terms of building 'interpersonal credibility' (i.e. "this guy seems to be alright"); it was also important for building 'impact credibility' (i.e., "this guy seems to know what we need and can deliver it"). In short, I also needed some 'quick wins' to build momentum and the programme; some tangible outcomes that would allow me to show what I *could* bring to the table (rather than what I couldn't). In this respect, one of my early aims was to rebuild the relationship between British Gymnastics and the English Institute of Sport (hereafter EIS), who were our main sport science and medicine provider. To do so, we quickly appointed a Head of Sport Science and Medicine, who also wasn't a 'gymnastics lifer', and embedded them within the EIS (who are UK Sport's sport science, medicine and technology arm). From this one appointment we therefore achieved 'multiple hits': the coaches and technical staff benefitted from some much-needed co-ordination of our support services; they also saw that 'non-lifers' (who were trickled in) could *add value* to their work (rather than distract or dictate), and the relationship with the EIS took a key step forward. In fact, this individual is still working for the sport and, I think it is fair to say, has played a significant role the programme's recent and ongoing success.

Building and promoting cultural and philosophical alignment

As another implication for 'what you have to able to do' as the PD, the ability to generate 'cultural and philosophical alignment' has also been reinforced during my own and many of my peers' experiences. In other words, the ability to build and promote a shared set of beliefs on performance and how the whole team, athletes and staff, needs to work together to achieve it. Importantly, this alignment needs to be with both internal and external stakeholders. Internally, this was always at the forefront of my mind when interacting with staff – especially those in the leadership group. To achieve this, much of my early work at British Gymnastics was to help us identify the aspects of performance that we had absolute control over, up until a gymnast raised their arm at the start of their routine on competition day (at which point, everything was effectively handed over to the athlete). In this way, we created a shared model on the pillars of performance and then used these as our frame of reference for all subsequent decision making. To promote consistency in these pillars, new members of staff were also carefully recruited on a 'philosophical', as well as the traditional 'skills' or 'knowledge', basis. Indeed, if the programme was to be as coherent and consistent as possible then it wouldn't have made sense to bring in individuals who were on different pages philosophically; for a collaborative effort, they had to be advocates of the pillars.

As well as 'downwards alignment' from PD to staff, it is also essential for PDs to seek, develop, and sustain 'upwards alignment' with their CEO. In short, the importance of the PD-CEO relationship cannot be understated: if you can get this right and the CEO 'has your back' then it can make a massive difference to your ability to do the job. In my case at British Gymnastics, it was clear that the CEO who appointed me believed that I was the person to deliver the mission. However, 20 months later, and just ahead of a European Championships (at which we performed well), another CEO came into the sport from overseas. Naturally, they had their own views on how the sport needed to evolve and work towards its objectives, whilst at the same time learning the nuances of the UK high performance system too. It became apparent that there was some fairly immediate scepticism around the philosophy of the performance programme and maybe my personal abilities too – which became an ongoing challenge. It also felt like the new CEO was challenged that the UK system invested so much power into the PD role, in terms of channelling the financial investment in from UK Sport and running the performance programme. Indeed, many of the 'spikes' during my tenure were around managing upwards to the CEO and Board rather than downwards to the staff within the performance programme. This was particularly challenging given that the 'noises' from within the sport were contrary to those from of UK Sport and, on reflection, ultimately contributed to my eventual departure from this role.

In terms of lessons from this experience, my main reflection is that I could have perhaps been more giving of information; as well as placing even greater emphasis on explaining where the performance programme had been before. In this sense, it would be fair to say that the sport had been at a relatively low ebb and we definitely weren't a finished product – this was only likely to occur in three or four years' time. Perhaps another factor to note was that I was never required to attend board meetings in my time with the sport; instead, the performance programme reported to a committee that transferred information to the board. Despite the benefits of this structure, in terms of allowing me to fully commit to leading the system and not be dragged into matters that were largely irrelevant to performance, as many PDs experience, this way of working potentially did breed a level of disconnect; or at least a limitation in how connected we were. In sum, it was always difficult to judge the mood of the whole business and, therefore, promote the *philosophical alignment* that was bringing so many benefits within the programme itself.

Protecting and prioritising the performance programme

Of course, it is inevitable that there will be some degree of 'noise' or distractions for the PD to manage from structures and agencies that operate 'above' the performance programme. In fact, many points of friction can be useful for progressing a sport when they generate critical and constructive conversations. However, the extent to which the staff within the performance programme need to be aware of these dynamics and events is also something that PDs need to be particularly mindful of. For example, in my time with British Gymnastics, UK Sport could feed information in bucket loads but, to help the staff remain focused on the key aspects of their role, I often shared this information on a 'need to know' basis; or, even more accurately, a '*really need to know basis*'. In essence, a pillar of my own approach – as I had learned from other PDs – was to avoid filling up staff members' heads with things that simply weren't relevant to them. As a result, my aim was to act as an incredibly dense filter to make sure that little noise came in from 'the outside'; that nothing was said or done externally that negatively affected my staff. In sum, there is an element of a 'game' to be played with external agencies and partners as a PD; you need to respect and manage their interests and actions but, at the same time, make sure that these interests and actions don't distract those in the sport.

As well as this more protective mode of leadership, there is also clearly a need to find ways to get the best out of your staff. In many respects, you may argue that the PD role is simply about man-management; or at least *more* about man-management than anything else. Indeed, once your credibility to do the role has been established, managing people certainly becomes the greatest challenge and no sport is the same. For example, part of the challenge in track and field was that I had to deal with so many coach-athlete pairs; whereas coaches in gymnastics and swimming tended to work with multiple athletes – which presented its own challenges in terms of the reach and influence of those coaches. Similarly, it is also common to work with staff from a variety of countries and cultures, who can go about things in very different ways. In keeping with best coaching practice, you really have to treat individuals as individuals and there is no one set way to bring them on board and continue to develop them. Often the relationships that take longest to build can also be the most productive and rewarding in the long term. My perspective here is primarily based on my coaching experience: the moment that you think you've got '*the* solution' or a 'one size fits all' model then you'll come crashing down. For example, before the 2012 Olympic Games, we made decisions around what the men's and women's teams needed in terms of their preparation: the men wanted to go somewhere quiet out of the country; the women wanted to be somewhere familiar in the country. So we made different decisions for different teams; and also for different athletes and staff within these teams. As simple as it sounds, this approach can often be overlooked in high performance sport; yet it is one of the most effective ways to protect and get the best out of a programme.

Working against a long-term vision and a 'nested plan'

As the final implication on what PDs need to be able to do, working against a long-term vision and 'nested plan' are, in my experience, crucial. Regarding the former, and in line with the 'performance pillars' described earlier, a long-term vision provides another constant frame of reference against which day-to-day decisions can be made. In the case of my time with British Gymnastics, I never saw 2013 as 'the end of my road'; which, on reflection, meant that my thinking was always on what was going to happen beyond this Games. As such, not many short-term decisions made: they were primarily based on what was in the best interests of the programme in the long-term.

In terms of 'nested plans', this principle relates to the PD's ability to identify the series of progressive steps, or phases of action, that the sport needs to deliver to achieve its vision. In other words, a 'Russian dolls' approach whereby the actions today fit into the actions that are needed tomorrow, that fit into the actions that are needed for the next week, month, quarter, or year. In my own case, this was reinforced during my time with British Para-Athletics – whereby lots of difficulties were faced by *not* being able to build in progressive steps or phases ahead of the 2008 Games in Beijing. This was due, in the main, to a large degree of uncertainty over the 'end target'; more specifically, there was little information or insight available on the events that would be in the final schedule and how classification might make our athletes eligible or ineligible to compete. Indeed, as we started to understand what events would be included, we could tell that it wasn't going to go our way. In this respect, and despite only having a small group of athletes, I was perhaps a little naïve in terms of anticipating and planning for the number of factors that would influence whether we could be successful or not. This learning on the need and benefits of a phased approach – as locked to the demands of the actual competition – was certainly something that I was mindful of in my time with British Gymnastics.

For example, and picking up on the investment of sport science and medicine mentioned earlier, this was one of the first phases in setting up 'the end game': i.e. to be able to select the athletes that we wanted to select for the Olympics. Indeed, while there was a bit of noise around how much we had committed financially to sports science and medicine, we felt that it was critical for being able to select an injury-free, as well as the healthiest, best equipped, and best prepared, team for the event that would ultimately count most. We were subsequently vindicated on this call: in particular, after two key athletes picked up injuries early in 2012, the quality of the team and processes we had in place played a crucial role in helping them to return in time for London, and most importantly, tangibly add to our medal count.

As an example of a later phase of our preparation for London, we also planned in the tough conversations on team selection as early as possible, so that individuals knew what our stance was. In the long run, this meant that the final six months leading into the Games were as noise free as we hoped it could be. We also developed a way to manage and engage with the media before big events – another area that we had proactively planned for and progressively worked on in the lead up to London. Overall, all of these separate phases and targets were designed to help us to perform 'on the day' at the Olympics: we wanted to come into the Games prepared, confident, and with appropriate expectations. In this respect, the final phase of our plan was to come into the Games under the radar. So rather than the 'fanfare entry' adopted by some others, we instead planned to 'sneak' into the village with a settled team and settled procedures without creating a mountain of expectation. Of course, we knew that we could perform, but we did what we always did and avoided getting caught up in the spectacle and the 'what's going to happen?!' As a result, it felt like the Games was our moment to grow and shine – rather than shrink and fade – in front of a home crowd that could give us a significant advantage on the day.

The present and future of the PD role?

Having focused on some important approaches and skills for PDs, I conclude this chapter by taking a look at the present and future of the PD role. More specifically, this consideration is made against current trends in the environments that many PDs operate and reflects some key challenges that they encounter; namely: *managing culture and the 'talent gap'*; *'role positioning' and balancing with 'the lifers'*, and *learning to lead*.

Managing culture and 'the talent gap'

Elite sport, especially at present in the UK, seems to be becoming an increasingly volatile system in a lot of respects; not just in terms of the pressure to deliver results to maintain funding or public/media support, but also because of the attention that is being paid to the *way* in which these results are achieved. In this vein, one of the most notable challenges for PDs in the UK – and a challenge which others have and will continue to face around the world – is their sport's culture (or reported culture). For example, UK Sport are now placing significant focus on this aspect after recent media coverage and government enquiries that exposed questionable practices (actual and perceived) in the elite sport system; a focus which has, quite rightly, brought some important issues to the fore. However, it has also brought many challenges for the PD; especially as the agency who is now challenging sports on how they are working to win medals is the agency who have set this objective as the primary means to secure future funding (as have other funding systems in other countries). Additionally, and despite its common usage in elite sport, 'culture' is one of the most vaguely-defined and measured constructs in performance. In short, the focus and politics of future 'PD-ing' seem to be becoming increasingly complicated!

A further challenge for PDs in the near future, if not already, will be managing the 'talent gap' that many elite systems are contributing to; or at least not addressing sufficiently. More specifically, by directing funds to 'the best of the best' athletes that a sport *currently* has, the 'con' is that most who sit below this are either missed or under-supported. This is an even greater issue when other funding agencies or sources in that country, such as in the UK, prioritise different objectives (e.g. participation- and health-based) over talent development. Consequently, a focus on individuals at either end of the continuum (i.e. participation/general health or elite athletes) means that a fracturing of the pathway is occurring in many environments, whereby talented individuals who sit in the middle (with the potential to reach elite level *or* return to amateur or participation-based sport), aren't being sufficiently catered for. Of course, this may not be a concern for PDs who are working for short-term objectives (e.g., medals at Tokyo 2020), but it certainly will be an issue for those responsible for their sports thereafter.

'Role positioning' and 'balancing with the lifers'

As described in the early part of this chapter, the first version of the PD in a UK context was generally a sport's 'master coach', who had been working in the system for a number of years, achieved the most credible results with their athletes, and acquired a breadth and depth of technical understanding of performance. As the system developed its' understanding of what skills were needed to lead modern Olympic and Paralympic programmes, the 'second wave PD' was generally someone whose expertise lay with the development and management of overall systems, structures, and processes. Notably, this second wave saw the increase of PDs who were 'outsiders' to their sport. This trend reflected a strength of the 'cross-sport conversations' that the UK system can encourage; but one which also presented a challenge for the 'outsider PD'. Now in the UK, it would seem that we are witnessing a 'third wave PD'. More specifically, a number of recently appointed PDs have, or have previously had, close ties with UK Sport; typically through being employed or trained by them. This progression from the 'first wave' to the 'third wave' PD in a UK context is conveyed in Figure 22.1; which indicates where these PDs are typically positioned in terms of their developmental history and connections (at least at the time of their appointment).

As an important point to keep in mind when reflecting on this trend, both UK Sport and NSOs are, fundamentally, independent of each other. By definition, both UK Sport and NSOs are therefore highly likely, at least in part, to work to different agendas. Indeed, UK Sport are, as it stands, primarily interested in winning medals at the next Olympics or Paralympics and require staff in the NSO who can deliver these outcomes. However, the primary interest of the NSO, who employ the PD, is the entire sport; which is made up of athletes in their per-formance, talent, *and* participation spheres. In short, each NSO has to ensure a connection and balance between all areas of their business, regardless of whether they are granted funding for elite performance by UK Sport.

Accordingly, there is a need to ensure that a sport's 'lifers' – or at least the needs and views of these lifers – are at the forefront of a NSOs operation and decision making. Indeed, lifers are the custodians of any sport and an imbalance means that performance is unsustainable; especially if funding or expectation levels change significantly. As such, sports need to be aware of their 'tipping points', in terms of where the interests lie amongst those leading an NSO, as well as throughout their staff. More specifically, each sport needs a core of 'lifers' to balance the 'transits', who are typically there to achieve short-term impact; and each 'transit' needs to compliment the central thread provided by the 'lifers'. In this vein, I often have difficulty dis-cerning why some sports, especially those with limited funding, have lots of 'transit' staff and 'career administrators' in key roles; especially when we know their likely employment patterns. In fact, an argument could be made that the lifespan of a PD should be limited as the longer they spend in a sport, the more they tend to lose their ability to stay 'history/politics-free', to challenge shortcomings, and see issues and tasks for what they are. Regardless of this, however, a

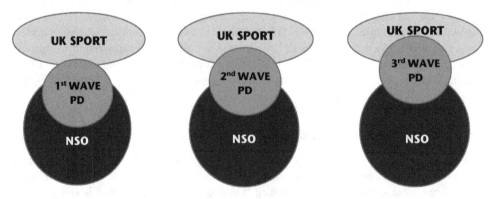

Figure 22.1 The apparent general trend in PD 'positioning' across funded Olympic and Paralympic sports in the UK

key challenge for PDs in the future is how to keep the elite arm of the organisation from floating too far off from the rest of the sport and, ultimately, its future athletes, staff, and leaders.

Learning to lead

As my final consideration on future challenges, efforts to 'fast-track' individuals into the PD role seem to becoming increasingly apparent. In this vein, there is a trend (within the UK at least) for individuals to acquire PD appointments who have had more specialised training and education on being a PD than their predecessors, but who have spent less time working and performing in leadership positions. In short, there are now more PDs operating at the sharp end of performance who might have had relatively little experience of doing it before, or seeing others doing it. In this respect, I don't think that there's a 'manual' for being a PD; but there *is* a large element of 'time on task'. In my own case, I felt that the roles that I undertook for the 10 years before Para-Athletics then British Gymnastics provided me with the incremental exposure to challenge that helped me to deliver when it became my time to lead. Indeed, my best learning for the PD role came from the time that I had spent coaching and then managing under three PDs over a ten-year period; effectively building my knowledge on how I would (and wouldn't) want to lead a system if given the chance. Of course, academic qualifications, formal training, rubbing shoulders with established PDs, and reflecting on lessons from other domains can play a role in helping individuals to take on the PD challenge. However, in my view at least, leadership ability is fundamentally driven by leadership-relevant experience or, more specifically, intense leadership-relevant experience. In this respect, I don't think there's a shortcut for learning to be a PD. Indeed, if we know that the development of sporting talent takes a significant amount of time, then why would this not stand for a PD? You can, of course, accelerate parts of that development; however, we know that expertise requires a high degree of *purposeful experiences* and *purposeful practice* that you simply can't rush.

Concluding comments

In concluding this chapter, I hope to have painted a picture of the PD's role – primarily in Olympic and Paralympic sport – and some of the skills and approaches they require to lead effectively. Specifically, these skills and approaches were: *managing the early phase well*; *building and promoting cultural and philosophical alignment*; *protecting and prioritising the performance programme*; and *working against a long-term vision and a 'nested plan'*. Moreover, I hope that the coverage to some current and future challenges helps to convey what might be coming next for those in the PD role; as well stimulating thought on what skills and approaches they might need to take these challenges on. Of course, and as noted at the start of this chapter, these views have been mainly informed by my experiences in a UK context. However, given the parallels in elite sport systems around the world, I hope that these views have provided a useful source of comparison for those operating in other countries and cultures; and perhaps an indication of what opportunities and challenges may lie around the corner if similar paths are taken.

23

Leading a national system

Alex Baumann with Andrew Cruickshank

Introduction

When it comes to overseeing the performance of a national elite system, it is a common view that leadership is different to management. More specifically, leadership is often felt to relate to the more aspirational and inspirational aspects of work in this role, whereas management is typically associated with 'doing what needs to be done'. Despite their apparent differences, however, those responsible for national systems are required to both lead and manage and so these terms will feature throughout this chapter. It is also fair to state that the *general* principles of leadership can be quite similar across different national systems. However, the application of these general principles can – and in fact should – vary in relation to the *specific* needs and goals of each environment. In this vein, my primary goal in this chapter is to offer a personal view on some general principles of leadership when leading a national system; covering both 'what to do' and 'how to do it'. Throughout, I also aim to demonstrate how these principles need to be tailored to 'match the context'. In doing so, I draw on my experience of leading various systems over the last 20 years, but with a particular focus on my time as CEO of High Performance Sport New Zealand (hereafter HPSNZ) between 2012 and 2017, as well as Canada's 'Own the Podium' from 2006 to 2011.

National systems and the responsibility of the CEO: a brief overview

To provide some further context to this chapter, many countries around the world now have purpose-designed organisations that are responsible for funding or investing in (more on these terms later) elite-level sport. Many of these organisations are also responsible for channelling a host of other linked resources, such as staff, training, and technology. In some cases, this channelling of money and resources is focused on sports that are traditionally classed as professional, whereas other systems might focus primarily, or exclusively, on the Olympic, Paralympic (both Summer and Winter), and Commonwealth Games. For example, in the case of HPSNZ, our remit was to support Olympic, Paralympic, and non-Olympic Sports. With Own the Podium in Canada, our remit here was Olympic and Paralympic Sports.

Despite these similarities in their broad focus and goals, differences across each country's geography, history, culture, politics, and media, mean that national systems do, of course, differ in lots of ways. For example, some nations need to co-ordinate activities across various regions or provinces (such as Canada), whereas others have more centralised models (such as NZ); both of which present their own unique needs. The manner in which sports are funded (or invested in) – as well as the volume of money they receive – is also shaped by a unique mix of norms, expectations, and agendas in each nation's government and society, particularly so when this money is derived from public sources. However, the common thread throughout most, if not all, national elite systems is the pursuit of sporting achievement. In fact, most sources of money, such as national governments, demand this; requiring the system to set specific medal targets for each Summer and Winter Olympic and Paralympic Games, against which decisions on future funding (or investment) are consequently based. Against this context, my overriding responsibility as CEO for Own the Podium and then HPSNZ was to effectively establish and evolve a system where each sport was: (a) capable of consistently delivering results and medals for themselves and the nation; and (b) as self-sufficient as possible in pursuing these outcomes.

Delivering outcomes for the nation: some principles on 'WHAT to do'

In the pursuit of sporting achievement, it is important for a leader of a national system to be guided by certain principles; principles that provide a framework or reference point for all of the work that they do. In this respect, I feel that six core principles have driven the performance of the systems that I have led to date. Specifically, these are: *strategy, people, culture and environment, planning and monitoring, immersion and integration of the entire system, innovation*, and *intelligence*. In my experience, these all play a significant role in long-term success. However, in this chapter I have chosen to focus particularly on the role of *strategy* and *people, culture, and environment*, given that these can often be the building blocks of any system. It is important to note that these areas are not mutually exclusive. Indeed, strategy depends on the people, culture and environment; and people, culture, and environment depend on the strategy. For purposes of clarity, I will cover each separately here but hope that the links between both can be clearly seen.

Strategy

In short, developing a clear strategy – and as early as possible – is vital when leading national systems. In fact, it's very difficult to lead without one, even if you've got the skills to empower people. More specifically, the strategy should drive *all* activities on a day-to-day, week-to-week, year-to-year, and cycle-to-cycle basis. In this respect, a strategy should provide the framework against which all decisions are made in the system: so simply put, if it's not in the strategy then don't do it! Part of the reason for this is that, in elite sport, you have got to contain interests because sometimes people do things for their love of doing it; but if it's not in the strategy then that effort is not supporting what we fundamentally need to do. It is therefore important that the strategy itself is clear and succinct; so much more an 'eight-pager' than an '80 pager'. Of course, there is a lot of complexity in what national systems do but, essentially, high performance isn't rocket science and so there's a need to keep things as simple as they can be to channel focus and effort. Importantly, this applies to systems at all stages of their development. For example, as a system grows it inevitably gets more complex and there is a lure to start looking for the 'silver bullet'. However, the risk is that you then lose sight of the basics as there is no substitute for hard work – we know that. As such, a clear and simple strategy can provide the anchor for all times in a system's evolution.

In terms of the components of strategy, the way that finance is allocated is clearly a central factor. In my view, there has to be a targeted investment approach as a system can't be all things to all people given the limitations on national resources. Importantly, however, targeted investment is also a positive strategic choice as ambitious goals help sports to strive for more and continually raise the bar. Additionally, reducing investment can often be the stimulus or lever that some individual underperforming sports require to make the required changes to their strategy, structure or personnel. That said, there does need to be a balance between broad and specific investment as relying on a couple of sports is a very dangerous strategy (i.e. more eggs in fewer baskets). In this way, decisions on where to allocate money across the full spectrum of sports can't be based exclusively on previous results as, over the course of multiple cycles or years, some sports will underperform (or be perceived to have underperformed) in certain periods or moments for a host of different reasons. In this respect, sustainable systems require leaders to evaluate a sport's future potential as well as past performance; including what those sports have meant, or will mean to the culture and narrative of the country. For example, in my role with HPSNZ, our investment in both cycling and rowing had to be cut based on their results at the Rio Olympics in 2016, but this was still of a level that could enable success in Tokyo given their potential to perform at the next Games. Of course, the balance between investing resource for 'now' or 'later' is difficult; especially as national governments tend to focus on one major event or phase at a time. However, if success is to be sustained, then this balance is crucial.

As a broader example on the nature and role of strategy in a national system, my own approach with HPSNZ for the Rio Olympic and Paralympic cycle tried to channel many of the principles listed above. Overall, the ambitious goals of 14+ medals from the Summer Olympics and ten to 14 gold medals from the Summer Paralympics drove our strategy. This latter focus on *gold* was a particularly key driver as it put Paralympic sport at the forefront of peoples' attention in the NZ government and society. More specifically, one key challenge that we had to address was "why does government invest in high performance sport?" I had also experienced a similar challenge in Canada, where targeting funds generally went against the grain of society. In the case of NZ, being successful on the world stage was clearly part of the motivation but another part (that we integrated within our strategy) was that such success was important for its broader potential to inspire the nation. In this respect, the government in NZ understood that you won't always improve your medal count; it inevitably has to plateau, so, something extra was needed behind it and that was the goal of inspiring the nation. That said, the medal counts were always going to be the most significant factor in how we would be judged after both Games, but this focus on inspiration provided some balance and was an element in our decision-making. In the end, we invested in 13 different sports in the Olympic programme and five different sports in the Paralympic programme as well as some targeted campaigns from a small group of other sports that all had the potential to win medals *and* inspire.

People, culture, and environment

As noted above, a key enabler of a national system's strategy is that system's people, culture, and the environment. With respect to people, you can have a fantastic strategy but if you don't have the personnel to deliver it then it doesn't really matter what the strategy is! Accordingly, checking, monitoring, and managing each individual's fit across the system's goals and strategy is essential – for example, you can have the world's best physiologist but if they are not a team player then there is no place for them in a system that aims to succeed via a collaborative approach. Of course, some individuals are particularly important for enabling strategy; namely those who lead and coach in each sport. Indeed, high performance directors and coaches (even more so) are typically the key enablers of an athlete's success. Given this emphasis, world-leading sports science, medicine and technology support should also reflect the sport's coaching goals; not the other way around. Certainly, a key approach at HPSNZ, and a critical feature of effective HP systems in general, is the customisation (or tailoring) of servicing and support based on individual sport need and the areas with the greatest impact on performance: not a 'one size fits all' or 'cookie cutter' approach! In many cases, there is therefore no need for every sport to have every type of practitioner; in fact, less is often more when it comes to support. In short, national systems and their individual sports require the 'right people', not necessarily 'lots of people'.

In terms of culture, or 'how we do things', this is also clearly linked to the people in a system and grows bottom-up, laterally and top-down. Despite what many people still appear to think or do, culture isn't something you 'do' on a staff away day; it has to be continuously worked on through the promotion and reinforcement of day-to-day behaviours that are linked to the system's values. Another important consideration on culture is that a 'happy culture' isn't necessarily a 'performance culture'. More specifically, performance requires a level of challenge and tension that means that the environment can't, by definition, be an inherently 'comfortable' place. Externally, a performance culture also needs to be outwardly facing and understand what everyone else is doing around the world; taking the good points to move the system on, confirming what can be overlooked, and validating what is already being done. As such, a system can't be so insular to expect that it knows it all, or not to let others come in from outside to assess and comment. In the end, it's the execution of the strategy by your people that matters when it comes to competing in elite sport; not just the strategy itself.

Delivering outcomes for the nation: some principles on 'HOW to do it'

While having principles on 'what' needs to be done is important, my experience to date has also emphasised the importance of 'how' national systems are led. In this respect, the role demands a host of qualities and skills. However, a number do stand out for me that I have chosen to focus on here. These are: *adopting a partnership approach, providing and promoting challenge,* and *embracing and enabling urgency.*

Adopting a partnership approach

If a national system is to be successful, then bringing people with you is clearly a key objective from a leadership perspective; especially when you need to drive changes quickly and, in the long-run, enhance the capacity and capability of each sport to be self-sufficient. In this sense, I've always believed in a partnership (rather than a compliance) approach: the relationships with sports cannot be 'here's your money and get on with it'; but it also cannot be 'do this with your money and only this'. Instead, I feel that a 'how can we work together to reach our shared goals' approach is needed because, in simple terms, each sport's goals are the national system's goals. Against this approach, I've always made a conscious effort to prioritise the term 'investment' over 'funding'. In short, for me, 'investment' denotes a partnership approach; that 'we are in it together'. On the other hand, I believe that 'funding' tends to denote a compliance or transactional approach; one that, at worst, can lead to a 'hands off' mentality. So as ever, language can be crucial.

One of the most significant benefits of promoting a partnership approach is that sports then come to you with their challenges, which you can help them to solve for the benefit of everyone, rather than them hiding them for fear of funding cuts. In this sense, the alignment of a national system requires an environment where individuals can share thoughts and concerns without retribution. I've therefore always tried to have visibility and be 'in the system', as well as encouraging staff to get out on the ground too. For example, at HPSNZ I tried to emphasise the importance of our staff understanding the pressures on each sport and what could and couldn't be done to achieve our shared goals. Additionally, the goal for my performance consultants (i.e., the main contact point for each sport) was to try and understand the sport more than the sport themselves so that they could add value rather than be 'compliance managers'. Overall, relationships need to be two-way if they are to deliver optimal, mutual benefits.

In terms of other benefits, such 'two-way work' is the cornerstone of individuals feeling involved and committing to the system's goals and journey. It is important that individuals feel like they have a voice and that leaders operate an 'open-door policy' to encourage staff to proactively share their views and questions on the various elements of programme delivery. Of course, such a proactive approach is also required of the leader and the leadership team. For example, the initial period in the CEO role is intense but, in the majority of cases, it's important not to come in all guns blazing and instead listen to people and help them feel that you're engaging them. Clearly, not all of these views will be equally relevant or actionable, but at least they've been heard; a factor that can build credibility and limit the potential 'kick back' when it comes to the inevitable time for tough decisions. When these two-way relationships are missing, it's far more likely that these tough decisions are going to rile people before they're even made!

When it comes to building these two-way relationships, recognising that you are not the fountain of all knowledge, what each individual brings to the table, and who is best placed to make performance-based decisions are all important factors. In this sense, system leaders can often make mistakes through getting bogged down in the operational elements of the role and losing sight of what's going on within the organisation; in other words, not 'being around' enough to build and sustain relationships with key individuals and groups. In this respect, I've learned to be more personal across my leadership roles to date – developing what a lot of people call the soft skills (albeit I wouldn't necessarily class these as soft given the how significant they are). For example, understanding your staff as individuals is important: you need to appreciate where they're coming from, both professionally and personally; put their perceptions, decisions and actions into context; and then use this to inform how you can interact with them in a respectful way. For a truly collective effort, leaders also need to surround themselves with the best people and then, crucially, empower them to get on with their jobs.

This challenge isn't easy however, as there are often a lot of people involved in a national system – with increases in investment often leading to even more appointments and roles. Certainly, a key requirement for leaders of national systems is the ability to foster positive, two-way relationships with a diverse range of individuals: including influences that come 'top-down' (e.g. government ministers and officials), 'bottom-up' (e.g. high performance directors, coaches, and athletes), and 'laterally' (e.g. commercial partners). For example, one increasingly salient 'lateral' influence is the media given that they can shape national views on investment, medal expectations, and the evaluation of performance at major events. In response to this, I've tried to be open with the media, such as when explaining investment decisions, and proactively helping the public to understand what the national system does (as most just focus on the Olympics and

Paralympics every four years). Of course, media interest also brings benefits that should be harnessed as well. For example, the media are a powerful tool for selling the stories of athletes and forging links back to communities, as well as building the 'national system brand' to encourage additional investment from commercial and philanthropic sources.

While positive relationships with the full, 360-degree range of stakeholders are important, generating a positive impression and, equally, a flow of information from 'above' is often a particular focus for national systems. In some countries, those 'above' are primarily the system's Board, whereas in others, such as New Zealand, government agencies are also involved in delivering one of the system's major inputs – money. As such, if the political will isn't present in the latter then sports will struggle; or even more precisely, political will from those with appropriate influence. In this sense, successful national systems are often those where relevant ministers are highly ranked in cabinet. They are also those where these ministers are 'on the ground' a lot of the time to feed in information as, if they are not, it becomes far more difficult to get the base or additional investment that is needed to keep evolving. As governments themselves evolve, it is also crucial that the national system's chair is engaged with all political corners. Once again, however, these relationships are not static and one-directional. Instead, you have to proactively manage upwards to the board and chair to optimise their knowledge of the system, given that these individuals often act on the system's behalf in some of the most important conversations or events. For example, I always brought my management team to board meetings at HPSNZ so that the conversation was as robust as possible; so that the board could be provided with all of the detail that they needed or requested. This also enabled an added sense of responsibility and accountability for my senior managers and fostered a united board and senior management aligned to our agreed strategy and targets.

Providing and promoting challenge

As stressed, two-way relationships and a partnership (rather than a compliance) approach have been central to my experiences in leading national systems. However, and in line with the need for a 'performance' culture, partnership doesn't mean that you don't challenge. Part of this challenge lies in constantly framing individual, group, and the whole system's actions against the ultimate goals and strategy. More specifically, a continual question within the system should be "will this have a performance impact?" If the answer is "no" then the response must be "then why are we doing it?!" In sum, if a national system is to maximise its potential and deliver the best return then all actions, as a non-negotiable in my eyes, need to be performance-driven. However, for a number of reasons, we're often too soft on people and compromise strategy; as a result, I've tried to consciously present quite an uncompromising approach when it comes to upholding our goals and plan. In other words, you need recognise, engage, and manage the people, groups, information, events, and noise that are not critical to achieving the mission, but you can't be distracted by them. For example, an analytics company predicted that NZ would win 20 medals at the Rio Olympics in 2016 but we kept saying "no", our target, as set at the start of the cycle, is 14+ medals (ending up with 18 across nine sports); a message that was particularly important when the Prime Minister was a key supporter of the high performance system and often spoke of the performance goals and wider benefits of success on the international stage.

Once again, however, challenge should not just be a one-way process and set by the leaders of the system. Instead, challenge needs to be role modelled and leaders have to themselves be challenged. Challenge should be a feature in all relationships and flow to and from every individual and group if a system is to really operate at the cutting edge of performance. For example, the CEO needs to be challenged by the board – you don't want a box-ticking approach as many board members have knowledge and abilities that can be drawn on to stimulate thinking, planning, and action in the system itself. It also makes sense to bring in, or consult with external individuals or groups who bring new ideas and impetus for progress. Overall, I don't mind tension at all; in fact, I think it brings the best out of individuals and simply being 'happy' isn't necessarily going to maximise performance. Of course, the ability to challenge needs to be learned and takes time to become an established feature within a system. For instance, the level of debate and challenge improved over time at HPSNZ but we still had issues with people calling each other out if behaviours weren't aligned to our values. From my own perspective, I also used to hold my cards close to my chest and be quite stoic but then increasingly put things out there as I appreciated that challenge was essential for progress. The level of challenge in a system can also come and go if it is not repeatedly pushed and reinforced. For example, some big nations have recently lost a large part of that challenge as they're scared of offending people or a negative story coming out in the media; fundamentally, however, a challenging environment can lift the system to push its boundaries.

Embracing and enabling urgency

Linked to 'providing and promoting challenge', the need to embrace and enable urgency is also crucial when leading national systems. Indeed, decisions in elite sport usually have to be made quickly as opportunities and progress can be quickly lost or slowed down if they are not. Additionally, you always have to be thinking of "what's next?" In this way, working with speed is another key qualification of the 'partnership principle' identified above; in sum, regular consultation can help to bring people with you but, in the end, a decision has to be made without undue delay.

Significantly, this challenge is not static: as national systems grow, so too can the 'over-structuring' of processes, which compromises your ability to be agile. Agility and responsiveness to new performance opportunities, or the ability to quickly address areas of challenge or underperformance, is essential for any effective HP system. As such, a threat to the functioning and performance of a national system, as far as I've experienced, is that we have too many steps for information to filter through, consult too much and, as a result, take too long to make a call. In the majority of cases you don't need 100% of the information; 80% of the information is often enough on balance as, by the time you wait for the other 20%, you lose focus. For example, I felt that a massive strength at HPSNZ was getting the right balance between data/information and expert opinion to inform future strategy and investment decisions. For as well as the risk of over-structuring, systems can bury themselves in data, information and analysis as they evolve and become more complex. The gathering and analysis of information is of course important: BUT, there is a threshold when there is *enough* information to justify a decision or change of direction rather than continuing to go and chase more and more data which costs time and money.

Of course, working with urgency is not simply a personal preference of the leader. In particular, this ability – and the means to enable urgency in others – is shaped by the model, systems, and processes which the national system operates. Most broadly, and as mentioned earlier, national systems typically work from a centralised or federal model. For example, HPSNZ operated a centralised model in which all key strands were overseen 'in-house'; from investment to performance support to training environments, we employed all of the staff and so could move quickly on a lot of matters. It was also easy to bring key people together, such as high-performance directors, given the size of the country and the fact that sports were located in relatively close proximity. Another positive feature of HPSNZ was that the organisation was a subsidiary of Sport NZ but had its own board and so enjoyed a large degree of autonomy and the potential to take quick actions. Significantly, Sport NZ would also deal with many of the briefings to the sports minister, which meant that we were freed-up from a large part of the bureaucratic process and could focus our attention on leading the system. Additionally, urgency was also enabled within the system itself by streamlining the reporting structure and process. More specifically, when I arrived at HPSNZ there were up to eight individuals working with each sport. Subsequently, this was changed to one point of contact (i.e. the performance consultant) who understood the whole relationship with the sport and so enabled a more co-ordinated, efficient approach. With most staff and stakeholders also looking for change at the time that I was appointed, all of these factors allowed me to drive change quickly; which ultimately became a defining moment in my own career.

In contrast, and reflecting its size, history, and politics, Canada operated a federal model where the national system had to co-ordinate activity across a range of provinces. As such, the Canadian system – and others like it – was characterised by extra layers and numbers of stakeholders. For example, investment was provided from a number of entities (rather than a single source like in NZ), coaching was overseen by various associations, and performance support was delivered through centres in each province, which, perhaps inevitably, reflected different approaches and standards. In sum, federal models present a more complex challenge in some respects and their layers mean that change often takes more time. In this model you can therefore run the risk of consulting and consulting and consulting, leading to a 'watered down' decision which invariably doesn't support high performance. More layers also tend to mean more egos; whereby individuals often want to gain or keep control over their 'part' of the system. Another key factor to recognise is that there is often a duplication or overlap in roles in federal systems, so individuals can often go beyond their remit (and therefore the system's strategy) to carve out their own, unique contribution. As a result, leading a federal system requires much management of the frustrations that stem from the system prioritising national over provincial interests. It also requires an acceptance that the rate of progress can be slowed down at times.

However, this challenge isn't insurmountable and there are still numerous ways to generate urgency; you just need to find a different way to the approach in centralised models. For example, committing additional time to build relationships with the most influential stakeholders early on can lead to greater speed in the future. In this respect, you have to pick and choose who you try to get on board, as based on the strategy and who can add value and impact the outcomes. Certainly, the distribution of people and workload in federal systems means that upward management becomes a particularly key focus (given that those above can shape the agenda for the whole nation). Streamlining the bureaucratic process and allowing for sufficient 'give and take' is also important, as is simply getting staff out on the ground as much as possible; or using Skype or phone instead of email. For example, while high performance directors could be gathered in two weeks within NZ, the same process could take four months in Canada, so finding alternative channels to optimise contact were vital.

Concluding comments

In this chapter, I hope to have provided a useful insight on leading national sport systems as well as some principles that, in my experience, have driven enduring impact. Specifically, these principles were *planning and monitoring, immersion and integration of the entire system, innovation, intelligence* and, in particular, *strategy* and *people, culture and environment*. As well as these 'what to do' principles, I also presented some 'how to do it' principles which I've found to be useful in my roles to date; focusing on partnership, challenge, and urgency.

To conclude with some overarching comments, leading a national system is a sizable task and challenging role. On a personal level, this type of position can certainly impact your work-life balance, ability to 'switch off', and longevity in one environment. Given the fast-paced nature of high-performance sport and the limited chances for 'white space' thinking, plus the number and scale of people that you need to bring together, it's also inevitable that you will have to take calculated risks. You also have to accept that you won't always make the best call – and often not the 'perceived best' call for every individual or group with a stake in the system. On this basis, the ability to learn (and quickly!) is vital for making the most of your time in this leadership role; whether that's about 'what to do' or 'how to do it'. Indeed, the best leaders that I've encountered are like sponges – they continually absorb information and lessons and use these to deliver positive future outcomes. The value of this ability is emphasised even further when we recognise that, despite the apparent similarities, no two systems are alike.

24

Managing a professional football club

Frédéric Paquet with Geir Jordet

Editors' introduction

In this chapter, Frédéric will describe his perspective on managing a major professional sport organisation with an emphasis on the challenge of managing different groups of people. This includes people involved in the performance (players, coaches, and support staff), and the business side of the organisation (administration, the board, and the owners) as well as external people such as media, player agents, other clubs, and fans.

Introduction

I am currently the CEO for AS Saint-Étienne football club in the French top professional league (Ligue 1), and my role is to manage all the departments of the club and build a link between the owners (we have two owners) and the employees of the departments. This means that I am in charge of defining the strategy for the different activities of the club, which are sport strategy, commercial strategy, and administrative strategy. I also propose global projects to the board, and make sure this is accepted. If it is accepted, I implement it.

The CEO role of a football club is not necessarily typical in France. That depends on the club, and sometimes you have a CEO or a general manager for the business and administration at a club, and other times the CEO/general manager is more for the sports organisation. Sometimes the head coach is more than a coach and also functions as a general manager. Different organisations have different organisational charts, and the format for the CEO position really varies from club to club.

My path

I think I am the first generation in France involved in this kind of job. 20 years ago, there was no CEO in a professional club in France (and I guess in Europe as well). Before, there were presidents and a coach, but there was no sports director or CEO. My generation, the people of my age, have created this role.

My start to being involved in professional sports took place in rugby. I was a general secretary of a rugby club in Paris, and then I met people who wanted to be involved in football and they made me come with them. I started in Lille OSC when they were in 2nd division. At the time, there were only ten employees who handled the sports team. Still, from nothing we created everything to win the championship and the cup 11 years later. We also built a brand-new stadium and new accommodation.

We were the first generation to start professionalisation of the organisation in professional sports. At least in France we were first, I do not know the history in other countries, but probably it is something of the same. I started as a marketing director. After that, I created the operations department. I have been director of the academy, sports director, and CEO. I have done all the jobs in the clubs at different periods of time, and I have been director for every department of the club. This way, I know all the major jobs within a professional club, and it has effectively taught me how to become a CEO. I know exactly what everybody does in the different departments because I have done it all before.

Type of leadership

There is not only one kind of leadership. Leadership is linked to the behaviours and personality of people. You do not just decide to be a leader. You become the leader and you need to be accepted by people to be a leader. You need competence for this job. You need credibility. And you need the capacity to gather everyone around a project.

Specifically, you have to be able to present to all of the employees in the club a vision of what you want to do with this club. With this, people can see why they are here, why they must work, what they work for, and when they have to do it. You have to be able to explain and help people get there. My philosophy is that the more responsibility you have, the more you have to take time to help people to work. It is not that I am the boss and they work for me. My philosophy is the opposite. As a boss I need to help people working for me to be as efficient as they can. You are only as good as the people working in the group, so you need to make them be good. To help them, you have to know people, understand what they do, and you have to help them achieve the goal you give them.

To achieve this, they need to trust you, so you have to be trustworthy. They need to trust your competence and your loyalty. You have to give them all the tools to work. You will take care of them. And you need to show this. When a situation is difficult, do not hide! Be in front of them. Propose solutions. Protect the people who are working for you. Protect them by giving them solutions, and by designing who is responsible for what. But sometimes, also be able to say, "you are not good anymore for the group, for the club, so you cannot stay". Make decisions! You have to make decisions to build this unit as best as you can. For me, it is very rare that you have one, good, solution. To me, what we try to do is to get the least bad solution. It is really difficult to find the best solution for everything. So, you have to work, and anticipate, to think of all the options you can have, and take one. In this way, you have to involve people. They have to be involved in the project and be informed about what they are supposed to do, so it is a very participatory way of working. At the same time, you need to be clear about what you want to achieve, and what you are supposed to do. Then, you help people do it! You can have all the help from me to do that. But be good! Because in a professional club, expertise and excellence is key! Our job is to be prepared, and to produce performances. Not only because you are good, but because of who you are. You have the spirit and you want to always be better. You always have to ask yourself if what you have done is good enough. And you have to improve every day.

It is essential to improve and go deep in your analyses to find good solutions. And as a leader you have to be an example of that. You cannot ask people to work hard, to be efficient, and to be loyal, if you do not do it yourself. That means that you have to work and you have to show this. You lead by example. You show everyday your capacity to decide, to shoot away in the direction where we want to go, and propose this in a realistic project with realistic specifications to reach that project. All those kinds of things make you a leader, and this makes people want to follow you. People are ready to do this because they trust you, and they believe in you.

Why is football specific?

An interesting question is whether being a CEO of a football club is different than being a CEO in other businesses, other industries. For me, there are two specifics to leadership in a football club. First, you are managing only human beings. There are material products. Your main material is the human being. And you have two kinds of human beings. You have normal human beings, who are in the administration, so the officials. And you have the stars, who have an ego. You cannot manage these types of people in the same way.

The stars are sport people, but they are also entertainment or media people. They have a show every week, or every third day depending on the competitions, in front of an audience. These are public people. You cannot have the same management for the players and the coach as you have for other people in the administration. But some of the things are still the same. There are some fundamental philosophical things that are the same, like trust and loyalty. The values you have are the same. But the way to manage them can be different. So, this is the first thing. We only have human beings in our company.

The second thing is that this is a media world. Everything we do is in the newspaper and in the radio. We are always in front of the camera. So, this is not the real world. We have to be aware that everything we do is scrutinised and everyone is watching. To me, this is a big difference from normal companies.

About managing these special, highly talented stars, you first have to respect and love what they are. These kind of people for me are the same as actors, all these people who make a show in front of an audience. They are highly skilled because there are only a few of them in the world. Not everybody is able to be a part of a division one team, or coach a team at this level, whatever sport it is. The characteristic or feature for these people is that they need to have an ego. There are few people who can do what they do. They are in the media, and are treated like special people, like stars. Those people give, not their life, but they give of themselves every time they enter the field. If they play a big game, everybody loves them. If they play a bad game, almost everybody hates them. So, it is very emotional. And despite what you might think from reading newspapers etc., these people need to be loved, because this is a very emotional world. They need to be taken care of, and we need to take care of them, have a structure for them and so forth. From the youngest age they do not live in the real world, because we take care of everything for them. At the same time for them, everything is difficult, because in their world it is a lot of sacrifice and hard work. It is hard, it is tough, it is mentally difficult. There are two parts. Most people who read newspapers or sit in front of the TV would say, "wow, their lives are easy. They have money, they have girls, cars, and they are always featured in the newspapers". But to reach that status they have worked a lot. They work every day. Every day! They make sacrifices. So, for them, this is not an easy job. I think we need to love these people. If you are a CEO or a sport director, you first have to love them. Whatever the faults they have, you need to respect the work they do. And you have to accept all the greatness and the skills they have and also respect the celebrity-based benefits that they have access to. This is a part of working with talented people. And this is why you need to be aware of that and adapt your way of talking and how you treat them. At the same time, there are some things you cannot discuss, such as the values of the club, the value of human beings. You cannot negotiate on that. And the values will help to create a structure. They can then say, "okay, your values are not my values and I don't want to work with you". Perfect! If your values are clear, then you can easily have these conversations. The worst thing is to have a team that does not share the same values. Because it just cannot work. I have met some CEOs who said they do not like their coach, saying "our coach is bullshit". But I am thinking, this is your job, it is because you have talented players and coaches that you have gotten this job. This is your life. We live in these surroundings and this is why we are here, because we have players and coaches. People are people, and it is because of them that you are where you are, and you must respect that.

Obstacles to the job

Being the CEO of a major football club can be very challenging. In this section, I discuss some of the obstacles that come with this job. Above all, I think it can be dangerous for the club if I stop anticipating and start to react, because the consequences can be very serious. But, this is something that is up to you. The main thing for me is that obstacles are mainly coming from yourself. If you are careful enough, if you do everything you have to do, you will decrease the risk of any obstacles. When the management of the team is going outside your club, so, the media or whatever, and you lose the control, the smallest thing can become a tornado. And when you lose the control of the protection of your group that can be very difficult to solve. The main idea is to anticipate the problem that you can have, and to then solve it before it becomes very bad.

One example could be when people start talking to the media. The voice of the club is coming from different people, the coach, the players, people in the administration. And when you lose control of that, it can make a big mess in your club.

After that, another type of obstacle is when you do not win games. Even though your work might be going really well, losing games can make things difficult. Because, at the end of the day, the question that provides your most important assessment is, how many games have you won at the end of the season? You can do a bad job, but, if you win the game you'll become the hero. At the same time, you can also do a very good job, every day, but if you still don't win any games, for whatever reason it is, you will be shit. Of course, if you do really good work, you will have a higher chance of winning games. And if you don't work well, the periods where you win games will not last for long. But the performance of the team is there because of reasons. So, when you lose games, not just one, but many games in a row, there is usually a problem in your management of the performance of your team. So, again, it is up to you. Because, if you do not work well enough at the beginning to avoid this kind of problem, you might end up with this problem.

Conclusions

This job asks of you to be accurate and aware, every day. Every day! You cannot say, "yes, this worked pretty well, so let's do it like that and we'll see in one or two weeks". No! If you are not aware every day, you're very soon dead. Every day you have to say "okay, this worked well, but can we do it better, and this did not work, so how can we fix it now?" Every day. This is a "never-stop job". That could be an obstacle as well because you have to be in check and all the people within the club and offices have to be prepared for that. Don't stop. Don't rest. Just be aware! Constantly ask yourself if there is a way in which you can improve. Ask yourself if there is a small problem you can solve right now. That is the philosophy.

25

Managing impressions and relationships when speaking to the sports media

Kieran A. File

Introduction

At first glance, a chapter on speaking to the media may appear out of place in a handbook on elite sports performance. We typically associate elite sporting performance with what is happening on the pitch, in the pool, or on the track rather than what goes on in the interview booth or press conference. It is also a widely-held belief that you cannot talk your way to a win and that actions speak louder than words, especially words spoken in the media. Additionally, for many elite performers, speaking to the media is an unwanted distraction that can take them away from their teammates during times of celebration, interrupt important recovery routines, be an invasive presence during preparation, or take messages and meaning out of context, innocently or perhaps for strategic effect. So, why would elite performers, or an elite performance handbook for that matter, dedicate any time and space to it?

The simple answer is that speaking to the media is now an obligatory component of the elite sporting experience and it is a space where elite performers can achieve important goals relevant to a life in high-performance sport. Two of these goals are *the management of your impression* in public with fans, journalists, and other interested over-hearers, and *the management of important professional relationships* that can be affected, for better or worse, by media performances. Both of these goals are important considerations for elite performers. Having a positive impression can, for example, increase your fan base and open up potential sponsorship opportunities. On the contrary, having a negative impression can attract scrutiny which may prove distracting or detract from your accomplishments. Potentially problematic media behaviour also has the potential to create tension for the close working relationships many elite performers need to work hard to foster. Conceptualising media interview performances as a relationship management opportunity also opens the door for strategic action to be designed and taken, whereby a range of interpersonal goals like defending other's reputations, motivating one's team or particular players, or even attempting to plant the seeds of doubt in the opposition's head can be performed by skilled interviewees in these public conversations.

In order to achieve these important goals in media performances, elite performers need to develop healthy attitudes to the media, awareness of what they can expect in media interactions, and an array of strategies to help ensure they negotiate their media interview encounters in a professional manner. This does not mean elite performers need to like the media or the people behind the microphone or the keyboard. Rather it means understanding and respecting the role the media play in the elite sporting experience and developing strategies to manage everything they can throw at you so you can work towards managing your impression and your relationships when being interviewed. In some cases, elite performers may also wish to develop a greater awareness of the media's practices and processes so they can be harnessed and manipulated for strategic gain.

In this chapter, I elaborate on these two goals drawing on my experiences as a media educator for elite performers and my own research into media communication and language use in the sports media interviews. In Section 2, I consider how elite performers typically attempt to manage their impressions in the sports media and the importance of understanding your context when thinking about impression management strategies. In Section 3 I unpack some of the key interpersonal work elite performers do when speaking to the media in order to protect and have a positive effect on important professional relationships. In this section we also consider the notion of playing mind games in the media which is a different kind of interpersonal strategy some elite performers may wish to engage in. It is hoped that for elite performers reading this chapter, the discussion of these two key goals will help them reflect on how they can manage their impression and their relationships in their media interview performances.

Impression management in the sports media

Managing one's impression or coming across well in the eyes of others is a pervasive human concern in any social setting. We all want to come across well and we take steps every day to appeal positively to others. However, what this entails is an extremely complex question. Understanding how to generate a positive impression requires careful consideration of the context you are operating in and the social attitudes, norms and values that are shared by people involved in this context.

Researchers have identified some of the broad underlying values that elite sporting performers appear to orient to when speaking in the media (Caldwell, 2009; File, 2012, 2015, 2017; Rhys, 2016). File (2015), for example, found in an analysis of 160 post-match interviews with professional football and rugby athletes that athletes shared a concern with constructing themselves as modest and humble, as respectful of the opposition and officials, as emotionally balanced and as a team player. These values may reflect, in part, perceptions by elite performers of what the fans, the public, or journalists reporting on sporting events typically consider socially appropriate for athletes speaking after matches have been completed. This study analysed post-match interviews from two different sports but also two different regions of the world suggesting that, at least in a team sporting context, these values reflect some of the more general concerns of elite performers when presenting themselves in the media. These values were most visible when elite athletes were faced with a question that potentially threatened their claim to being modest, humble, respectful, emotionally balanced, or a team player. For example, interviewer questions that aimed to highlight the individual accomplishments of an interviewee during a match, that aimed to elicit an interviewee's reaction to a controversial refereeing decision, or that tried to capture of the emotional highs and lows of a sporting result were often met with a range of evasive or downgrading strategies as the player attempted to navigate any potential pitfalls to their impression.

Humour is also a strategy that elite performers can draw on in their media interviews to help manage their impressions. Possessing a good sense of humour is seen as a universally appreciated social attribute, and is one elite performers can utilise in order to come across positively. File (2017) found that football managers would employ humour attempts in post-match interviews, in some cases to negotiate questions about controversial refereeing decisions. An example reported on in this study was Garry Monk's (manager of Swansea at the time) "I didn't know you were allowed two goalkeepers" response when he was asked about a missed handball decision that went against his side. Depending on how they are delivered, humour attempts like this, at a moment of great frustration for a football manager, can give the impression of someone that is in control of their emotions while at the same time allowing you to register your displeasure at a refereeing decision. They are also quite indirect and can therefore help elite performers to avoid sanctions often associated with directly criticising referees (see File, 2017 for further discussion of this).

However, while humour delivered well can facilitate a positive impression, humour that fails can leave an elite performer picking up the pieces, defending themselves or even apologising. File and Schnurr (in press) found that athletes' and coaches' humour could fail and the repercussions of this could be damaging to one's impression. One example from this study that gained some recent attention was a humour attempt by Sam Thaiday, a professional rugby league player for Brisbane and Queensland. Thaiday, in a post-match interview, likened a recently completed match to losing one's virginity – "not pretty but we got the job done" (see Hunt, 2016 for a report of this interview). This strategy was seen by some as an amusing and unique way to answer questions in an interview genre often criticised for its generic responses. However, others found the joke distasteful. This and the other examples presented in this study suggest that humour which can be deemed as sexist, racist, or that makes light of issues like domestic abuse may be edgy and can win you some fans, but it can also draw negative attention to your impression and activate a wider audience that is likely to condemn such humour attempts.

Bear in mind your context!

The above reflect some general values and strategies that elite performers appear to orient to when attempting to construct themselves in the media. However, the specific context an elite performer operates in will also require some careful consideration. Fans listening to your interviews may draw on a number of social and cultural ideas that have become associated with your sport or the way elite performers who play your sport typically behave. For example, how a boxer is expected to speak pre-match may be very different to an equestrian rider, rugby player, gymnast, or tennis player due to the sociohistorical and cultural values that reside in the fabric of these different sports. As an elite performer you have a choice whether to draw on or resist these expectations and associations as you go about cultivating your impression.

In some cases, though, certain social values and ideas can have an overbearing influence on how your media interview strategies are interpreted by fans and therefore constrain your behaviour. File (2018) demonstrates this in a study that showed how managing a big club like Manchester United can create certain expectations about how the manager should speak. In this study, an analysis was carried out on the way David Moyes spoke in media interviews during his tenure as Manchester United. During his tenure, Moyes was the target of criticism by Manchester United fans not just because he lost a number of matches but also because his media interview performances did not appropriately capture the way a Manchester United manager should speak (Stone, 2014a, 2014b). This study compared the answering strategies Moyes employed with those used by his predecessors, Sir Alex Ferguson and Michael Phelan, and found that Moyes spoke quite differently to his predecessors. Some of those differences included Moyes' tendency to compliment fierce rivals (i.e. Manchester City and Liverpool), to mitigate strong criticism of his team and team performances in losing efforts, to reduce or avoid talk that highlighted the expectation surrounding the club, and to avoid over-promising with respect to the future and the response expected from the team. Many of these differences between the way Moyes and the way his predecessors spoke were highlighted by fans as problematic because they rubbed against the norms associated with being manager of a club with high expectations (Jackson, 2014; Stone, 2014a, 2014b).

Media strategies like being complimentary of the opposition, being less critical of your team, and trying to avoid over-promising are used by football managers and managers of other sports teams across the world every day to generate the impression of a manager who is respectful and careful not to create too much pressure on his team. So why did they not work for David Moyes? In some contexts, like being the manager of a big club with high expectations (like Manchester United), these strategies could take on different hues of meaning. For example, compliments directed at a rival after a loss may be interpreted negatively as admiration of the opposition team which might upset fans that have a hegemonic position to uphold. Or, by being less critical of his own team's performance in a loss, the manager may be coming across as accepting of mistakes and bad performances which could raise questions about a manager's ability to be able to handle a club with high expectations. What this study highlights is the importance of understanding your context and that decisions about how you present yourself can be constrained by the context you are operating in. At a practical level, this may mean that some of the general media interview strategies elite performers typically draw on (like being overly respectful to the opposition or not promising too much) may not be appropriate to the specific context the elite performer finds themselves in.

Your context can also throw up very specific and unique challenges that require careful thought and consideration. For example, what is the best course of action for a player upon returning from a performance-enhancing substance ban? This is certainly a challenging context from an impression management perspective, one that should involve a range of strategic decisions from identifying a particular publication to share the story with through to working out what you want fans of the club to know about your return. Other specific cases I have been involved in include helping a player negotiate the fallout after signing for a rival club (and seemingly betraying fans of his current club), and helping coaches and players find the best way to deal with public scrutiny surrounding their appointment as manager or captain of a team, especially in cases where their appointment is seen to be a controversial one. Managing one's impression in relation to specific issues like these can require a detailed unpacking and understanding of the context, the clear identification of the underlying threats to one's impression and the design of the best course of action with which to go ahead.

In summary, while there do appear to be a number of general values the sporting public seem attached to with respect to professional athletes, particularly when speaking after a sports match or event, successful impression management requires attention to one's own context. In some contexts, the general strategies elite performers typically draw on may need reconsideration as they may indirectly create meanings that negatively affect your impression. For any elite performer that is experiencing increasing levels of media exposure, it is worth considering what values sum you up and/or are evident in your sporting context and getting help on how you can orient to them in typical sports media interview genres.

Relationship management in the media: protecting your working relationships

Elite performers also need to understand that media interview performances play a key role in the ongoing management and maintenance of professional working relationships in high performance sports teams and organisations. While the primary audience for sports interviews is the fans and sporting public, it would be naïve to think that media interview performances are not available for teammates, coaches, squad members, or opposition athletes and managers to access at some point in time. If you have said something that is or could be interpreted as particularly inflammatory or critical of an individual then some form of wider coverage is almost guaranteed as media sites are increasingly publishing stories based on controversial interview performances. This, therefore, means it is important for elite performers to have their key relationships (and the maintenance of them) in mind when approaching a media interview or press conference.

One of the biggest threats to professional relationships is being interviewed after a loss. In losing efforts, interviewers will often ask elite performers to evaluate things that have gone wrong and this can prime listeners for any criticism or blame an interviewee appears to be attributing to others for the loss. One of the biggest regrets or concerns for an elite performer is that they have said or will say something that is or can be understood as overt criticism or blame of someone in their team or circle which, in turn, causes a rift in that relationship. Being able to carefully negotiate your evaluative messages in a losing effort is a skill elite performers need to develop if they are to be successful at managing their professional relationships in the media.

Many of the elite performers I have worked with or interviewed as part of my research have alluded to the need to be delicate and careful when speaking to the media after a loss. Richie McCaw, World Cup winning captain of the New Zealand All Blacks rugby team, was particularly conscious of the way he was coming across in the media in losses. In a research interview I conducted with him about his experiences when speaking to the media, he alluded to his underlying relational concerns and the strategies he tended to employ to manage relationships when speaking after a loss.

Research interview with Richie McCaw
1 March 2012
Extract theme: relationship management, not 'having a crack' at your team or the referees

Richie McCaw

1   Some days you just don't turn up but you're not going to say that are you + so==

Kieran File

2   ==Why are you not going to say that even if it is the truth?
3   Why would you not come out and say we just didn't turn up?

Richie McCaw

4   Well that's having a crack at your boys isn't it, you know
5   So you might do that behind closed doors
6   But that's not something to air out in public you know

Kieran File

7   But you do do that behind closed doors?

Richie McCaw

8   Oh yeah definitely + definitely

9   You point out things with people and you're pretty frank about it, you know

10 Um, but [in the media] it's not the time to air your dirty laundry and, especially as a captain, blame guys for not fronting, you know

11 You say "hey we're all at fault here, we've got a few things we can get right and we've got to go and sort that out"

12 That's why rugby players get accused of being pretty boring interviewees

13 But they don't want to be a front-page headline

14 You know you make an outrageous comment about "the ref is an idiot" or you know, that just gets you nowhere

15 Because next week you've got the same ref or the week after you've got the same ref

16 You ain't gonna get anywhere

17 And that's why as a loser you've got to be gracious with it and just say "oh we're going to fix it"

18 And when you win you sort of say "we're not going to get ahead of ourselves"

19 And that's the general picture especially in a competition

20 So {laughs} I think you can see why probably boring is the right word

This extract, from a very experienced and respected elite performer, reveals a concern with avoiding publically 'blaming his guys' (lines 4 and 10) as well as the avoidance of critical comments about the referee in a losing effort (lines 14 to 15). While the reason for the avoidance of blaming his players is left implicit, a reason is offered for avoiding blame of referees: that you need to have an ongoing relationship with them and critical comments may negatively affect this relationship. This is almost certainly the case in team circles as well, where public shaming, or causing a player to lose face with the sporting public, not only has the potential to affect your own relationship with the blamed or criticised individual, but may also affect that individual's standing with other members of the team or circle, especially if you are the leader of the group and your opinion carries weight with others (as alluded to in line 10). Neither of these outcomes is relationally a good one, as a mixture of unconfident, unhappy players and bad relationships could negatively impact team work and cohesion.

The notion that such comments can become a front-page headline (in line 17) also shows that the media are particularly interested in professional working relationships or any apparent pressure on them. Overtly emotional remarks that hint at problems behind the scenes contribute to the drama that encapsulates interest in professional sport by the public and is therefore an interest media outlets are keen to probe. While avoiding criticism and critical feedback is not possible in professional sport (something also alluded to above, lines 8–9), as it performs an important function in the correction of on-field issues, the media does not appear to be the best forum to offer extensive or overt criticism, especially immediately after a match or event. This is why elite performers often look to avoid comments that could be perceived of as blameworthy and to modify or soften any critical commentary that they do offer in media interviews. Even in cases where a critical comment has been softened, the practices of the media, including the shortening, adjusting or repositioning of quotes to remove softeners and to fit particular narratives can also alter the effect of a comment. This can have the effect of heightening the illocutionary force of a critical comment which may in turn put even greater pressure on a relationship.

McCaw also alludes to the potential for such concerns to result in an unengaging or boring interview experience for fans. It is often the need to manage relationships in the media that drives the generic or 'boring' media interview performances, whereby elite performers draw on a range of safe platitudes in an attempt to negotiate potential threats to their relationships. Skilled elite performers will always be looking for opportunities to engage audiences in the media (as this can help improve your public impression), however, they are also adept at identifying situations when more careful management of relationships is a priority which may mean authoring a less engaging media interview performance. Of course, elite performers then run the risk of being labelled boring or generic; however, the reason such strategies are frequently drawn on is because they serve important interpersonal goals for elite performers like the protection of relationships.

Other interpersonal goals: praising and playing mind games in the media

Beyond protecting your relationship with your team, skilled practitioners may also use their media opportunities to achieve other interpersonal goals. Praise and positive remarks given in media interviews are an example of this. Players and coaches are often required to positively evaluate their own performance or the performance of their team in media interviews. Ex-All Black captain Anton Oliver referred to this process as "handing out the goodies" (research Interview, 04/06/2011). The act of praising can be conceptualised as a strategic one whereby high performers use it to positively impact another individual's feelings of self-worth or their standing in public. Examples of this include a coach motivating an individual player through the media by praising them or members of the team throwing their support behind an embattled manager. These actions suggest the use of praise is an important tool an elite performer can employ to have an impact on the way others feel.

Another interpersonal goal experienced practitioners might attempt is to use the media to get under the skin of competitors. For the most part, elite performers are at pains to illustrate the amount of respect that they have for their opposition when speaking to the media. This is often driven by a desire to not provide any additional motivation to the opposition before a match. However, media opportunities can be strategically used to try to unsettle an opposition team or an individual – a practice that is often referred to as mind games. The goal of mind games is to innocently or directly raise doubts about the abilities of an individual before the match and/or to undermine the confidence of the intended target or the confidence in the intended target by team mates. The use of the media in this process helps to improve the likelihood that a message of this kind, that aims to unsettle, will get to its intended target.

One elite performer that is often associated with mind games is the current England rugby team head coach, Eddie Jones. A recent example of this came in the lead up to 2018 Six Nations rugby match against Wales where, in a pre-match press conference, Eddie Jones questioned the ability of opposition first five, Rhys Patchell, to be able to handle the occasion (Jones & Williams, 2018). The quotes attributed to Eddie Jones from this pre-match press conference have been provided below:

1   When Alun Wyn Jones and the guys go down for breakfast on Saturday, they'll be
2   looking at him [Rhys Patchell] thinking, "can this kid handle the pressure?".
3   It's a big ask.
4   It's easy to play when the ball is on the front foot and going from side to side, but
5   when it gets a bit cut and thrust, nip and tuck, this will be a proper Test – then we
6   will see if Patchell has the bottle to handle it.

7   He hasn't played much Test rugby at all. He is going to have [Chris] Robshaw at
8   him, [Owen] Farrell at him, [Danny] Care at him – all guys that have played a lot of
9   Test rugby.

A number of strategies are employed in this example that can be read as an attempt to under-mine the confidence of and the confidence in the player in question. For example, he highlights the player's lack of experience (lines 7 to 9) and refers to him as a kid (line 2), both of which implicitly function to question this player's credentials and therefore chances of success on the big stage. He also raises the possibility that the player's own team and captain will be questioning his ability to perform and creates a story about what will be going through the Welsh captain's mind (at breakfast) before the event (lines 1 to 2). Such a strategy could also plant seeds of doubt across the team. He also cites specific actions and events that the targeted player is likely to expe-rience during the game (lines 7 to 9) which, when they occur, may act as a primer or reminder for such comments (and associated doubts) to resurface in the player's mind during the match.

Of course there is no guarantee such comments will achieve their intended outcome. However, by using the media in this way, they are at least likely to reach the player or team tar-geted for the psychological barb. Experienced practitioners know that comments that are marked or untypical in media interviews (like the public questioning of an opposition player) make for an engaging news stories, and the subsequent flurry of interest in such comments can make avoiding these comments difficult for the intended target. Journalists will often want to follow up such reports and stories by asking the targeted player, or other players in the team, for their reaction to these comments. In this regard, the media, in their desire to elicit a reaction and give a story legs, inadvertently act as the messenger, delivering the comments to the player or team in question. And, even if it is publically rejected as ineffective by the intended target, the message, and the ideas inherent in it, have at least reached the target and therefore have the potential to impact the psychological preparation of that player or team.

In some sports and some media interview contexts, mind games are commonplace. The pre-match interviews and press conferences before boxing and mixed martial arts matches, for example, frequently involve public questioning and criticism of an opposition fighter, sometimes with the target of such mind games sitting in the room. In other sports, certain personalities or teams may become associated with such behaviour. The Australian cricket team have been an example as this is a sport that is culturally recognised for its values of respect and politeness (often referred to as 'gentlemanly' behaviour). While there is technically nothing wrong with playing mind games, some sections of the media, particularly those covering the opposition you are attempting to unsettle, can use these comments to portray you in a devious and/or malicious light which can leave you open to accusations of being a bad sport. Considering the extent to which any unwanted attention from the media will affect your team is an important factor in deciding when and how to use this particular technique.

Conclusion

What this chapter has argued is that elite performers need to develop skills for negotiating their media interviews so they can both manage their impression with the public and manage any potential threats to their professional working relationships that can be (inadvertently) caused by media interview comments. Speaking and communicating is an interpersonal activity whereby people design messages in an attempt to make a connection with others and come across well and also make choices that aim to protect and maintain good relations with the people they are speaking with or to.

These principles are no different for people who, as part of their profession, need to speak to a wider audience through the media, although the specific values speakers need to orient and the strategies they need to employ can be specific to this context. With respect to managing one's impression, appearing modest, respectful, emotionally balanced and, if relevant, a team-oriented player are all general social values shared by athletes, the media, and fans, and are therefore brought to bear on interview performances by those who are listening and interpreting an elite performer's performance in a media interview. At the same time, an elite performer's specific context may constrain their behaviour which can require a more careful consideration of the interview strategies employed in order to successfully negotiate a positive impression. When managing relationships, being particularly aware of and prepared for difficult interview situations, like speaking after a loss, is time well spent. Being careful to mitigate criticism that could be blown out of proportion by the media and threaten relationships is one consideration elite performers should engage with.

In conclusion, because of the potential value associated with a good impression and strong relationships for elite performers, developing skills for speaking to the media in ways that foster and protect your impression and your relationships is therefore a worthwhile endeavour and should be a component of any elite performance development programme.

References

Caldwell, D. (2009). "Working your Words" Appraisal in the AFL Post-match Interview. *Australian Review of Applied Linguistics*, **32**(2), 13.1–13.17

File, K. (2018). "You're Manchester United Manager, You Can't Say Things Like tThat": Impression Management and Identity Performance by Professional Football Managers in the Media. *Journal of Pragmatics*, **127**, 56–70. doi: 10.1016/j.pragma.2018.01.001

File, K. A. (2012). Post-match Interviews in New Zealand Rugby: A Conciliatory Media Interview Genre. *New Zealand English Journal*, **26**(1), 1–22

File, K. A. (2015). The Strategic Enactment of a Media Identity by Professional Team Sports Players. *Discourse & Communication*, **9**(4), 441–464doi: 10.1177/1750481315576837

File, K. A. (2017). 'I Didn't Know You Were Allowed Two Goalkeepers': How Football Managers Negotiate Invitations to Criticise Referees in the Media. In D. Caldwell, J. Walsh, E. W. Vine, & J. Jureidini (Eds.), *The Discourse of Sport: Analyses from Social Linguistics* (pp. 71–91). New York, NY: Routledge

File, K. A., & Schnurr, S. (in press). That Match was "a Bit Like Losing your Virginity": Failed Humour and Identity Construction in TV Interviews with Professional Athletes and Coaches. *Journal of Pragmatics*

Hunt, E. (2016, June 2). State of Origin 2016: Sam Thaiday's "Losing your Virginity" Quip Splits Opinion. Retrieved 6 June 2016, from www.theguardian.com/sport/2016/jun/02/state-of-origin-2016-sam-thaidays-losing-your-virginity-quip-splits-opinion

Jackson, J. (2014, March 14). David Moyes: Manchester United are Underdogs in Liverpool Game. *The Guardian*. Retrieved from www.theguardian.com/football/2014/mar/14/david-moyes-manchester-united-underdogs-liverpool

Jones, C., & Williams, R. (2018, February 8). Six Nations 2018: Rhys Patchell's Team-mates will Doubt Him, Says Eddie Jones. *BBC Sport*. Retrieved from www.bbc.co.uk/sport/rugby-union/42989860

Rhys, C. S. (2016). Grammar and Epistemic Positioning: When Assessment Rules. *Research on Language and Social Interaction*, **49**(3), 183–200.doi: 10.1080/08351813.2016.1196546

Stone, S. (2014a, April 22). Moyes Can Have No Complaints Over Fan Reaction - Mitten. *BBC Sport*. Retrieved from www.bbc.co.uk/sport/football/27113751

Stone, S. (2014b, April 30). Aura of Authority: How Van Gaal Differs from Moyes. *BBC Sport*. Retrieved from www.bbc.co.uk/sport/0/football/28542835

Part V
Fitting systems to societies

Up to this point, our contributors in this book have shared insights on a number of important factors in elite sport systems; covering aspects of coaching, science, and medicine, and the leadership and management of these and others. Through these contributions, we also hope that a number of common themes have become apparent, especially with regards to *how* and *why* individuals and groups work and interact the way that they do within this high-profile and high-pressure environment. However, we also hope to have highlighted that these common themes are not identical themes: in other words, while some general principles may apply and prove to be effective in lots of different elite sport systems, optimal impact arrives when these principles are specifically tailored and woven into the deeper fabric of the team, department, organisation, or culture. Indeed, the majority of the messages so far have been delivered on an 'it depends' basis: there are few, if any, automatically 'right' or 'wrong' ways to help performers and teams to develop, prepare, or perform; rather, there are simply 'more appropriate and effective' or 'less appropriate and effective' ways relative to the context and challenge. Accordingly, the purpose of this section of the book is to further emphasise how leaders, coaches, and practitioners work to fit their work to each unique environment.

As an important point to elaborate on, these environments are shaped by a multitude of factors. Some are more directly related to the sport, some are more directly related to the culture of elite sport in the specific region or country, and some are more directly related to the culture of wider society in the specific region and country. Indeed, the way in which a team, department, or organisation works will be shaped not only by the nature and demands of the sport itself and how most competitors train, prepare, and perform, but also to what is perceived to be normal, appropriate, and aspirational in the wider elite sport *and* regional or national community; especially when there is a strong media involvement. In this respect, social identity and expectations are significant factors in how elite teams, departments, and organisations approach their work and harnessing them can be a powerful driver of progress and performance. On the flip side, there have also been plenty of cases of difficulty when elite systems have been more imposed, or 'copied and pasted' into different societies or cultures, including within the same country or region. Or, additionally, when these systems have found friction – either early or later in their development – with the evolving values and perceptions of their surrounding society.

So, to consider this key challenge in more detail, our contributors in this section offer their experiences of applying their general philosophies and ideas across very different – and often very unfamiliar – cultures and societies. Sticking to the overall objectives of the book, these perspectives are again intentionally diverse in terms of the sports, roles, and societies considered, so to encourage a focus on the implications of *how* and *why* elite sport tends to work as it does. More specifically, the first contribution is provided by Mads Davidsen and focuses on his experiences of working as a technical director at Shanghai SIPG Football Club in China. In this chapter, Mads reflects on his professional journey and outlines his current role, before describing how he has tailored his work to his Chinese context. As part of this account, Mads summarises the organisation of Chinese football clubs and at Shanghai SIPG and then outlines some of the cultural challenges, language-based challenges, some typical mistakes, and how to adapt when working in the country. From here, Tynke Toering then presents her perspective on the challenges of working in typically male-dominated settings. In her reflections on this topic, Tynke considers the role and influence of gender stereotypes and gender bias, how these impact on the experience and progression of women's careers, and steps that can increase gender diversity in elite sport moving forwards.

Building on from Mads and Tynke's views as 'hands on' practitioners in different contexts, Chapter 28 then sees Anne Pankhurst and Rosie Collins present a position on the development of players and coaches around the world. In their contribution, Anne and Rosie focus their thoughts on the nature of 'elite-ness' in a performer sense, some imperatives of athlete development policies, issues in the development of elite athletes and associated coach education and development, and the impact of historical, cultural, social, and structural factors on this development. As another opportunity for comparison and contrast, Guus Hiddink then presents an account of a 'coaching nomad', based on his wealth of experience and successes around the world with various club and international football teams. More specifically, Guus focuses on how to adapt and work as a professional football coach in different countries and under very different cultural, linguistic, and societal circumstances. As part of this perspective, Guus provides an overview of his journey in football and outlines his approach in terms of working with other staff, bosses, and, of course, players. Guus also offers some reflections on challenges around language and the personal factors and consequences of working in diverse settings. Finally, this section then concludes with a contribution from B. J. Mather and Dave Rotheram, focused on the societal contrasts between England and Australia in the context of talent development in rugby league. In this chapter, B. J. and Dave outline some of the history and organisation of the sport in both countries, before considering some key contrasts across both environments through some of their recent research work, including reflections on the influence of academies, politics, and finance.

Overall, we hope that this section is useful for emphasising the importance of tailoring approaches to specific contexts and societies. In this respect, we again recommend that some points are kept in mind as each chapter is considered. In particular, notice the extent to which our contributors work out (or refer to the need for) a balance between *delivering* and *tailoring* their pre-established, or generic ideas and principles. Also worthwhile to note is the extent to which this tailoring works to manage expectations and build relationships, but also to harness as many of the positive, 'natural' features of each different context or society. In this sense, it is worth recognising how each coach, practitioner, or leader has come up with their solutions or principles for aligning to the values, standards, and goals of those they work with or for.

26

Fitting within the social milieu

Mads Davidsen

Introduction

During a radio-interview in Denmark a few months ago, the interviewer said there were thousands of young coaches who "would give their right arm to be in your shoes". I said "I don't think they would". A bit cocky, yes, but it's a comment I stand by because I don't think many people are willing to sacrifice enough to achieve what they actually set out to do. Indeed, if I look at one area where I have done something that sets me apart from other professionals in my field, it has been my willingness to make sacrifices. I personally don't view the choices I've made as sacrifices per se, but sacrifices they have definitely been. Deciding to not drink alcohol so I could allocate all my time, energy, and focus towards my career as well as working for free when you just want to learn. You use all your money on study-trips, and every time money does come in you use it on something that can develop you. When you travel around to different clubs, just to visit and get inspiration, and you don't have any money and have to stay in shitty hotels and B&B's just to be there. Postponing starting a family so as to first build up your career. All of these things have I done for ten years to get to where I am today.

Back in 2010, I vowed that I would go abroad and take the first chance of the career I dreamt of that came my way, regardless of where in the world it was. And that is exactly what I did. In my book, when people want something, they do what it takes to get there. I have every respect for those people who say they just want to live in their home town or country, make good money, and enjoy a good work-life balance. I am not saying my path is better; I am just saying, don't talk about ambitions and dreams if you don't want to sacrifice to reach them. My dream has always been to make a difference for people and projects. To lift others, achieve and to fulfil our potential together with others.

My journey

My coaching career began in 2005. Before that time, my own playing career had been on the third tier of Danish football; I had suffered from a lot of injuries and lack of talent, so I quit. It was then that I was invited to do a little bit of coaching, which I did for six months in B.93, a team based in Copenhagen. At the end of the six months I was asked to become head coach, a position which came as a real step up as suddenly I had to train more than I actually did as a player. It was during this time where I really felt like I could improve the players I was coaching; that I could actually help them to achieve something. Despite also studying for my masters degree at the same time, I started to focus more on my job in football. I was also studying for other development courses at the time, and this is where I met Ebbe Sand (a former Danish professional football player) back in 2008. Our conversation one night in the hotel I was staying at for a coaching course is what started my journey towards his academy in China. I was clear about my professional ambitions and desire to go abroad, and explained that I didn't have anything holding me back as I'd never bought a house or an apartment, and owned few possessions so I was ready to move quickly when the right opportunity came along. After that night we spoke many times, and when the job offer came in 2012, he still referred to that conversation and how I had made a lasting impression in terms of how far I was willing to go.

At the time of our initial conversation, Ebbe was the striker coach for the Danish national team. But when in 2012 he came to open this football academy in Shanghai, he asked me to run the academy as its technical director. It was a tough, but good year. After nine months, we had a good academy, but I was missing the higher-level football content and wanted to go into a Chinese club. At the same time, Chinese football really started to progress, and it felt like this was my chance. I took a trip with a Chinese agent and we visited different clubs, with me spending all the money I had on dinners and meetings. Then, as if by coincidence, I received a call from Sven-Göran Eriksson who was about to get a job in Guangzhou, south China. The general manager from that club was someone I had already met one month before. So I joined the club along with Sven, and was just doing scouting for him the first six months; finding players, looking at opponents, conducting analysis, and whatever else he needed me to do. I became one of the assistant coaches at the end of this six months, and we had a really good year. With a team that had the 13th highest budget, we finished third – an outcome which probably will never happen again! And from here followed what so often happens in football; we become attractive to other opportunities because we'd over-performed.

Shanghai had never been big on football. Historically this had always tended to be Beijing and Guangzhou. But the Shanghai government wanted to make a big new club, so they put together the government and Shanghai International Port Group (SIPG FC) and they took over a minor club's players called Shanghai East Asia, with the goal of driving football forward in Shanghai. SIPG contacted Sven and asked him to be the head coach of the team. When Sven was subsequently sacked in 2015, the club promoted me to the position of technical director, with the task of setting up the whole philosophy throughout the club.

Current role

My role as technical director at Shanghai SIPG FC has been to create, develop, and implement a football philosophy and strategy in the club. This extends from the first team right down to our U5 academy-team, and covers everything in terms of methodology, style of play, coaching, training curriculum, coach development, communication, player development, and staff recruitment. This all comes with the general goal that I ensure we develop as a club over time; trying to reach our targets of being constantly in the top flight of Asian football and having the best academy in China, as well as developing our younger players to the top level so they can go on to make up our first team.

My journey in this role began with the need to build everything in the beginning, because the club was started completely from scratch. I'll never forget sitting down in our first meeting, and the General Manager and Club Secretary asked us how many goals and cones we needed.

Absolutely everything was being taken from ground zero. For these first two years we spent a lot of time focusing on the first team only; making sure we got league results immediately, and that we established the right recruitment set-up, the right training, and the right philosophy. After this initial phase, I started to focus more on the academy side. This involved building up the U23-team, U21, U19, and U16, and we are now in a position that we go down to U14. This again involved ensuring we used the same philosophy and style of play as with our first team, and building a methodology for delivering these across all age groups. At this stage, we had to ask a lot of questions in order to get things right, such as "if we want to play like this, how do we train on Monday for the U14, how do we train on Wednesday for the U19, and how do we coach?"; "What do we analyse? What is our analysis model?"; and "What is our recruitment strategy? How do we find players? What kind of players are we searching for?"

All of the above together makes up what I view as phase one, of three. Now we are in phase two, I am in more a position of overseeing the running of the club, and trying to look for opportunities to make important marginal gains. My work has been less practical for the last year and more strategic. In the beginning things were quite the opposite, as I had to train and coach every single age group twice a day. I had to show everything by doing, because I had to show everyone how it *should* be done. Now the coaches can operate themselves with me standing behind them and whispering them in the ear.

The Chinese football club as an organisation

Every football club in China has what we call a president. A position which in Europe would be known as the CEO. It is the president of our club that I report to. Under the president are four general managers, who act as day-to-day leaders of different areas; one is focused on marketing, one oversees the more football operational side (e.g. taking care of logistics for trips and tournaments), one is responsible for finance, and then you have me, on the same line, as a technical director. Under us is an academy director, who in a way is on the same hierarchical line as me, but who still reports to me. Beneath the academy director, every football team at the club has a team leader, and normal staff, coaches, and such.

Outside of the day-to-day club environment, we also have four youth scouts working for us to recruit Chinese players. We don't have any foreign scouts searching further afield; the rule in China is that a team can only include three foreign players, so few that we actually decided that it simply wasn't necessary. That said, through my own personal network we do have partners around the world who update us on players that might be of interest to us. If they help us we pay them, but they don't work for us contractually.

Working specifically with the first team, is head of medical, Eduardo Santos, who works with the coaches with regards to training, rehab, and general organisation. There are also two fitness coaches for the first team, and this set-up extends to the whole academy; with an academy head of fitness and each team having its own fitness coach.

The culture in China, is that for the first team a head coach will often bring his own staff. This is something that I have been fighting against. In recent years, some clubs have been known to hire ten coaches one year, then sack them and hire ten new ones the year after. I believe that this is an unhealthy model for any club to follow. Instead, we have decided to have certain positions that are always covered by the same people. For example, last year, the head of medical, goalkeeper coach, and head of fitness remained at the club, even though our head coach changed. Rather than bringing their own team with them, the new head coach had to adapt to our staff, and make use of the knowledge and the philosophy in their work that they had already. One could say this has been my biggest change I've made to the club's ethos in my time here, but it hasn't been easy at all due to the existing culture. I can understand why coaches prefer to travel with their own team and the people they trust; they know exactly how they work, but I stand by my opinion that this practice is simply not healthy for the club in the long term.

Cultural differences

There is no doubt that culture is very different between my native country, Denmark, and my home for the last six years in China. It can almost feel like a different world. The differences extend across many different levels, but perhaps first and foremost in terms of leadership and communication. In the Danish society, organisations have a very flat, hierarchical structure, involving close dialogue and relationships between the boss and their workforce. This is very different in China as communication from the boss, who sits in the decision-making position, is very one-way towards those who work for him. In China, employees either won't or indeed often can't ask questions to their boss, and they are also not interested themselves in having any involvement in the decision-making process. So when it came to working as a leader in China, it was clear that I had to adapt to my working environment and learn how to operate within its culture. I believe that the key to succeeding in this task is to adapt. This does not mean to completely change yourself or to simply go with the flow, but to adapt to the existing culture and then try to slowly push it towards your own way of doing things. For example, I changed my feedback strategy because the Chinese don't like to be criticised publically or in front of others. To be fair, no one likes being criticised, not even us Europeans, but there exists another level of embarrassment in China if a person is publically offended. With this in mind, I decided to split up my feedback procedures, so the general performance feedback for the team was given to the team together, with a focus on the more positive elements, and the more negative/room for improvement points were given individually or in smaller groups. This was for me a way to adapt to the culture without changing the way I work and lead people, and represented the best way I could find to succeed within the environment.

Another way I have adapted to the Chinese culture in my work has been that I felt it was important to involve the leaders above me a bit more than maybe they were used to. Club owners in China tend to stay away from team affairs; you generally don't see them and they don't interfere, they just make decisions and let a general manager implement what's decided. By contrast, we involved them when we were buying players. I'd explain to the owner in detail why we knew this was the right player for the club and show him my analysis; sometimes he was impressed and even surprised at how meticulous we were in our detail about why one player was more suitable than another. I felt this change of general protocol was an important means of adapting with a view to bringing more success to the club over time. A clear and transparent strategy and consistency within the management group and in the squad. Focus on the process and not the results. Then you win – over time.

As much as anyone in a fresh, exciting position is keen to bring about change, I cannot stress enough how important it is when working in a different culture to 'play the game' and adapt. I sometimes say that China has a 5,000 year-old history and that it would be naïve to think I could change that in my time here. Indeed, my contract doesn't stipulate that I am here to change the culture either, but I feel this is probably where most foreigners fail. I've seen foreign coaches come here, grabbing what they think is easy money but, trust me, they're out again in a short time as they become very unpopular in the culture faster than they realise.

When it comes to football more specifically, one issue felt in China is that football culture is still to be properly established. China is a football development country and needs time to understand and educate its stakeholders to take the right decisions on and off the pitch, in order to become a more progressive football nation in the future. One element in need of development is the country's sports system; despite many years of successful Olympic programmes boasting several hundreds of medals the last 40 years, a closer look shows you that most of these medals are won in individual and closed-skill sports, where athletes are often successful through many repetitions and quantity training methods. Football is, by contrast, a team and open-skill sport with decision-making happening all the time, and this is an issue which I have noticed exists at the grass roots level in terms of how training and coaching are understood, which needs to be reviewed and opened up as the demands in football are so different to where the country's sportspeople have historically found so much success.

Another sport-specific example of cultural differences I have found from working with the Chinese players on a daily basis is their motivation. To those from more rough and underprivileged backgrounds, football is often seen as 'a chance in life', an opportunity to fight against poverty and feed the entire family through a successful career. This is further compounded by the fact it is a norm in Chinese culture for the child to act as the hope of the family's future, needing a good career in order to pay for their relatives' lives. For me, coming from a privileged country such as Denmark where we often discuss how to 'create hunger in paradise' this couldn't have been more different. In Denmark, the living standards enjoyed by the players mean they generally all are there because they simply love what they do, so much as to continuously work for ten to15 years in their chosen career every single day.

In support of this approach, there is evidence which shows that internal motivation has a longer lasting effect than external motivation. Arguably, if you play football to survive and secure your pension, you will lose your drive and meaning when that part is secured – so what do you play for then? With this in mind, I set out to create a culture of excellence in my daily environment, where the main purpose and motivation was to improve the players' learning every day. I wanted to 'trick' those players with the external motivations to understand that this more internally motivated way of working would also benefit them in the long run financially; as they will earn more money the more successful they are. I selected the players with internal motivation and ran extra sessions with them, while the externally motivated players were ready to leave the training pitch or just as they arrived for the normal team session. In the beginning, they barely noticed the extra sessions going on, but after a while they started to hang around watching, later on asking about what was happening and eventually joining in, coming to my office asking for more. By this time I had all the players putting in additional work and feeling an internal drive to do so, something which culturally was not there from the beginning.

Looking out beyond sport, I think it is also important to understand and respect the country you live in, in order to successfully adapt to its culture. And I have found through my time here that cultural differences can also exist within the country itself. For example, Shanghai is a very international city, not hugely different from many major western cities, meaning that some things here are similar to my life in Copenhagen. Chinese people call Shanghai the 'Chinese Paris'. Of course architecturally there are no straightforward similarities, but when people who live in north China come to Shanghai, they see this city as different. The Shanghai people view themselves as international people, whereas if you go to Beijing, they view themselves as Chinese. This difference in mindset makes a big difference for foreigners, like myself, living here. If you visit a coffee shop in Beijing they assume you speak Chinese, whereas if you visit one in Shanghai they hope you speak English, because they want to talk English. Some people I have met from other cities tell me they don't like people from Shanghai because they see them as arrogant. Indeed, it is said that people from Shanghai think everything around Shanghai are simply farmer cities, because they see Shanghai as the centre of China, even though Beijing is of course the capital. This international mindset is why I have heard from other people that it is easier to work in Shanghai, because not only do people there understand slightly better what you mean, but they also *want* to understand you better.

Language

I believe that Chinese is probably the most difficult language in the world to learn. And I'm not on my own with this opinion, many scientists and linguistics also believe this to be the case. When I studied German I could find there was some logic to what I was learning, "ah, that's the same as in Danish" or "this is the same in English". But the Chinese language has its own language code, which means there is nothing a person learning it can compare with. Added to that, the Chinese system of every word having four different meanings; the intended meaning is only determined by the pronunciation, which means you can really easily mess it up! When I found out what it would take to be fluent, I said to myself "I simply cannot do this, with the intensity of my normal work, so I will only focus on the football side". I videotaped myself in training in order to determine the 100 words I most commonly use in my philosophy and training. I then took the list to a teacher asked her to teach me those words as fast as possible. You could say that my football Chinese is now of a decent standard, but if I was to try and speak about politics, for example, I would be in trouble! After starting with these basics, I took some further lessons to be able to order a coffee and to be able to small talk, but I am certainly not fluent.

The issue of language is certainly an important one. New coaches come in to the club all the time, and you cannot expect them to learn the language when they are here only for a season or two. Translators are very important, but this is still complicated as the Chinese language has a lot to do with pictures and is therefore difficult to translate directly into English words. If, for example, someone wanted to say that they are happy today, the Chinese translation would be something like "the sun is standing high on the sky". Differences in meaning and inference such as these have taught us that the translator needs to understand what is being said very specifically. As a result, we are not able to use translators like we would in Europe, where a knowledge of languages but no football understanding is acceptable, instead we need translators to be able to understand as much about football as possible, because they don't just translate, they *explain*. Therefore, the best translators we have found are actually the coaches who are able to do so as an additional part of their role.

Another way I have learned to get around this problem is that because we cannot always talk together, it can sometimes be more valuable to see the same pictures. I began to use far more video analysis and show the footage instead of just talking about what I meant. This change has had a huge impact on the players; when we saw the same picture I could see them grasping the idea much faster than when someone was just saying something. I believe this visual communication is so much more efficient when you can't speak the same language.

Typical mistakes when working in China

Generally speaking, I would say that the biggest mistake foreigners make when coming to China is that they come in thinking that they have to change everything. This problem is not only the fault of the coaches, but also the clubs. As I previously discussed, the hierarchical structure of the clubs in China means they typically give too much power and freedom to the coach. They often say to the coach that "you can buy the players, you decide all your staff". The coach then of course thinks that they have all the power, but they have to make sure that the Chinese environment around them is working with them, because without it the players won't stay. Again,

I believe this comes down to not accepting the Chinese culture, but most importantly that the Chinese culture when it comes to football specifically is still emerging. Imagine if we travelled back in time and watched training sessions in Denmark in the 1970s. Assume that we knew what we know today about tactics, technology, nutrition, conditioning, etc. – you would laugh. But those 30 or 40 years of development were needed to bring Danish football to where it is today, so why would anyone think they can change Chinese football in one or two years? And yet I find this wrong assumption to be one which many coaches coming over here have. They come in and start to blame and point fingers at everything, because it is too behind the times. Coaches push too much, have too many complaints, make too much noise, and what I have seen is that rather than driving things forwards, slowly the environments moved against them.

That said, the Chinese football culture is changing, but slowly. Change isn't just coming about in things such as the exercises used in training, but moreover in the mindsets of those involved. The biggest change which is taking time to come about in Chinese football, is the progression from what one might call 'formal training' to more 'functional training', a point which comes back to my previous discussion of changing the approach to more open-skilled sports. Young players may have done inside passes more than 20,000 times without any opponents or any pressure, and there's nothing wrong with that basic technique, but what they are lacking is sufficient exposure to functional training. This means that when they turn 18, and are suddenly told by a Spanish coach to play 4–3–3, with triangles and moving around, they cannot deliver because it is so far from the formal training they are used to. You don't go from passing from A to B, to suddenly play 11 versus 11. There needs to be a building up of skill; starting to play one versus one, two versus one, two versus two, four versus three, and so on.

Another specific case on how foreigners often misunderstand the communication which exists in a professional Chinese environment is the lack of answering. There is a saying in China that the word 'no' does not exist, and this is reflected in the way you are met with a negative reply. I myself have had several meetings where I came out thinking things went really well and soon a deal would be done, but I never heard from the other party again. This is typical in Chinese culture that they won't necessarily tell you their full opinion in the meeting, but will make a decision afterwards and if their answer is no, often not contact you again. This can be difficult for us Western people to read/understand, so it's important in meetings that you listen carefully to any signals you can detect, and have a good understanding of the relationship you are building up with the person that you wish to do business with. I have known several coaches come here and believe that they had already signed a contract, but the feeling wasn't mutual and when I had to tell them that things wouldn't work out as they expected, they thought I was crazy. They would say things like "What are you talking about? We just had a great meeting" and I would tell them "I'm sorry to tell you, but you will never hear from them again". Then after three months they would call me to say that they haven't heard from anyone, just as I'd predicted.

The real challenge is now to make sense of and navigate such meetings. The most important question you have to ask yourself is, "what power does the person you are meeting with actually have?", because things may not be all that they seem. A classic mistake many foreigners make is that they go in thinking things are positive because they are meeting the general manager. However, where in Europe a general manager would have, let's say, 80% of the decision power within the company (with perhaps the last 20% just asking the board if they can go ahead), in China the hierarchy is extremely top-down, meaning that you are unlikely to meet with the right person to make any decisions or take any action, such as the owner. An owner will never be part of an initial meeting, nor do they probably even have a public e-mail so they can be contacted directly. Add to this that they very likely cannot speak English, so you can't call them either. Indeed, the only person often available to meet with is the general manager, and they are happy to meet with you, not because they are lying or being evasive about who holds the 'purse strings', but rather because the Chinese are humble towards you because you are a foreigner. It is out of respect that they will not turn down a meeting or say no to you directly, even if what you propose is a straightforward no-go. Instead, they will just let you introduce your idea and allow you to assume that you are on the same track. This is where the majority of misunderstandings occur for Europeans; a meeting with the General Manager in Denmark, Norway, or Italy would almost certainly lead to a done deal, but in China it is akin to proposing a big strategic plan for a company in Western Europe and having a meeting with the people who sweep the floors. They would probably also listen to you and be nice to you, but they do not have any power. It is also important to note that in China the professional hierarchy is so extreme that even that after the meeting, the General Manager will 90% of the time not even report it to the owner, because he will probably assume that the owner isn't interested. Unlike in Europe where reporting is keenly encouraged, in China you don't speak up, and everyone above you speaks down.

Adapting to a new culture

I believe that my experience shows that you need at least 12 to 24 months to really understand the culture and country that you are in. During this time it is important to be curious and open-mindedly listen to their way of doing things and from there try to adapt and develop it towards what you think is the best way. Too many foreigners fail to spend this time simply studying the culture and environment, and I believe this mistake is a reflection of a massive underestimation of what successfully doing so could bring over time.

Being a backpacker will never enable you to understand the world, is my thinking. I read some books by people who had worked in China and I conducted some of my own interviews with people who had lived, worked, or operated in China; I also wrote down some things that I wanted to achieve and, most importantly, how I could achieve them. It was a personal anthropological study and my aim was to understand Chinese culture and the way of leadership in China. I needed to know how I could take my philosophy of leadership into China and work most effectively.

If you want to work in China with Chinese people, adapting to and respecting their culture is what's most important. Whether you fundamentally agree or disagree with their culture ultimately doesn't matter, but if you don't try to adapt to it, you won't have success in the long-term. Understand the culture, respect the culture.

It is after spending six years in China, studying not only my own journey, but also others' success or failure in adapting to the culture (or not), that I have developed my own cultural intelligence philosophy:

> You have 0% chance of succeeding without adjusting, respecting and accepting the culture of the country, business and/or organisation (club), you work for/in.

I believe that you must learn how to behave in a certain culture in order to survive. It's a word I don't actually like because for me it's my choice to be there and I never have a job just to have a salary. I have a job to make a difference, but that basically is what it's like. It is funny how it really is so simple. I would claim that 75% of the foreigners who come to China don't follow this approach, and that is why they fail. When taking a job in a foreign country, the basic questions you need to ask yourself are:

- Adjust or adapt?
- Respect or force?
- Accept or change?

For me, my approach means that I don't have to be Chinese. I don't have to do everything they do, exactly like them. But I do have to adjust my own approach toward them. For example, some people feel the need to always eat with chopsticks because the Chinese do, but then they look like a mess because they don't really know how to eat with sticks. It's OK to say that I am European and I like to eat with a fork and knife. Don't misjudge the small things when you actually should be focusing on the big factors instead.

Conclusions

In general, for me having cultural intelligence is not only the day to day differences about moving from a life in Denmark to a life in China. Those changes are obvious, and I think anyone could appreciate what initial challenge they could bring. But going one layer deeper, the cultural intelligence I'm interested in is the differences relating to the business environment overall. If I went from working in football and to a job in the insurance industry for example, I am sure I would have to adjust again. Even if I wasn't changing country, I would to adapt to a different business. There is a fundamentally different way of approaching one another; I am sure that people working in insurance don't scream at each other like we sometimes do on the football pitch! But even if I stayed in football and changed club, from Guangzhou to Shanghai, it's still a big difference! It is still important to adapt and adjust, even when moving within the same industry, and in the same country.

27

Vive la difference

Perspectives on the challenges of being a woman in high-level sport

Tynke Toering

Introduction

When I started playing football, I was the only girl on my street, school, or club team. Most of the time, I greatly enjoyed playing. However, it has also happened that boys got sudden 'injuries' when I dribbled them, that same-age kids and some of their parents supporting an opposing team shouted things like "Kick her down, that shrew!", and that a boy with whom I regularly played football called me a transvestite. Only the latter got me angry because I felt let down by a friend. As opposed to this, in the other situations, I felt strong because I apparently played a good game; otherwise, these people would not have responded in the way they did. I absolutely loved playing football and, in my mind as a kid, football never was only men's business. It was incidents like the examples above that made me aware that I was perceived as a girl before anything else, and that this had consequences for what I was and was not 'supposed to do'.

Taking a broader perspective, the recent #MeToo discussions indicate that the beliefs about what are appropriate behaviours for men and women are quite depressing if you are a woman with ambitions. Even we, as women, do not seem to fully grasp the extent to which our minds have been intoxicated by such normative beliefs. Who has decided that we can't be whatever we want? Although, fortunately, times seem to be changing and important progress has been made thanks to the generations of women and men before us, it still is a men's world. This chapter describes some of the challenges for women working in elite sport. Its intention is not to recapture all we know about gender research, but to connect some research findings to practical experiences of women in the elite sport workplace. This will generate suggestions for how ambitious women, men, and organisations could contribute to more gender diversity in the sport workplace.

Men's world

So, who created these behavioural guidelines? And what makes it 'legitimate' to punish people who violate society's unwritten rules? The work by Madeline Heilman at New York University indicates that gender stereotypes and the extent to which we fit these are at the core of the issue. Stereotypes are heuristics or rules-of-thumb that human beings use to quickly estimate a situation. Such automatic judgements enable efficient functioning in many instances; that is, if we carefully weighed the pros and cons of every little decision we make in daily life, it would take an inefficient amount of time to make up our mind and act. However, in situations that require more thorough evaluation, heuristics can lead to several cognitive biases (Kahneman, 2011). Gender stereotypes are generalisations about the attributes of men and women. Quick and unconscious judgements based on gender stereotypes lead to gender bias in situations where women take a position perceived as more suitable for men, often to the detriment of their career progress.

Let's take women in science as an example. In her book *Inferior: How Science got Women Wrong*, research journalist Angela Saini presents a convincing case for how research findings regarding gender differences have been explained in a stereotypical way throughout history, usually by men, and unfavourable to women. In particular, the professionalisation of science towards the end of the nineteenth century (when it became serious business) seems to coincide with sexism in science. As an example, Darwin thought that women were intellectually inferior to men. It has been suggested that the psychological differences (as opposed to physical differences) between men and women are much smaller than the gender differences in terms of the roles and behaviours seen in society (e.g., Fine, Dupré, & Joel, 2017). This means that the characteristics we assign to men and women and the expectations that are a consequence of these, seem to be the reason that the genders are treated differently, even in the same situation.

Gender stereotypes

Research shows that gender stereotypes do create gender bias in the workplace. Being competent and qualified does not guarantee a woman the same steps forward in her career as an equally competent and qualified man. Heilman (2012) indicates that gender stereotypes can be categorized into *descriptive* and *prescriptive*. Descriptive gender stereotypes tell us what men and women *are* like. Prescriptive gender stereotypes indicate how women and men *should behave*. Both stereotypes can complicate women's career progress. Descriptive gender stereotypes typically create a 'lack of fit', between what women are thought to be like and the qualities perceived as necessary for success in traditionally male positions. This leads to negative performance expectancies of women's performance. Violation by women of the normative expectations created by prescriptive gender stereotypes, for instance by taking a traditionally male job, often leads to their devaluation and social punishment.

Elite sport is an occupational field traditionally regarded as male, a fact that is illustrated by the small number of women on boards in the sports industry. A report by Women on Boards (2016) based on publicly available data from websites across global sports indicated that female representation on elite governing bodies of the Olympic movement is below 30%, and is 16.6% on National Olympic Committees and close to 18% on International Sports Federations. Furthermore, female coaches have been and still are severely underrepresented in elite sport; Fasting, Sisjord, and Sand (2017) recently found that only 14% of coaches in Norwegian elite sport were female, despite similar social backgrounds to men. Another example is the gender pay gap with women earning less than men (particularly in football, cricket, and golf), that is starting to be addressed as more sportswomen start to take a stronger stance against this inequity (e.g., Women on Boards, 2016).

Descriptive gender stereotypes: the cause of negative performance expectations

Heilman (e.g., 1983, 2001, 2012) suggests that the male stereotype is often characterised by agency (e.g., competitiveness, dominance, rationality), while the female stereotype is characterised by communality (e.g., concern for others, focus on relationships, emotional sensitivity). In addition, men and women are not only regarded as different, but also as opposites, meaning that women are likely to be what men are not – with the reverse also being true. These conceptions are quite consistent across culture, time, and context (Heilman, 2012). While the female stereotype in itself is positively valued, conflict arises when the beliefs of what women are like do not fit with the characteristics thought to be important to successfully perform in a job. In this situation, *both women and men* tend to have negative performance expectations of (other) women. Do you think about a man or a woman when thinking about a 'leader'?

The Lack of Fit Model (Heilman, 1983, 2001) describes how a perceived misfit between the conceptions of what women are like and the attributes perceived as important to successfully perform a job, can negatively affect performance evaluations of women. High-level positions are thought to require assertive and tough behaviours, which deviate from our beliefs about what women are like. As a consequence, women are not expected to be equipped to successfully handle the job requirements. Heilman argues that this can distort several cognitive processes involved in performance evaluations, such as selective attention, interpretation, and recall.

Selective attention means that we often look for information that confirms our expectations. In the case of a woman doing 'a man's job', women are expected to fail. Selective interpretation occurs when the same behaviour is interpreted differently when it is performed by a man rather than a woman. An example of this was given by Lean In (2018): "When a woman asserts herself – for example, by speaking in a direct style or promoting her ideas – she is often called 'aggressive' and 'ambitious.' When a man does the same, he is seen as 'confident' and 'strong'". Selective recall refers to the fact that we are better at remembering expectancy-consistent than expectancy-inconsistent information. This means that it is more likely that a woman's stereotype-consistent behaviour is recalled than her stereotype-inconsistent behaviour, which of course can have negative effects on her performance evaluations when the job she performs is perceived to require mostly stereotype-inconsistent qualities.

Connecting gender bias research and experiences of women in elite sport

I've been working in elite football and sport science for over ten years now, starting with my master's and PhD research. After taking a masters in psychology, I studied human movement sciences and wrote a masters thesis on self-regulated learning in young promising football players, gathering data from players in professional youth academies in the Netherlands. This was a great experience and, fortunately, I got the chance to continue doing research on the topic for a PhD at the University of Groningen. Thereafter, I've been working as an associate professor at the Norwegian School of Sport Sciences in Oslo, teaching various subjects in sport psychology and coaching, and following up on my research in self-regulation and talent development in football. During this time, I worked for several years as a consultant for the Norwegian Centre of Football Excellence, an institution that provides knowledge from research and best practice to all professional clubs in the country. At the same time, I also did different types of sport psychology consulting work in football organisations, in different European countries. Here, I worked with both management, coaches, and players. At the moment, I am a Senior Lecturer at the Institute of Coaching and Performance of the University of Central Lancashire in the United Kingdom, undertaking performance psychology consultancy in addition. As described in the introduction, I first experienced the consequences that violating society's normative beliefs could have for girls by playing football as a kid. I have experienced various similar situations, but nothing really prepared me for the challenges I faced as a woman working in the men's world of elite sport.

Possible challenges: "just because you're a woman"

As a woman in elite sport and football specifically, reading up on gender research and finding out how just the fact that I am a woman may compromise my career was new to me. Some findings resonated more with my practical experiences than others. Being a woman in such a 'male' position can in itself lead to negative performance expectations (and this of course affects one's career). Moreover, the greater the misfit, the more negative the effect on performance evaluations; that is, the degree to which a job is seen as typically male and the degree to which the female stereotype is activated by the perception of the woman in question increase the 'misfit'. Women may encounter more negative reactions and performance evaluations when a job is regarded to require male qualities and the field of work is typically male. The extent to which a job is perceived as male is, in addition to the job description, determined by "occupation (e.g., the military vs. education), subfields or professional specialties (e.g., surgery vs. pediatrics), academic fields (sciences vs. humanities), and function and level within an organization" (Heilman, 2012, p. 118).

Furthermore, I suggest that factors facilitating the perception of sport as masculine have an effect, as the perception that women have only recently 'seriously' started performing sports (particularly 'male' sports), and that men are physically stronger than women, which often means that men perform at a higher level in sports regardless, persists. Men may therefore be more valued in sport and be expected to have more expertise, even in jobs that do not require the same physical abilities as athletes. If the 'maleness' of the professional specialty and/or academic field matters, it may be less complicated for women in elite sport teams to serve as a doctor, physiotherapist, or mental coach, rather than as a head coach or technical director. In quite masculine cultures women tend to be accepted at the elite level in positions that are perceived as supportive roles. However, even within these roles, the level of her position does matter.

An often-mentioned example of negative performance expectations for women is the gender pay gap when starting in the same job as men. Although nowadays women in top jobs are more likely to have salaries equal to their male counterparts compared to decades ago, there still is a gender pay gap (Women on Boards, 2016). A woman who was the first to perform a certain top job in a major sport worldwide several years ago, and who has been in several high-level positions in elite sport since, explained how she once, early in her career, found out that she had been underpaid. It was only when she got a raise in order to keep her in the organisation that she found out that her male colleagues had been earning this amount of money from the start.

The second factor that can increase perceptions of a misfit between gender and type of job is women's personal characteristics. It has been shown to have negative consequences in terms of performance evaluation if these characteristics make her 'womanness' more salient (e.g., Heilman & Okimoto, 2007; Johnson et al., 2010). That is, if you are a mother or perceived as physically attractive, it is more likely that your performance is evaluated negatively in a 'male' job. To illustrate, a friend recently shared an experience where a relatively young woman had been hired as a leader. One of the first things discussed by her new subordinates in the hallways was the way she looked, implicating that she probably got the job because she was pretty. In addition, they suggested that she would not have the competence required.

Heilman (2012) suggests that other factors which increase the likelihood of more negative performance evaluations for women are those that enable speculation. In these situations much is left to the rigour of the evaluators, and in that case, women are often worse off. Examples of the latter are when there is little information, irrelevant information, strengths and weaknesses are known (because these must be weighed), and unclear performance evaluation criteria are employed. Based on this, it seems that the more professionally an organisation is run, the less likely are potential problems related to gender bias.

A woman working in elite sport often is the only girl in the group. Literature on group work does not make for positive reading. As an example, in mentoring relationships, it is often unclear how much of the credit (or blame) should be placed on whom. This means that the success of a woman mentored by a man can easily be attributed to his expertise, which may mean that the woman at times does not receive the credit she deserves (Heilman, 2012). A valued male colleague support can open doors and help a woman build a good network (Lean In, 2018). A potential downside is that the woman could end up being regarded as nothing more than the mentor's sidekick. This means that, although the intentions of both mentor and mentee are purely positive, the relationship could at some point possibly back-fire in terms of career development. It is important for both women and men who mentor women to be aware of these processes and negotiate their relationship in a smart way. Again, the professionality of the organisations they work for will have a great impact on positive outcomes for both these women and men.

I believe that it is important to mention here that being the only woman in the group is not always problematic; at least, I have also experienced a positive side of it. Given the 'adverse conditions' for women in male-dominated workplaces, a woman who does get the chance to work within such an environment can be quite sure that she has been hired because of her competence. This should add to her belief in her own capabilities. Furthermore, she has a chance to influence the decisions that are made. If you are not at the table, you will not be able to affect what is going on. She will also have a chance to show the value of female stereotype consistent behaviours (soft skills) to performance. Lastly, she will most likely be a role model for other women. This provides an opportunity to show men that women indeed are competent, and opportunities to inspire and maybe support other women, which can be very giving and may contribute to greater gender diversity. Although navigating one's position sometimes is challenging, even difficult, experience teaches that what it comes down to for the only woman on the team, is to perform well now that she gets the chance and to show that she wants to be there. Enthusiasm is a big thing. After all, most of us in such positions pursued our specific careers because we love the job and the elite sport environment, so why not radiate that? This drive is one of many things we have in common with the guys in the group.

Prescriptive stereotypes: the cause of devaluation and social rejection

As described above, prescriptive gender stereotypes produce norms that dictate how men and women are supposed to behave. The female stereotype prescribes emotionally sensitive and caring behaviour, while radiating confidence and dominance are regarded as appropriate behaviours for men but not women. Violating these norms can lead to punishment, such as social disapproval and other negative responses. To work effectively and be successful, however, women in high-level functions and/or in traditionally male fields, such as elite sport, must engage in behaviours inconsistent with the prescriptive female stereotype. It turns out that engagement in such gender stereotype-inconsistent behaviours often is a catch-22 for women in the workplace: women lose some either way. Much depends on the professional behaviour of both colleagues and the organisation. Several examples will be presented below.

Possible challenges related to behaviour

Men expect women to act in a feminine way. A woman in a 'male' job is often regarded as less of a woman if she acts professionally. At the same time, a woman should behave professionally at work. A personal example of this was when a male colleague in elite sport approached me during an event and we had a friendly chat. One thing we discussed was how it is to be the only woman in a room of nearly 100 men. He suggested that I should be more "naughty". I am sure none of my male colleagues has *ever* been told, at work, to show such behaviour. While the remark amused me – it so clearly confirmed the strength of gender stereotypes – at the same time, it annoyed me because I was there as a professional person, not as 'just a woman'. Neither laughter nor anger will bring changes, but it is not possible to ignore such behaviours in the workplace, at least if we aim for more gender diversity in the workplace. Individually, women need to consider how to smartly juggle the biased impression of colleagues. Possibly, acting more flirtatiously may bring some women progress, but others would regard this as submissive behaviour undertaken at the cost of personal respect. It may be worthwhile to discuss such issues with male colleagues, but the potential downside for women of bringing up such issues could be to make them more vulnerable to accusations of being too sensitive or lacking humour. Situations like this must be on the discussion table if anything is going to change. Such a simple example clearly shows the complexity of women's position in the workplace due to gender bias.

The gender pay gap has been mentioned earlier. A behaviour related to this and considered inappropriate with respect to the prescriptive female stereotype is negotiating one's salary. Women are supposed to be modest and, in addition, money is often regarded as a 'male issue'. However, salary is one of the main measures of one's worth at work, and if women do not ensure their worth is rewarded financially, they could appear to agree with the notion that women are worth less than men doing the same job. Further, research shows that both men and women may be less likely to want to work with or hire a woman who is willing to negotiate her salary (Heilman, 2012). As women generally seem to negotiate their salaries to a lesser extent than men, this means that women in elite sport may benefit from informing themselves about effective salary negotiation and how to apply this knowledge to their specific context. Particularly now that times appear to be slightly changing, women may want to consider this.

Self-promotion is another example of behaviour inconsistent with the female stereotype. Given that women are expected to be uncompetitive and modest, explicitly drawing attention to one's skills to get ahead of others can be perceived as something that women should not do. Although self-promotion is beneficial for both women's and men's careers, only women are punished for it (Heilman, 2012). So, although it seems recommendable to everyone to volunteer for certain tasks and to maybe even suggest certain tasks one could do, women may need to take a more nuanced approach to be taken into consideration at all. I am aware of female colleagues who decided to suggest tasks and projects they could do, in a presentation to their boss, but making sure that a senior male colleague would be present to back them up. In this way, *they* made the suggestions, keeping that 'power', but they came across as less ambitious or assertive than when they would if they did the presentation alone without the senior colleague attending, which increased their chances of being heard. This *can* be an effective strategy if a woman is not being heard or considered at all.

Related to self-promotion, speaking up at seminars or meetings is consistent with the male gender stereotype and inconsistent with the female one. Men tend to talk more in meetings and seminars. They more often take 'central' seats, interrupt more, and ask more questions than women. In addition, women get interrupted more often by both men and women (Lean In, 2018). However, to be successful, you do need to make sure that your voice is heard. This in turn may lead to negative social consequences, which probably is why many women hesitate to raise their voice. Personally I have at times applied the strategy of asking at least one question during a talk I attended and/or sharing at least one or two comments during meetings. Barack Obama made a point of this in a speech at the MIT sports analytics conference in 2018:

> Early in my administration I found that guys are loud mouth, and often times brilliant. Women would not always share their perspectives around the table in the same way, or as aggressively, or talk over people. I think that that is not unique to women, sometimes that is true for minorities, at times it just had to do with status. Washington tends to be a status pound. So one trick I had was that I would call on people, I would not just wait for folks to volunteer. Because if you wait for who is talking the most, then it is going to be the same folks, over and over again . . . So I made a habit of calling on these people on the outer rim, because I knew they were doing all the work and they are writing the memo's for the people on the inner rim of the table. But that is what I mean with being intentional about it. If in fact you want a broad set of voices, you will get them. And in today's culture, if you are not deliberately doing that, then you are going to fall behind and somebody is going to beat you in whatever they've been trying to do.

Leadership and communication style are relevant topics too. The perception persists that effective communication and leadership mainly require directness and assertiveness, both of which are incompatible with the female gender stereotype. On occasions, the term 'ice queen' is applied to women in this respect. Some fellow women in elite sport who have a direct communication style indicated that they did not let such perceptions get in the way of doing their job, but they did sometimes feel that it was unfortunate to be perceived in that way. One strategy some of them used was to show a bit more of themselves at work, so that it would become clear that it *is* possible to be many things at the same time *and* be effective. The latter, over time, provided them with a broader range of potential communication styles. Nevertheless, it should be much more strongly recognised that women with their stereotype-consistent feminine, 'soft' approaches and skills bring something different and valuable to the workplace that men typically do not. Qualities such as listening, showing empathy, and having a team focus do contribute to better performance, for instance by generating a wider range of considerations and contributing to more constructive group dynamics. The fact that women are a minority in a team makes them more salient, which actually increases their potential power. This could automatically emphasise to the men in such groups how feminine leadership and communication styles can contribute to performance. Seen in this way, being a minority does not always have to be disadvantageous. Another aspect I suggest that women pay attention to is to make sure that they radiate enthusiasm regardless of their communication style, that they show they wanted to be there. This is of course always a good strategy to get people on one's side.

The mere fact that a woman is successful in a male job can lead to negative reactions (Heilman, 2012). Successful women are often regarded as too assertive (male) and not nice enough (non-female) at the same time. In general, as described by the Lean In (2018), "success and likeability are positively correlated for men and negatively correlated for women. When a man is successful, his peers often like him more; when a woman is successful, both men and women often like her less". The main reason for negative reactions to successful women in 'male' jobs appears to be that these women are perceived as less of a woman (Heilman & Okimoto, 2007). When women successfully perform a job that requires more feminine gender stereotypic behaviours, they are not disliked or disrespected. I have often considered that both men and women attribute the success of women in a male job not to her competence, but to her 'womanness', exactly those qualities that cause more negative performance evaluations for women to begin with. As an example I remember a discussion about a club in a large professional sport. A central position in this club was held by a woman. This woman clearly was very competent in her work. However, she was also perceived as physically attractive. Some male colleagues discussed her competence, and one of the topics crossing the table was that "the chairman probably had additional interests in her". I think that such remarks hardly are made when we talk about the competence of men in similar positions.

Social challenges

Being part of the team

Not every male-dominated field has an extremely masculine culture, although it appears that such a culture is less likely when jobs are divided more equally between men and women. There obviously are large differences between different sports and teams. An often-mentioned challenge is that, when there is only one woman in the group, she will never fully be part of the team, however much she may want to be. It is probably not the case that men just don't want women on their teams, but men in these cultures seem to bond in a different way. For example, a female colleague in elite sport told me that she once ran a clinic with two male colleagues. Afterwards the two men went to the canteen and had a coffee together, leaving her to pack and put away the materials. The men didn't seem to think about asking her to join them or help pack the equipment. Other examples are when the group constantly is referred to as 'boys' or when small-talk mainly contains topics men typically are interested in (which the woman could try to influence). It is of course debatable if some of these behaviours really represent masculine cultures or if they depend largely on the individuals involved.

On a positive note, there may be male colleagues, who see the challenges for women on the team and who try to do something about it. One female colleague reported that her boss once gave a short speech that started with "Well boys. . ." – and indicated how much he appreciated the work that the group had done that day, and how much he appreciated having dinner together as a team. After the speech, a male colleague spoke up and added that he also appreciated very much to have a woman on the team because that is not so common in their sport. Although a woman may not want to be singled out based on her gender, this was an attempt to be inclusive that I suggest the woman in question interprets as a positive response.

Social gatherings

A big challenge for many women in elite sport are social gatherings. It is important to attend social events, given that this is how groups bond. However, in many social situations, women can very quickly regress from being a colleague to being 'just another woman'. In very masculine cultures, men tend to drink a lot and enjoy jokes that are often offensive to women. For a woman who looks and behaves in a feminine way, such situations can be extra challenging. While she will have to accept the sexist jokes to some extent, since they often are part of the masculine culture, she also needs to decide what she believes to be acceptable and make it clear when the jokes are taken too far.

If the workplace culture is very masculine, women need to accept that this culture is ever present, so in social gatherings sexist jokes are likely to happen all the time. Again, many issues link to the professional (and decent) behaviour of the individuals involved, and the culture of the teams and organisations of which they are part. To illustrate the type of behaviour women who work in a very masculine culture *may* encounter, an example from social situations can be given. A female colleague related that, during social interlude at a work event, she walked from one pub to another with her colleagues. She and a male colleague walked about 20 metres behind the rest and as they did so he said: "I really don't understand why you want to work in this sport. I mean, it's not a nice world. . . We talk about you. . . Those guys in front, I'm sure that they are talking about the two of us". Although the guy may have been speaking the truth, most women in a very masculine culture know such offensive comments are made, and try to ignore them. Furthermore, when the woman in question confronted her colleague with what he said, he realised that it indeed was offensive. However, this may be the kind of culture that women must learn to handle.

Other occupational fields and minority groups

This chapter discusses gender stereotypes, gender bias, and how these can compromise women's careers in elite sport. However, gender stereotypes in other traditionally male-dominated fields probably work in similar ways, as may stereotypes related to other minority groups. Examples of the latter are race, ethnicity, age, social background, and religion. But prejudice related to occupation and the country/region from which a person comes, can also play a role. It can be challenging to be the only academic in an elite sport environment, simply because practitioners (and especially those without an academic education) have certain expectations with respect to academics. Similarly, academics may be prejudiced towards elite sport practitioners. Further, coming from a country that does really well in the sport in which a person works can help create positive expectations around the job that person does. The reverse can also be true: people can be negative towards those who come from another country because "you're not one of us".

It is clear then that stereotypes related to gender roles are not the only expectations affecting career pathways. I believe that organisations and their members should embrace diversity and find synergies, instead of looking at diversity as a problem where one group lose something in favour of another.

What can we do in the elite sport workplace to increase gender diversity?

It is essential that the topic of gender stereotypes and gender bias in the elite sport workplace is on the discussion table. We may not like talking about gender bias, because some aspects are sensitive and/or unpleasant, but if diversity is to be increased, we must try to understand each other better. This starts with the willingness to make changes and an open discussion of potential challenges and issues. Once these are on the table, greater understanding will be created, as will the possibility to take concrete action. Pretending that gender bias does not exist, for instance by women who prefer to enjoy their job and their exceptional position and/or men who do not want to 'burn their fingers' and rather keep the status quo, will not help to change the elite sport culture. There are several things that women, men, and organisations can do to increase gender diversity in the sport workplace, some of which are presented below.

What can women do to improve their position?

I believe that women must follow their dreams and try to be whatever they want to be. Women are often advised to behave in a 'more manly' way in the workplace in order to be more effective. Personally I do not believe that lowering my voice when I speak, pretending to be really tough, or trying to be 'one of the guys', will lead to greater respect from my male colleagues. I do believe that I can earn respect by doing a good job, so I will work hard, do what I need to do to perform optimally, and so prove people wrong if necessary. If that means that I have to be assertive and direct, I will do so. On the other hand, if the setting requires that I use my typically female qualities, such as listening, I will also do so, and try and show the benefits of having such soft skills on the team. I won't be able to change the culture on my own and I am aware of possible negative reactions from colleagues, but I won't let this prevent me from doing well in a job I really like. This drive is an important aspect that my colleagues and I most likely have in common. I do believe it is essential for an ambitious woman to gather some people around her that support and advise her. Having such people around me has been a very positive personal experience, and I certainly would not have seen and capitalised on part of my potential and some of the opportunities that I have had, just by myself. I believe it is smart to have such people in the workplace but also outside of it, so that you get a more 'distant' perspective in addition.

While performing the balancing act between gender consistent and inconsistent behaviour, women need to be aware of the different sentiments that exist among colleagues (both men and women) and smartly navigate their career to suit their individual persona. Some women will be more affected by such sentiments than others, which often also has to do with previous positive and negative experiences. When a woman does not fully succeed, she should revaluate what has happened in a realistic way. It is important to be critical to oneself, learn, accept, and move on. However, there also is a risk that women blame themselves for failing to withstand powers that no individual would be able to fight on her own. Sometimes, part of the issue just is that she did not get a fair chance, whether she likes it or not. Ambitious women must realise that gender stereotypes and gender bias are part of much larger societal problems that have evolved over centuries, and it would be unfair to put the weight of a societal problem onto the shoulders of one individual. Although specific career advice for women, such as the advice given by movements like Lean In, may help a great deal, Grainne Fitzsimons and colleagues' (2018) findings indicated that this sometimes also gives the impression to a woman that she can solve the large-scale issues she encounters on her own. While such a 'do it yourself' approach is popular, it is society that needs to be fixed. Let me be clear that the latter does not at all mean that women should not read about or follow career advice specifically for women. What I mean is that they do have to put all of this in the context in which they are or have been working. As an example, much advice comes from women who already are in high positions, which is different from being halfway the career ladder. Furthermore, if we, as women, want to make a change, we must accept other women moving up the ladder.

Being successful and making good career progress can and does lead to negative reactions towards women. Given the existence of gender bias, ambitious women must be aware of the possible consequences of their success, so that they can put things in perspective. "It is lonely at the top" may apply more to women than men. These women must be prepared that people who have not been in a similar position will not always understand, while they may think that they do. When working in very masculine cultures, women should not be too surprised by sexist jokes. In social situations, women should be mindful of what's happening, and adjust their behaviour and if they feel that someone's behaviour is not acceptable, make it clear to that person. Each individual in the workplace deserves to be treated with respect.

What can men do to contribute to increased diversity?

The first thing men can do is to imagine, and understand what it is like to be the only woman on a team of men in elite sport, while having to handle the stereotypical views that women have to deal with on a daily basis. What would it be like:

- to have your competence questioned, based on characteristics that are irrelevant and impossible to 'hide' (women look like women)?
- to never fully be part of the group?
- to have to put overly much thought into how you are perceived by your colleagues?
- to have your masculinity questioned as soon as you try to perform well at work?
- to work in a culture where jokes offensive to men would be the norm?
- to know that you may not get the chance to be whatever you want to be?

Men could also ask themselves in what ways they, as a man, keep the cultural status quo intact, and in what way they could contribute to a better and more equal culture. What is your attitude to women at work? What language do you use in their presence? This might increase men's understanding of a woman's perspective and perhaps it make it easier for them to contribute to gender diversity.

Many men are unaware of many of the challenges described in this chapter, so these must be brought to their attention. Additionally, when you as a man are not sure how you can support women at work: read up on the topic and ask them! Similarly, when you don't know how to best respond to or deal with a specific situation: ask the woman involved! We will not be able to effectively handle such issues by pretending they do not exist and hoping for the best. I am sure that it will also make men's jobs much easier and more fun.

Third, I think that men need to learn to regard diversity as an opportunity to improve their own and their team's performance, rather than as men 'losing out' because of an increased number of women in the workplace. Research has also shown that business units with a more diverse workforce perform better (e.g. Badal & Harter, 2014).

Seven suggestions for organisations

- Discuss the topic in all layers of the organisation. It has to be on the table, out in the open. This enables constructive changes to be made.
- There is a lack of female role models. Make sure that you bring forward role models who represent the kind of woman today's talented young women aspire to be like (based

on the research discussed in this chapter, perhaps particularly feminine role models). This ensures a talent pool to pick from. Use these role models as mentors for the young and promising.

- It should be possible to combine a top job with family life. Make sure that it is possible for both women and men to balance work and personal responsibilities. It enables both men and women to combine work and family.
- Hire more women to key positions. This will contribute to making 'male' jobs less male. It will also lead to a culture change, and thus make it easier for women to perform well in their job. It will probably improve men's performance too, because of increased diversity.
- Pay men and women equally for the same job, period.
- Have a thorough hiring policy with performance criteria that minimize ambiguity so that competence is valued before anything else.
- Develop behavioural guidelines for the workplace and work-related social events.

Conclusion

This chapter illustrates the complexity of the situation that women in high-level positions and/or working in a traditionally male field need to navigate. As the start of the chapter indicates, women learn very early in life that, if they violate the rules prescribed for the female stereotype, disapproval will follow. The question then is how much disapproval she is aware of, how much disapproval she is willing to endure, and how she can act smartly, so that she stays out of gender stereotype trouble as much as possible while maximising her job success. Complying to gender stereotypes can easily lead to unfavourable outcomes in terms of performance. At the same time, social rejection because she violates the norm could go at the cost of both her performance and well-being. For elite sport, women, men, and organisations alike, it is extremely important to be aware of possible sentiments related to gender stereotypes to be able to proactively deal with these in a proper way and make sure that both men and women can be successful in their job.

References

Badal, S., & Harter, J. K. (2014). Gender Diversity, Business-unit Engagement, and Performance. *Journal of Leadership & Organizational Studies*, **21**(4), 354–365

Fasting, K., Sisjord, M. K., & Sand, T. S. (2017). Norwegian Elite-level Sport Coaches: Who are They? *Scandinavian Sport Studies Forum*, **8**, 29–47

Fine, C., Dupré, J., & Joel, D. (2017). Sex-Linked Behavior: Evolution, Stability, and Variability. Trends in Cognitive Sciences, **21**, 666–673

Fitzsimons, G., Kay, A., Kim, J. Y. (2018). *"Lean In" Messages and the Illusion of Control*. Harvard Business Review. Retrieved 22 Oct. 2018: https://hbr.org/2018/07/lean-in-messages-and-the-illusion-of-control

Heilman, M. E. (1983). Sex Bias in Work Settings: The Lack of Fit Model. In Staw, B., & Cummings, L. (Eds.). *Research in Organizational Behavior (Vol. 5)*. Greenwich, CT: JAI

Heilman, M. E. (2001). Description and Prescription: How Gender Stereotypes Prevent Women's Ascent Up the Organizational Ladder. *Journal of Social Issues*, **57**(4), 657–674

Heilman, M. E. (2012). Gender Stereotypes and Workplace Bias. *Research in Organizational Behavior*, **32**, 113–135

Heilman, M. E., & Okimoto, T. G. (2007). Why are Women Penalized for Success at Male Tasks?: The Implied Communality Deficit. *Journal of Applied Psychology*, **92**, 81–92

Johnson, S. K., Podratz, K. E., Dipboye, R. L., & Gibbons, E. (2010) Physical Attractiveness Biases in Ratings of Employment Suitability: Tracking Down the "Beauty is Beastly" Effect. *The Journal of Social Psychology*, **150**, 301–318. doi: 10.1080/00224540903365414

Kahneman, D. (2011). *Thinking Fast and Slow*. New York, NY: Farrar, Straus and Giroux

Lean In (2018). *7 Tips for Men Who Want to Support Equality*. Retrieved 2 May 2018 from: https://leanin.org/tips/mvp

Saini, A. (2018). *Inferior: How Science Got Women Wrong—and the New Research That's Rewriting the Story*. London, UK: 4th Estate

Women on Boards (2016). *Gender Balance in Global Sport Report*. Retrieved 22 Oct. 2018 from: www.womenonboards.net/womenonboards-AU/media/UK-PDFs-Research-Reports/2016_Gender-Balance-in-Global-Sport.pdf

28

Developing coaches and players around the globe

Anne Pankhurst with Rosie Collins

Introduction

In many ways, the world of sport is no different to the world in which we all live. Within each sport every country has its own culture. That culture is seemingly underpinned by a combination of long held beliefs, tried and tested approaches, and a differing stance on the inclusion of 'innovation'. As such, it is clear that the world of sport is a smorgasbord of interacting and conflicting cultures. As a consequence, applying the same athlete development system to the different sporting cultures would be difficult. It appears, that given the different (but linked) journeys of both athletes and coaches, our progress in both, in any sport, as has much to celebrate, but also still faces challenges.

What is an elite athlete?

In sport, the term 'elite' is a quantifiable one because it is outcome-based (i.e. competitive results are the indicator of elite status), but elite performance is also identified by the perception of an athlete's potential. Taking tennis as an example, elite tennis players are generally considered to be those in the top 100 in the world (even though international ranking lists exist for 1000 players!). The rankings are quantifiable because the sport has a common international tournament structure that can, and does, deliver an accepted international ranking system that can then be linked to player ranking in each nation. The top 100 international players, in both men's and women's tennis, therefore have a national ranking that links to their international ranking. Conversely, nationally ranked players are those best placed to progress through the rankings, (possibly reaching the international top 100), and then hopefully progressing to the top ten in the world – or even to the number one spot. Similar ranking systems can be seen in many (especially individual) sports. Even in team sports, ranking systems exist. Rankings give national governing bodies a framework, both for the development of individual athletes and teams, and to underline what success is, both within the sport and for each individual.

In terms of athlete development in any sport, it is necessary to understand the links between the governance of a sport (both in international and national terms), and its process for developing athletes. Clearly, success in any sport is determined by additional factors and not just a ranking. Elite athletes have a wide range of skills and characteristics, both of which ultimately classify them as elite. While many of these skills are sport-specific, they are developed from a combination of personal attributes, specific circumstances, and relevant opportunities. The combination of these three enables an individual athlete to develop, reach, and maintain elite standards of performance. Further, success and elite performance in any sport also depends on superior (compared to lower level athletes) competitive skills, physical abilities, psychological skills, and technical and tactical expertise.

In addition, what often puts an elite athlete ahead of others is the ability to plan and work to a personal training and competitive schedule over a specific period of time; often 12 months, but also in many sports over a four-year Olympic cycle. Long-term planning has become an integral and essential part of the development of elite performance, but hitherto has largely concentrated on physical, technical, and tactical periodisation. Recently, psychological periodisation has joined the list! Psychological periodisation is a term birthed from the original principles of training, which allows athletes to segment their physical preparation to be physiologically ready to perform. For example, they might load in the off-season, taper off in the run up to a big competition, and engage in active recovery post-competition. All of this will be carefully planned out over 12 months, or four years depending upon the sport. Psychological periodisation follows the long-accepted periodisation principles of micro, meso, and macro cycles, but this time for the expenditure, conservation, and recuperation of mental and emotional energy; something that is very necessary in a long season when athletes are also travelling, in order to train, develop, and maintain elite performance.

Of necessity, in any sport, a holistic and multi-faceted support team is necessary, but the financial cost of such a team is (understandably) high. High-level performance opportunities cannot be accessed without travel because of the need for an athlete to take part in both established and new competitive opportunities and experiences at the right level. In addition, high-level sport takes place in different conditions and on different continents throughout the year. In addition to the cost of travel, interdisciplinary sport science support is an essential, indispensible (and expensive) requirement for elite sport. Finally, good, experienced, and knowledgeable coaches are essential for success. This myriad of expertise and expense has to be provided for, and met, in some way and on a consistent basis. Consequently, the financial input of the appropriate national governing body and/or sponsorship is essential for an elite athlete. Financial support is but one of the issues confronting national governing bodies – another important one is how the next generation athletes can be developed? In other words, what are the requirements for future and continuous success?

The imperatives of athlete development policies

The identification and development of the elite athletes of the future is an imperative for all sport organisations and national governing bodies. Elite athletes are in many senses the ambassadors of a sport, with them the profile of the sport is raised and without them vital publicity for the sport is missing. The requirement for any sport is to provide a high quality and sustainable route through which young athletes can develop the skills and abilities needed to continually move up towards elite status. Without a continual throughput of talented athletes the public profile of the sport itself is lowered.

Sport organisations

In many sport organisations conflicting goals are evident. This can be because of conflicting philosophies among the people in charge, but it could also be because of the management structure itself. Often the key aspects of high-quality athlete development policies have not been identified, despite the fact that many components of them are obvious. Further, even pre-supposing that the key aspects have been identified, often implementation is problematic, frequently because of the structure of the sport organisation. In every sport, high quality corporate management must exist to support clubs, and develop coaches and players. However, tennis, like many other sports, has a large number of volunteers who have risen through the voluntary structure to become powerful committee members. These volunteers often determine policy and, therefore, practice, but do not necessarily know what a sustainable athlete development policy looks like. A further consequence of sport governing body management is that even when clear policies are established, they frequently change or are replaced by another system in a short period of time.

A national athlete development plan that can be sustained for a long period is essential, if for no other reason than the supposed ten years that is often cited as the minimum time it takes to develop elite athletes! In recent years many governing bodies have demonstrated a great propensity to change systems after a short period of time. In our experience, this problem is not restricted to sport governing bodies in the UK! Commitment to a specific athlete development system/structure for a minimum of ten years is essential if athlete and coach development alike is to follow a coherent pathway. Indeed, not only is this essential for current athletes, but the sustained success of the support through the development of coaching expertise. Within this timeframe, there can and should be flexibility, with room for small changes. However, constant change and instability should never be present.

Athlete development systems must also be progressive, enabling the athlete to move seamlessly from club, to local, regional, national, and then international level. Naturally, the 'shape' of the system should be a pyramid – with the wide base constituting large numbers of locally-based young athletes who show interest and appear to have ability in the sport. Inevitably, and given the objective is to develop elite adult athletes, the numbers working in the high levels of performance will decrease as athletes get older. Many will find their limits in the sport quite soon, while others will take time. The goal for the governing body is undoubtedly to support athletes for as long as possible to ensure the goal of attaining elite status in the sport has been achieved. For those athletes who leave the group for whatever reason, it is of paramount importance that they remain in the sport. A pyramid structure enables athletes to develop, improve, and progress seamlessly to the next level. However, and sadly for the future of any sport, these policies and systems are more frequently presented as a ladder system, that appears to be based on the idea that those few athletes who join at the bottom of the ladder will inevitably 'graduate' to elite athlete status at the top. Experience and evidence over the years indicates that ladders rarely develop elite athletes, and indeed don't offer an avenue for those that inevitably wouldn't make it to the top! Essentially resulting in reduced participation on the whole.

Coach education and development

High quality coaches are essential to the success of athletes and are thus a vital part of any Sport Development Policy – but in many sports even the 'components' of a good coach at any level can be difficult to define! High quality coach education policies and practice thus become an imperative within any athlete development policy in any sport.

As such, these policies and practices will also inevitably develop a pyramid of coaches, because a comprehensive coach education and development system needs to develop coaches who can bring new athletes (and especially young children) into the sport, but can also coach future and existing elite players. High quality coaches are needed at every level in the sport, but inevitably those who work with children will be more numerous than those who work with elite athletes. National governing bodies need to ensure that ALL levels of coaches can coach to a high level with athletes of different ages and abilities. Whilst predictive systems exist, nobody knows which child in a group has the potential to be the next elite athlete, so the coach working with children is just as important as one working with elite performers. Too frequently, athlete development policies underrate the need to develop highly qualified coaches at all levels of athlete development.

Talent identification and development

A well researched Talent ID and athlete development system that operates on a national basis to identify and retain young athletes in a sport, is an essential component of every athlete development policy.

Importantly, the structure must accept, account, and cater for the wide range of development and maturation stages that young athletes go through. The evidence from many sports is that very few Talent ID and development systems are successful, possibly because they do not accept that rates and timing of growth and maturation processes play a large part in the identification and development of talent.

A strong network of sport-specific clubs across the country

Club networks are an important part of athlete development policies. The evidence is that the majority of young athletes start out in a sport in schools, but inevitably progress to clubs as they develop. These clubs should therefore have the facilities and resources to develop high-level athletes, or should be willing to redirect talented athletes to other clubs if they are not able to offer the training, competition level, or breadth of experience required. The club environment is known to be important in the development of young athletes – forming a 'home' or hub for them as well as providing a network of friends.

The key stakeholders

A national policy must show an understanding of the importance and integration of the key stakeholders (significant others) in athlete development. These 'significant others' include, but are not limited to, club/academy coaches, parents, teachers, and other coaches. This group forms the social and often emotional background 'constant' for young athletes. As 'significant others' they will frequently know and understand the athlete better than anyone.

Too frequently, parents and previous coaches are 'dismissed' and ignored as the athlete grows and matures. National athlete development policies must build in opportunities to work more closely with parents and key stakeholders (especially of younger athletes) and move away from the idea the governing body should 'educate' parents – often about their own children!

Complex issues in the development of elite athletes

Of major importance, and linked to the development of elite athletes, is the implementation of high quality and sustainable athlete development programmes. These must be at the core of every sport organisation's work – if only to ensure the longevity of the sport itself! Elite athletes often receive a great deal of exposure, but these athletes are those who have 'made it' and who (by definition) are closer to the end of their journey, than the beginning! Elite athlete development is an ongoing journey, one that could have started before the age of five or almost certainly before the age of ten, in many sports. So a wide-ranging, long-term athlete development plan is essential. Importantly therefore, the finances of the sport organisation must be closely linked, not only to the elite programmes, but to programmes that introduce young athletes into the sport.

Athlete development

Within elite sport, National Governing Bodies (NGBs) are faced with a variety of challenges. Logically, they must decide what success looks like and then set strategies to deliver that success. This is paramount to allow coaches to direct their efforts appropriately through the athlete pathway. However, the quantification of success will inevitably be different for different sports. For the rugby football union success could be a strong talent pool that develops players who can win the Rugby World Cup, conversely for British cycling success may be the number of medals won in World Championships and Olympic Games. For a tennis association, success at the elite level could be reflected by the number of Grand Slam champions and players in the World Top 10, while for golf it could be having the winners of Open Championships. Common across all these definitions of success shows winning at an elite adult level, notably not through junior competitive success (i.e. winning at Under 9s). However, to achieve these dizzy heights, success for many NGBs could encompass an increase in the number of people taking part in that sport – in other words, the number of grass roots participants or the number of athletes taking part in competition.

If success is measured by the number of champions or world titles then, in a link to talent identification and development policies, many sports will know that the athletes who find success at the elite senior level are very often *not* those who were the best at junior national or regional level, as teenagers. Thus the question for many NGBs is how to prioritise their goals? How do they link athlete development processes and systems to the development of successful youth athletes AND then to successful adult elite athletes?

One answer is simple, given the (as stated earlier supposed) minimum ten-year time it takes to develop athletes the most important issue is programme consistency and longevity. Frequent changes of direction, and even of objectives, are simply not part of a coherent athlete development policy. However, in a number of tennis nations, multiple and frequent changes to player development programmes are the norm. A national player development policy needs to be developed, implemented, and sustained for a period of time of at least ten years so that a consistency of approach can be seen and understood. Such a policy can then work towards a clear definition of success, articulated to coaches and key stakeholders alike. The existence of clear, long-term and non-conflicting goals enables a programme, and the coaches within this programme, to develop elite athletes from a strong base of national, regional, and club level players.

Competitive development

Whilst player development could be viewed as a holistic component of success, it's clear there are many facets of a sport that can be developed. A hugely important aspect is the development of a quality competitive structure within a logical competition environment and philosophy.

However, this again raises the questions of "what is success?" and "how is it measured?". Should NGBs be developing a strong base of competitors from club to regional levels (capitalising on the largest number of athletes, or focussing on developing systems that support the top 1%)? Consequently the shape of the competitive framework is important, but it should link to the overall athlete development policy. The importance of *relevant* competitive formats for different ages, in relation to the appeal and longevity of a sport, cannot be overestimated. Governing bodies can 'make or break' the chances of young children developing as competitors, and staying in the sport, by having appropriate formats for different ages and abilities. As an example, across the world, and in keeping with other sports, tennis uses a mini version of the game for children under the age of ten. The format has children learning on smaller courts, with smaller rackets and a larger, slower ball. As children develop, the court sizes and ball speeds increase in specific stages. By ten years of age, most young players are ready to progress to a full size court, but possibly still need to use a slower ball. Such a system enables coaches to progress and develop the skills of their athletes seamlessly – but it also facilities appropriate competition for children to learn to compete. That competition must be appropriate, but too often sport governing bodies introduce competitive formats that are, quite simply, inappropriate for children and quickly put many of them off the sport. For example, whilst this structure within tennis seems appropriate, there is currently no scope for the players to regress in court sizes/ball speeds as needed once they have been successful once. Resultantly, whilst players are progressing through the system, they are often not progressing at a rate most suitable for the individual. In order to develop future elite athletes, as well as a strong base of national, regional and club level players, high quality and appropriate (to the age and ability) competitive opportunities are essential. Additionally, coaches should also consider that even in individual sports, team competitions are important, especially so for young athletes.

In terms of competition, every sport should have:

- a comprehensive and progressive competitive structure with sufficient numbers and distribution of competitive events and tournaments that are relevant to every age group and level;
- a nationally recognised and respected ratings structure that enables individual athletes and teams to progress to the next level.

However, the extent to which one nation can create such a system is challenging. In many sports, in order to experience the most diverse competition possible, athletes need to travel to the higher-level tournaments to push their abilities. As such, a *nationally* recognised and respected system is not enough – it also has to link to the international competitive structure in the sport. Coaches and athletes alike must be able to understand the requirements and expectations of competition at every level of performance. The international structure which sub and elite athletes need is often a role for the international sporting bodies, but the national competitive framework, must link seamlessly to it.

Coach education and development

It might appear that high quality coach education and development matters only to the coaches themselves. In theory, the higher the coach qualification, the easier it is to earn a living because athletes want good coaching. That is until not enough elite athletes are evident – and then a lack of good coaches is thought to be the reason!

However, one of the imperatives for successful player development is a quality coach education and development programme that is appropriate for, and specific to, the sport. Its objectives should be:

- to develop high quality coaches;
- to ensure that coaches at every level have ongoing opportunities to develop and improve their coaching skills, knowledge and abilities.

Evidence would indicate that in many nations, coach education systems do not deliver high quality coaches or sufficient numbers of coaches at every and any level. To some extent what is possible in terms of coach education practice links to government policy, as well as to internal changes by national governing bodies. As an example, within the UK currently, the tennis governing body outsources the delivery of Level 1 (beginner coach) to Level 3 of a five-tier process of coach education to private companies. These companies then deliver training (tennis modified) to non-sport specific National Standards (which are developed by the EU). As a result, the extent to which any national governing body can directly affect the information and training that its coaches receive is questionable. Following the basic qualifications at Levels 1, 2, and 3, Levels 4 and 5 (the levels deemed necessary for elite performance coaching) are then delivered by the national governing body through its own approved tutors. To date the content of Levels 1, 2, and 3 have been consistent for over 15 years. In theory at least therefore coaches have received a common set of information and training in what they should coach to whom and how – but only to beginner and improver level players.

Comparatively, Tennis Australia, the French Federation, and many tennis governing bodies complete all their coach training in-house. Interestingly, the United States Tennis Association (USTA) has no coach education structure at present, but does develop a number of elite players! The US does however have a strong collegiate system, currently run by two different organisations, neither of which is the national governing body. Many college coaches are unqualified, but the majority are ex-players themselves. But they do (or the collegiate system does!) develop many elite players who then go on to the international tournament circuit. The principle is that good ex-players can make good coaches. However, observation indicates that ex-players who then become successful coaches, have been able to use their experience and adapt their behaviours to work well with the next generation of elite players. As such, it is worth remembering that US collegiate sport has 'creamed off' the best players in their teenage years and of course that other nations do not have such a collegiate sports base.

With this in mind, it demonstrates that, in the likely absence of a collegiate talent pool, or the more likely want and need to capture and develop talent before these four late adolescent years, effective and coherent coach education systems should be a priority for all stakeholders, not just the coaches as previously suggested. With the added complexities of not just cross-sport cultural difference, but cross-country cultural differences, coach education systems therefore must be internationally recognised and applied (or at least as much as is realistic for the sport). Cross-pollination of coaches in this sense can be a brilliant way to drive talented athletes (and therefore the sport as a whole) forward, but athletes and their 'significant others' (key stakeholders) need transparency in terms of the qualifications and expertises of the coaches, as such, removing the potential stigma of ex-player to coach transition. A coach could and should be qualified in their own right, as well as being a talented player themselves, not utilised because of a preference for the latter over the former (avoiding the "I did, so you can" mentality).

Performance planning

The importance of planning for performance cannot be underestimated. Every elite athlete will use a performance plan and will revise and update it on a regular basis. The creation/development of a plan should be done by the athlete and the coach, with the input of significant others (e.g. strength and conditioning coaches, sports psychologists as well as stakeholders as appropriate), allowing the plan to be specific to the athlete, not just an accepted tour or circuit event list). Most plans are for a 12-month period (annual), but could be for four years if it is for Olympic preparation.

The plan is needed to meet the (clearly defined) goal of what the athlete will achieve in the period of time agreed (based upon what success looks like at their level in the sport). However, the plan will then have a number and sequence of clearly defined 'steps' or sub goals, all of which are put in place to build towards the attainment of the main goal.

Now, most importantly for us in this context, coaches clearly need training to develop sufficient expertise to construct a high quality, and hopefully successful development plan for their player or squad. Reflecting this, it is essential that annual and long-term planning skills (as well as physical and psychological periodisation concepts) are taught on the higher levels of coach education courses. While the construct will be similar whatever the sport, the detail should be specific to a sport, and the individual athlete or team member. Disappointingly, many higher coach qualifications do not appear to include this very important skill in the syllabus. Perhaps a potential cause of burnout, or 'wasted talent'?

Cultural and social impacts on elite athlete development: the issues for athlete development within the context of a nation

The ongoing evolution of coach and player development will always take place within the context of the nation itself. The following issues will inevitably impact both policy and practice.

Structural differences within and between national governing bodies

The structural differences within different national governing bodies can impact and even determine policies for coach education and development, player development and, to some extent, competitive structures. The structure and methodology of athlete development systems in any sport (i.e. ten and under, school and youth) and the identification and development of future talent are very much decided by the home nation. These systems do vary from nation to nation even within a sport. While that is conceivable, it is essential that the core issues of athlete development are catered for. These include the availability of, and access to, high quality facilities that are either publicly or privately owned and managed, on a planned basis.

Cultural and social behaviours

The cultural and social behaviours within the nation impact the development of elite athletes, but it appears to be rarely considered or discussed. In our experience there are, for example, cultural differences within and between different nations in terms of the role of women in sport. Cultural expectations do impact, for example, the role of women in a sport (in terms of the opportunity to play the sport or to work in a coaching or administrative role).

Again taking tennis as an example, while the number of females in the game has risen considerably, there are still fewer women players and women coaches at every level of the game in almost every nation from China to the US and also in Europe. While this is a long-term issue, seemingly based on cultural expectation or even habit, it is difficult to see how it will change.

While paying equal prize money to male and female tennis players does send out a positive message, it does not appear to impact the overall culture within the game very much. There are very few female coaches at the top level of tennis, despite the fact that in China, the US and some European nations, at least, the number of female coaches is increasing. However, many female tennis coaches only coach young children and reportedly find it difficult to be accepted as knowledgeable or competent enough to be given a coaching role with older or more advanced players. The picture is more encouraging in other sports, but they are notably team sports. Women's cricket and football are both now established in the public eye, at least in the UK, and women are beginning to be seen in senior management positions in different sports.

So while it is possible that the stereotype of male dominated sport is changing in some nations and sports, there is still a role for national governing bodies to ensure equal treatment and opportunity in the development of female athletes, coaches, and administrators.

Structural differences: the impact of macro (international) and meso (national) policies on the needs of the elite athletes in different nations

In the context of structural difference it is interesting to sports who are currently undergoing immense change. Rugby union has seen a wealth of rule changes to support the ongoing safety concerns, for example changes to the scrum. As a result of the raised profile of concussion in sport, it appears likely that 'heading', at least as we know it, will become a thing of the past in football. Again to rugby union, many are campaigning for the removal of tackling in school games. Reflecting this, in the US, in junior American Football, parents are increasingly removing their children from the sport because of the physical dangers they are told by the media exist in the game. Even within sports seen as less if at all dangerous, amendments are being made. For example, tennis has introduced heat rules and recently Wimbledon has set new rules to reduce the excessive length of matches.

One could consider whether these changes are needed, and it is clear that there is a school of thought that these changes are necessary for the continued safety of players. These changes could however alter the foundations of a sport, and the landscape of its future. Therefore, we may begin to create very different elite players, and coaches need to be at the heart of this (rightly or wrongly) inevitable change.

Coaching sessions for elite athletes are planned differently for micro, meso, and macro phases. With this in mind, national governing bodies could apply these principles to coach education and development. In this case micro policies operate on an internal level with individual players, coaches and clubs, meso policies on the national level for coach education, and macro policies on the international level. Through this lens, coaches would be better equipped to ride the ever-changing landscape of elite, and indeed junior, sport.

Furthermore, if we are looking to develop and progress our chosen sport internationally (be it for participation, or just exposure), this understanding and appreciation by coaches of the structural idiosyncrasies of policy would ensure their transferability across nations. Hopefully, encourage a consistent language, and shared understanding across coaches of all cultures, to the needs of sport evolution.

The challenges to developing a sport around the globe

Culture

While this has already been discussed in a previous section, in terms of challenges to developing elite sport it is worth revisiting from other angles. It is imperative to account for, understand, and work with the culture of the sport itself in every nation. Experience shows that, notwithstanding the key principles of coach and athlete development discussed in this chapter, what works in one nation may not work in another. Furthermore, while every athlete is born into a specific culture, many then move to another country to develop or compete. As an example: many young athletes, across several sports, move to the United States on college scholarships. For many of them this is a huge cultural shift in terms of the way their sport is organised, in the way coaching is conducted and maybe in the imperatives for winning. Similarly, some athletes follow a coach from a different country, whom they perceive to be able to help them move to the next level of performance. Additionally, the movement of coaches to another country is also a frequent occurrence. Coaches move to work with adult athletes, but also frequently with junior athletes. Inevitably they bring different standards, coaching practices, and expectations with them, which can be confusing to young athletes and parents.

Effective and ineffective coaching

Personal experience indicates that almost every coach wants to be a good coach (and many think they are already!). Sadly, (for the athletes) many of these coaches consider themselves to be better than they are. The best coaches however, realise they always have a great deal to learn and so will take notice of anything and everything that enables them to improve.

It could be assumed that every national governing body is able to identify good coaches and best practice in coach education. Again, personal experience indicates that poor quality and ineffective coach education structures exist in many sports, but are not recognised as such by the national governing body. Frequently poor practice in coach education and development includes the lack of research into best practice, inadequate and inconsistent training of the 'deliverers' (tutors), together with the continued use of old practices without regular updates.

Finally, it would seem obvious that coaches need regular, high quality, and appropriate support in updating their processes. The world of sports performance raises the bar consistently but many coaches work to the lower standard of the past. Whilst several nations do require coaches to update on a regular basis and operate a licensing system to ensure that updating is undertaken. However, sadly, and frequently, the updating courses are not reviewed or assessed in terms of quality.

The effects of history

The issue of constant and frequent change to athlete development policies has been highlighted in this chapter, with the discussion suggesting that constant change negatively affects both the opportunity for, and the process of, developing elite athletes in any sport. The recent history and/or mechanisms of elite athlete development (particularly in tennis, but in several other sports), suggest that systems and structures MUST be of a consistently high quality.

Reflecting this we suggest they should:

1   be developed with a holistic approach that views elite development programmes as a normal and natural progression from grass roots development and participation programmes;
2   be linked to the coach education and development programme to ensure that high quality coaches are developed;
3   be well researched, in terms of understanding the key issues for the path of athlete development from childhood to world class athlete;
4   embrace *every* aspect (culture, previous experience, physical development (including growth, development, and maturation), social and emotional development) that underpins the effective development of every athlete;
5   be well resourced in terms of facilities and adequate finance, but also in terms of high quality, knowledgeable, and experienced coaches, and physical and psychological skill experts;
6   have built in longevity to ensure a continuity of approach.

In addition, and obviously, over the time span of such programmes, there will be a need for constant re-evaluation and subsequent adjustments. However, those adjustments should be made solely to develop and improve existing systems, and not to move to a new one.

29

The coach nomad

Guus Hiddink with Geir Jordet

Introduction

Often when I was working, me and my partner went to Africa around Christmas time. In Africa, we met nomads. Coming from the west, you are thinking: "how do they survive?" They manage to survive under very difficult circumstances, in the desert and so forth. Of course they are concerned about their daily existence, or maybe also about tomorrow, but not so concerned about what will happen in a year or two ahead. For me, I love to travel and to look around. And I love to work elsewhere because I never had a big fear of how it will be tomorrow, or the day after tomorrow, or the week or the month after. I have never had a fear of this unknown. Not really. When the circumstances are okay, then I dive in.

It is not in the world of the nomad to go back, but sometimes you deliberate a bit before you go in. One example is when I was asked, after I had been in Spain, to work for the South-Koreans, on the other side of the world. At that time, they wanted me to come and give some advice leading up to them hosting (together with Japan) the World Cup in 2002. I said, "ok, I can give some advice", but I still kept my distance. Of course, the World Cup is very challenging and very attractive, but I was thinking, "what would I do in such a different world, the Asian world?" They then offered some conditions. I demanded, based on that, something I thought they would never give in to. It was some kind of self-protection. I said, if you want to achieve what you are aiming for, which was to be one of the best 16 teams in the world cup, naturally an unrealistic target because you're now 60–80 in the FIFA ranking, you must do a few things: hire a coach, and give him a full licence to work with the players at the club level. This means that the national team must be a club. Then, let the coach take the players for one and a half years around the world to give them experience. This was important because they were so closed in their own football society. And you have to have a budget to enable the team to travel to South America, Europe and meet very strong teams. South Korea at the time had a fully professional league. Not a big league, but still a real league, covered by Hyundai, Samsung, and all the big companies. I was thinking, they will never manage to get the players free from club obligations for 18 months. However, within ten days the guy came back – he later became my friend, and he said, "ok, on the conditions of having all the players whenever you want, we agree. Secondly, we have a budget from someone. And third, here's your contract". So I said "no, no, take it easy!" At the same time though, they did manage to put this together in ten days. This felt challenging, and it triggered me. So I accepted, and bombed my way in to this unknown world. I can do this only when the conditions are ok. If I would have gone there and not got the conditions where I could have my approach with the team, I would not have done it. It is not in the world of a nomad to go back. But I am not having that fear.

This chapter is about how it is to work as a professional football coach in different countries and different cultures. How do you adapt? How do you navigate and work with people in elite and professional sport, under very different cultural, linguistic, and societal circumstances?

My beginnings

Before I started coaching, I was playing professional football for 16 years. At the same time, I took a degree in physical education as a teacher. I did some training with a younger team on the side, which I loved. And in the mornings, I worked as a physical teacher with young boys and girls who could not adapt to normal school. They had to go to special school for different reasons. I did this for many years with a lot of joy.

However, once I got an offer to become a full professional assistant coach at PSV Eindhoven in my country, the Netherlands. This was after my professional player career. People around me then said: "Be careful, football is a jungle, don't jump in!" Yes, it is a jungle. But when you are in the jungle you have to grab the lianas, and then you can move around. I could have stayed in this rather comfortable zone, teaching in the morning and having a team in the afternoon, and I would have had a normal existence. But at that moment I said to myself "come on! If you want to challenge yourself, go for the unknown!" For me, personally, this was a decisive moment. Making a decision where I will have no security for tomorrow, or for the year after.

Since this, I have coached in Turkey, Spain, South Korea, Australia, Russia, England, and recently, China.[1]

My staff

When I go to a new team, and a new country, I do not like to bring in my own big staff. I could demand this if I wanted to, I could say: "I want an assistant, and another assistant. And I want a physical therapist, a masseur, a team manager, a video analyst, everything". I could easily ask for a five- or six-man staff. However, I do not like that because once you go for a staff like that, and probably it would have been a Dutch staff, you go into an isolated island. You enter into a new culture and with such an island you can be a little offensive or it can be very awkward with respect to the local culture.

I always have one main assistant who comes from the local culture. This person is more of a colleague, but officially is an assistant. Most of the time, this is a retired professional footballer who has come into coaching. Before I talk more definitely about the contracts and so forth I go searching for this assistant from the local federation or a club. And then I have several encounters with that man, so I can talk with him, more or less "feel and smell him", until I know how he is thinking and what he is doing. Then I have information about whether I can rely on this man, because he can give me a lot of information within a half a day about their culture, such as: what are the good things, what are the tricky things or bad things, and so on, in a club or federation. This is based on me trusting him after several conversations, of course. If I were to come with an island of my own staff, you need three, four, or five months to get adapted into that new environment. That is why I prefer to always hire a local.

From the outside, I can bring one or two assistants that are working together. Maximum. Other staff are local. I always talk very openly with them. Until I see that they cannot live up to the standards we like to have, whether it is a physiotherapist, physical trainer or what so ever, I always say beforehand, that after two months, I might have to bring in someone new. An expert, someone I have confidence in, that can come in and cooperate with them. Whether I do that or not I decide after I know if the experience with the local people is ok.

About my style and way of doing things, the president and the board hire me to reach some targets. The targets can be for example to get into the last 16, become champions or qualify for the Champions league. So, these targets are rather focused, and I can use my methods of working towards that.

My bosses

The cultural influence is what you have to try to distinguish. What is the culture in this club or this society? On top of that, I think for the targets there are political influences. I try to avoid always, in the bad sense of the word, the political things. That is why briefly, when I started in Korea, it was political. Of course everyone says, "Korea was wonderful". Yes, in the end it was. Because I was working for one and a half years before that. Or fighting. I do not know if it was to my advantage not knowing the language. I could not read, I could not understand the TV, or the radio, or the newspaper. They are so polite, and they did not tell me what was written in this, let us say, rough preparation time. I am not talking about the last two or three months, at the World Cup and the successful preparation for that, but before that. I was not told at the time, but I was given a nickname: "Zero-five". Because I had said something about the Korean team in the past, the team that was present for five World Cups, but never with a win. They always prepared with games against Malaysia, Singapore, and won, three, four, five–nil, and the country was always thinking, we are ready for the World Cup. And then they met the real teams in the real world, and they got smashed. So, when I came in, I wanted to go the hard way. I said: "We will have a rough time, and there we will be killed, but we will learn a lot from that experience".

This is also why I always want one person I make myself responsible to. And in Korea, he was also the president of Hyundai. I told him: we are going into a rough period now and we will lose. He replied: "You don't even have to report to me because the team had five world cups already, and nothing". He was a very intelligent, western-educated man. He told me he would cover me until the end. But if I had not made this contractual approach, it would have been a technical committee to report to. The technical committee made with other coaches, previous coaches, their selection. They were all representatives from north, east, south, west, from the whole country. Ten football regions. And they bring all their players from their region, shouting: "Hey, my player must be selected, my player this, my player that. . .". It was not on quality, it was political. So, that is why I killed the technical committee of ten men, powerful men. I said no. Those are the struggles you must go for.

Always, there needs to be just one person you report to. One, so I have this one channel. I tell this person I can come to talk to you and say what I am doing, and you can decide whether you like it or if you kill me, fire me, or whatever. I do not do this with a committee.

In Russia, there is also the influence of the football culture, which is dominating in the clubs by powerful presidents, and even sometimes, in some clubs, by for instance the army or the old

KBG, such as in CSKA Moscow and Dynamo Moscow. Lokomotiv is the state railway. Spartak Moscow is the only people's club. And this is important to know. Players behave differently when they are in Dynamo, the army club. The coaches are put in there by the generals. And the players are not stupid, they know. If you do not perform, you get punished. As a leader to be safe, you have to punish the worker. Even if it is illogical. So, those things you must know when you operate in Russian football. Spartak is more of a free club, that is why it is very popular. During the games, what I was taught, is that they could yell at everyone, politically. They were allowed to yell, swear, and whatever. During the game, not outside. In Spartak they could say that this politician or this person is so and so. Because, people are very creative in this. And all these influences you have to deal with. With me, they said: "First, we have to qualify, and then we have to perform well on the European stage". But then you get all these influences. I was put there by another authority, by the Russian federation. In Russia they accept authorities, but they do not trust them. They cooperate, because if they do not cooperate, they go to Siberia or you look for another club.

My bosses and I have the same targets. I had the target to qualify, they must have the target to qualify, so we have in principle the same target. Of course, I make decisions on who to play, how to play, and so forth, but first of all I have to win people's confidence – particularly your players. So, what do you have to do? Not say that you are different with long speeches and verbally asking them to trust me, because they know those stories. But you get offered situations where you can go in and show them. For instance, when authorities of the federation come and say they would like to talk with the players.

This happened once in Russia, before a game. It was a friendly game, and I said okay. You know how it is with the big guys, the presidents, holding speeches for 30 seconds or so. But this guy kept on talking for ten to 15 minutes. And the players got very tired. Afterwards, the next day, my boss at the federation said "next time, let's do it in a different way. We can come in and say 'Let's go! For the country and for the flag', you know, for 30 seconds. Next game". I do not remember if the fixture was against England or Germany, they came in one or two hours before the game in the locker room and started talking, so I would say: "Guys, listen! Our boss would like to say some words". And then he said a few things, and after around 30 seconds, he ended it with: "Fight!" Okay, good, so then we went out with him, out of the locker room. And all of a sudden, I saw him in the corner of my eye, coming back into the locker room. I waited for ten seconds and then he started talking again. So, I went back in, and this was a crucial point, I think. I said "Vitaly! (In Russia one always calls one by his first name. It is an honorful approach). Vitaly! Come". I grabbed his arm. And the players, they were looking. They knew our relationship, that he was my boss. So, I grabbed him, and I said, "Vitaly! Come on! What did we say the last time?" I took him and pushed him, and we walked out. And later, I would hear from my local coach that this was the moment where things changed. Afterwards I was thinking they could have killed me, because I was taking away, a little bit, my boss's authority. The players at this point were looking at each other and saying "shit!" This was a breaking point. Because he could have said, "I'm your boss! Get out!" That would have been a normal reaction. But, not being totally stupid, he was maybe thinking of the reaction of the others. So, those are key moments. You get offers, but you have to smell those moments. If I would have given in, he would have gone in and held a speech again for five or ten minutes. And I would had stood there. Then I would totally have, in my opinion, lost the authority with the players. Because they would have thought "hey, this is another coward coming here to guide us!" Those moments you get offered. Take them! With the risk that you might get killed. But

I would rather be killed than work under those circumstances. Authorities are sometimes a little bit scared. You think they are big, but they are sometimes scared because of prestige. And you can play with that.

The players

Coaching in different countries can be a very different experience. You come in to a different world, a different society. And also, a different football society and a different football culture. In my country, in the Netherlands, we raise youngsters so that they ask "why?" "Why should I, why should this, why should that?" That is totally different from many other cultures where they never ask this question. In Korea, they never ask "why". In Russia, they think "why", but they do not ask "why". In Australia, they say "ok, we'll do it". And in Spain, they also do not ask because of your authority and your position. Here in Holland, you have to win your authority by knowledge, experience, and quality, but it can be different in other places.

When I went to Australia, they said: "We have not qualified to the World Cup since 1974 in Germany, and we have to qualify for the World Cup in Germany in 2006". I looked at the players, and they were all playing in Europe. And I said, okay, I will take the challenge. But, we do not travel to Australia, because they had suggested to have the training camp in Australia. I said, 90% of the players are playing in Europe and there are two players playing in their league in Sydney. We had our practice here, in Holland. I said they could come here, and that is what I wanted.

When I started there, practising with them, the players were so committed in the first training session. I like to play eight versus eight, or ten versus ten, and so forth. They were so eager to play, and they kicked each other. Usually I like it when it the game is getting a little tough but they were literally kicking each other on the side of the pitch, having a fight. Later on, the players who were fighting came in and said "boss, we fixed the problem ourselves". And then you would think that these players would avoid each other, but no. Soon after there was another clash. So, there was a very open-minded approach to the game. But, the downside of that was that they said: "We are so committed! Australians are so committed, we fight, and we fight!" And I said: "Yes, but we haven't qualified for 37 years. Ever thought of why that is?" Commitment is not enough. You have to look at other parts in which you have to improve. Tactical and strategical elements of the game. Try to use your brain a bit more.

I always try to construct my teams in a spine, tactically or strategically. And I like to have players in the spine, who know the game and who also have the ability to transfer the ideas we are talking about in our practice sessions into our game. My opinion is that football is not really a coaching sport, if you compare it with basketball, handball, or other sports. Like in volleyball, you can draw the patterns, and you can practise those patterns in training sessions because there is a reduced number of players, and there is not always a physical opposition, so you can manage more as a coach in terms of patterns of play. But in football it is more complex I think. So, I need players in my spine who know how to play offensively, defensively, and in transitions. If I know there are one, two, three players in central defensive, midfield and maybe an attacking player, midfielder or striker, who can play: well, then the unit is more safe as a team. I can yell on the side. But I know, that if a coach is yelling at the side, as a player you don't understand because of all of the noise. And if the coach does that all the time, he will always be two seconds behind the situation. When I started coaching as a young coach, I saw myself sometimes on TV afterwards. I could see myself yelling after the situation and no one reacted. I was like a supporter on the stands yelling "you should do this and that!", but it had happened already. The situation is already history. So, I tried to think in advance of the situation that was about to come up. This is not easy, but you try to. And if you have some influence, you can have some contact with your key players, for example by saying "hey! We have to draw back" and so on. So, I always try to build my team with that spine. A spine of "coaching players".

In big clubs, you have always a culture. And in those clubs, although of course in lesser clubs as well, they have culture often guarded by big players. For example, when I worked at Real Madrid, and Real Madrid is for me the biggest club there is with respect to the culture, the pressure, everything. I got to my desk on a Monday, and this player had had a big game on Saturday. On Sunday night, he was going into a night club at 1am, left at 3.50am, and went to another club until 6am. And I got this information on my desk because they are followed by club people, spies, and they are followed by the press. So, I said to my captain: "I'm going to kill this guy. He has irresponsible behavior". My captain said "Boss! We did already, we did it already". The main culture guardians were at the time Hierro and Sanchis. And my captain said, "we know already, so we kill him!" This is the culture in this club. If you're at this club you know what to do within the borders of what is accepted. This is the culture outside the pitch, you know, and I find it very interesting.

Language

Language is an issue when coaching abroad. But I think sports, especially football, and music or maybe art, are without frontiers, without real borders. Everyone plays football, and basically, we already have this language together. If you put some international people, players, who know how to play football together, they will still play together even if they do not speak the same language. They have communication without language. But of course, you do need a lot of language. I need an interpreter. Most of the time I try to use my assistant coach. If I have a different language like Russian or Korean, then I use my assistant. Also, I pick my assistant, for instance when I was in Russia there was a player, a top player who had played in the Bundesliga and spoke perfectly German. So, I could speak German with him with no problem whatsoever.

Plus, always when I go someplace, like to Russia, Spain, or Turkey, I try to learn the language, also because I like languages. For example, I learned Spanish in two months because I studied it for 16–17 hours a day. I listened to audiotapes in the car. Spanish is a very easy language to learn. Russian is more difficult. My partner is very interested in society generally, so in Russia we hired a teacher and tried to learn some basic Russian language. In addition to the normal language, I always prepare a list of football expressions, offside and so on. Sometimes this is like in the early days when one sent telegrams with the principle notes. Of course, now you can write anything you want, but I would talk like a telegram in the early days, in principles.

When it comes to interpreters, I have learned it is best to have an expert – that is, a coach or a football player who knows football, instead of an official interpreter. I had once an interpreter at the beginning in Turkey. Of course I did not speak the Turkish language, and I had an official interpreter sent by the club. I talked in German, and he translated. I said something to the players on the pitch and my speech was more or less done in 30 seconds. And I said to the interpreter: "Translate!" When I talked 30 seconds, he talked for three minutes. I mean, with German, maybe it will take 30 seconds and when you say it in Turkish it will take 40 seconds, maximum 50 seconds. The first time this happened, I let it slide, but the second time, I was thinking, this is impossible. I then put one of my confidants in the back of the group the next time, and he told me the interpreter was telling a totally different story. This was a lesson for me to, beforehand, have very good talks with people you have in your staff, about trust and confidence. Also, football experts will know the principles you are trying to communicate. Even though language is a barrier, I can then say I want this principle explained, and he can use his words on what we are going to do, and what our targets are.

Personal factors

Coaching across the world has affected me personally in a few ways. My fixed ideas of other worlds, my prejudices, are disappearing. I am now less judgemental from a distance. People around the world are of course different, but they are not that different. We always have this idea that the Koreans are like that, the Australians, Norwegians, or the Dutch are like this. Get rid of this idea. I have met a lot of people all over the world who I still have contact with, which has broadened my concept of life. So this is not just about football.

I always defend when people are attacking Australians or Koreans or Russians. When someone says, "the Koreans, they look alike", I'm thinking "come on. Open your eyes and look. They are totally different". Of course they have their society and so forth, but people are different. I have gotten rid of some of my prejudices.

This is about curiosity. And it is about tolerance, in general, not just in the exact profession that we are in. Because it is not always healthy in this profession because we have these targets. You may have your limits for the players and for yourselves, and sometimes tolerance is not good, you have to focus on the outcome targets you are set to reach with your team. And that is why it is good to have people around yourself. Like my partner. My lady is always travelling with me. I can make things very narrow. I focus on my targets. I am hired to reach these targets. So, I close my blinkers like the horses and go there, not knowing or not being interested in what is happening around these targets. But she is going into normal life. She is very open. Within no time she knows people, whether it is in Russia, Korea, London, or wherever. In Korea, for instance, I set up this foundation. But that was not my idea, it was hers. In Korea, it looks like a perfect society, because they keep their face and prestige, which is very important. But behind the scenes, she discovered and learned about the society by talking, I mean real talking, not just superficial. In no time, she gets to know people and she goes: "I've heard stories about how women who are divorced here are degraded to second level citizens", for instance. The foundation is based on handicapped and sight-impaired children. Also, in Korea when the success began to come in the last three months, she said, "You're so popular in this country. You have to do something to pay back a bit". So, she was the initiator of this. It means that you are so focused, stupidly, on what you are asked to do, that you find an excuse to not open your blinkers. You need people around you to open them, and that is why we came to this foundation. So, you need people around you who are in touch with society in general. In the early days, you would think this one thing is important and the other things not so important. Which is true in a way, but sometimes you have to get a knock and wake up, "wake up my friend".

Conclusions

I think when coaches go abroad from their own country, they must in principle already have that adventurous characteristic to go abroad. On the other hand, you see coaches who are going abroad and come back in no time. Three or six months. I do not know exactly, but they might not have the ability to go into depth in society. Whether it is in the club or in a federation or in the broader society. And they are sticking to this, maybe a little bit too rigid, approach. I am not sure, but you see several returning coaches after very short experiences abroad.

Doing well coaching abroad can be about flexibility, respect, and tolerance. And it is important to go out with an interest for the culture you are going into. Of course, the target is in your club or federation culture, but there are many influences you cannot separate. And these influences are coming from within the club and in the surroundings of the club or from the national culture itself. I find this interesting.

You need the professional skills. But you also need the human skills, taught or from nature, when you go abroad. Of course, you are asked to reach targets. I am not hired because I am a nice guy. But you can use the influences from the outside as well.

This is my approach. It might not be the best approach, but it is my approach.

Note

1 Guus was formerly with Fenerbache (Turkey), Valencia (Spain), Netherlands (twice), Real Madrid (Spain), Real Betis (Spain), South Korea, PSV Eindhoven (Netherlands), Australia, Russia, Chelsea (England, twice), Turkey, and Anzhi Makhachkala (Dagestan/Russia).

30

The transition to elite performance
Societal contrasts in the same sport

B. J. Mather and Dave Rotheram

Introduction

Governments, National Governing Bodies (NGBs), and professional sporting organisations are forever searching for the 'golden bullet' that will bring international sporting success. In addition, but just as importantly, they seek the extra benefits linked to the generation of revenue, national pride, and increased sporting participation. This 'search for solutions' is situated against an environment of increasing competition, however; particularly evident in the Olympics where nations have invested heavily but are still competing for the same number of medals (circa 300).

In terms of rugby league (hereafter RL), Great Britain (or England) has not won the World Cup since 1972. The Great Britain Lions have not won a three match test series against Australia since 1970. Consequently, when major tournaments are reviewed, there are always recommendations made and countless newspaper column inches devoted to where it all went wrong. Since its inception in 1954, the RL World Cup has been held on 15 occasions, with Australia winning 11 titles. As such, it seems 'obvious' to the media and observers that all GB needs to do is copy the Aussie approach – an idea which has gained equal popularity but in reverse for sports such as cycling at which the UK dominates. We think this is a gross oversimplification so, accordingly, this chapter is a comparison of the talent systems of England and Australia, to explore the differences and similarities in approach with specific reference to the social milieu in which each nation operates. In short, to see if it really is as simple as just copying a successful system!

Pertinent to this chapter is a recently completed comparison of Canadian and Swedish ice hockey pathways. Ice hockey has some similar characteristics to RL in that relatively few countries play and there is limited opportunity to play as a professional club player, the major league being the National Hockey League (NHL) across North America. "Canadian and Swedish hockey systems offer two different approaches to elite player development, resulting in different trajectories regarding international success in the World Junior Championships and in the number of players drafted into the National Hockey League" (Ogden & Edwards, 2016, p. 312). This report offers a number of interesting parallels to RL and has furnished a useful template for the design and conduct of this chapter.

Background

The UK and England perspective

The sport of rugby league originated in England, in the first instance as a breakaway from the rugby football union (RFU). This 'breakaway' was strongly influenced by socio-economic factors. At the end of the nineteenth century there was no such thing as the five-day working week and, in order to play rugby, this meant that players would take time off work and not be paid. Clubs in the North of England wanted to compensate their players by providing 'broken time' payments. This was met with disdain by the so-called middle classes of the southern clubs and the RFU who believed that sport should remain strictly amateur (cf. Collins, 2006). By receiving payment in lieu of work, these players were perceived to be professionalised.

Another (not so well documented) reason for the 1895 break away was the demand from the Northern clubs for league and cup competition. Accordingly, soon after the split, league and cup competitions were created in Rugby League. These two socio-economic factors are significant in their impact upon the talent system. So, it is fair to say that competition is part of the sporting DNA of RL and accordingly, the sport is governed in the community game by its 'playing leagues' around the nation based upon a geographical split.

The aim of the talent system within English RL is for England to win the World Cup and every home international test series. Therefore, to reach this outcome, process goals are in place to ensure that there is a plentiful supply of elite athletes that progress through the pathway to be elite performers.

The talent identification and development (TID) processes employed in RL at the base of the pathway is via the community game and schools. Previous TID models in RL were aligned to a standard model of talent development (SMTD) (cf. Bailey & Collins, 2013) of early selection and arguably, subsequent mass 'de-selection' of potential future high achievers. Therefore, an alternative model was sought that widened the base of the pathway but also provided more athletes with access to appropriate talent development environments. The model provided for contextualised coach education, a progressive talent curriculum and a player profiling tool, allowing players to have some ownership of their learning journey.

In the UK system, the main responsibility for the development of talent sits with both the RFL and the 13 licensed Academies. The RFL, in its role as the NGB, holds the responsibility for age-banded international RL. These are national (i.e. England) player development programmes which operate at Under 16, Under 18 age and an England Knights programme for players considered to be two to four years away from the senior squad. These programmes select up to 40 players per year who receive further developmental and international playing opportunities. Players are drawn from the 13 Academies and Super League clubs, which have a total of 400 registered players (Under 16) and 300 registered players (Under 18).

The senior England international team is drawn from players from the Super League competition (circa 250 eligible), and England eligible players who have migrated to the National Rugby League (NRL) – the elite competition in Australasia, or others who satisfy international eligibility rules.

The Academy function is to search for, recruit, and develop talent for the Super League competition and England. These are funded by Super League (Europe) with a total investment of £1.8 million per year. Along with club 'match funding', the total annual investment into the Academies is circa £3.6 million.

The Academies recruit players into their formal programmes from the Under 15 age group. At Under 15 and Under 16, players are recruited to player development programmes known as scholarships. These are year-round development programmes with eight playing opportunities from February to July. At Under 19 level, there is a full playing season of 22 games and a play-off series.

The Super League competition is a 30-game regular season with play-offs. Additionally, all clubs enter the Challenge Cup (knock-out competition). Consequently, it is conceivable that players in successful club teams could play up to 37 competitive club games per season.

The Australian context

In Australia, the sport of RL is played nationwide but, as in England, centres around two major 'hotspots'; namely, the states of New South Wales and Queensland.

While Queensland is governed wholly by the Queensland Rugby League (QRL), New South Wales (NSW) has two organisations responsible for the delivery of Rugby League. The Country Rugby League (CRL) have traditionally been responsible for rugby league within country areas (non-Sydney metropolitan) of NSW and are a member of the New South Wales Rugby League (NSWRL), the overarching governing body within NSW. The NSWRL and QRL are members of the Australian Rugby League Commission, along with the 16 NRL clubs throughout Australia and New Zealand.

There are 11 National Rugby League (NRL) clubs based in NSW, eight within NSWRL boundaries, two within CRL boundaries (Canberra Raiders and Newcastle Knights) and one club that crosses boundaries due to it being a joint venture (St-George-Illawarra Dragons).

While the NSWRL, CRL, and QRL all run broadly similar development programmes, differing largely due to geographical distance and available funding, the information offered in this section is based on the 2017 season and historical situation regarding TID pathways in NSWRL specifically. The landscape has changed in 2018, following a review of the National Youth Cup (Under 20s competition) and associated pathway changes. Notably, however, the previous system has been in place since 2008 and is responsible for the current crop of NRL athletes. Australian talent pathways focus heavily on SMTD-like representative playing opportunities at Under 16 and Under 18. These 'junior rep' competitions (in NSW) began in 1970 and 1965 respectively.

For NSWRL-run competitions, each Junior League district club operates their 'junior rep' development programme through the spring/summer/autumn period, with an eight-game competition programme culminating in a finals series and grand final. This is replicated within the CRL at Under 16 and Under 18 with their Country Championship, a competition-based programme used to identify the most talented athletes. In recent times, NRL scouts have used the Under 16 Country Championship to identify and recruit talent, luring them to Sydney with the promise of a contract and an opportunity at an NRL club. Given that most NRL clubs are based within the Sydney metropolitan area, it is understandable why an athlete from the country may feel he needs to relocate to fulfil his ambition under the current model of development.

The NSWRL Under 16 and Under 18 competitions have 17 entrants in each, with the competitions running on a two-year competition draw cycle. There is no central funding allocated to any of the teams in order to assist with development, nor are there any minimum standards of delivery, development philosophy, core curriculum, or development framework imposed by either the National or State Governing body. Responsibility for this currently rests solely with each team, with varying degrees of success usually dependent on the level of funding and resources available to them.

Each team can register a squad of 25 athletes for that year's competition. Initial trial and talent identification events can begin as early as September and it is not uncommon for over 100 athletes to attend the early stages of selection. Furthermore, athletes may often attend more than one district's talent ID events to maximise their opportunity for selection. Final selection of the 25 takes place in January, with the competitions commencing in February.

Prior to the 2018 season, each NRL club had an Under 20s team that competes in the National Youth Competition in a full season of league fixtures and a play-off series. This replicates the NRL competition with most games being played at the same venue as curtain raisers to the NRL game. The pinnacle of the development pathway at Under 16 and Under 18 levels is selection for each state's State of Origin (SOO) team, with no national representative team being selected at Under 16 level.

Key contrasts

A summary of contrasts is shown in Table 30.1. Clearly, from the data and facts already presented, there are many differences between the RL TDE's of UK and Australia which offer two very different systemic pathways to becoming an elite athlete. As stated earlier, there has been a commonly held belief in the UK that, to beat Australia consistently, we simply must copy what they do and get better!

This is not necessarily so as highlighted by eighteenth century philosopher, David Hume. "Hume's law" states that many make claims about what *ought* to be on the basis of statements about what *is*. Therefore, in a RL context we must temper the use of the statement "Australia is doing this therefore we ought to. . .". Indeed, it is difficult to quantify exactly

Table 30.1 A comparative summary of the TDE in both the UK and Australia

Age	UK	NSW/Australia
12–14	Coach and player development via community clubs and schools. Assessment and monitoring conducted by Academies	Development Squads at Under 12, Under 13 and Under 14 run by District Clubs (NRL, not community). Games played on an ad hoc basis. No formal monitoring of athletes or assessment, beyond game play and traditional scouting
15–16	Selection to Scholarship. These are year-round player development programmes operated by Academies with six to eight playing opportunities from February to May. England Youth – a year-round development programme for up to 40 players and two test matches versus France.	Selection trials begin in September, development programmes with a large squad of approximately 40 athletes begin in October/November. Junior Representative competitions (nine games + finals) with 25 athletes, begins in February, finishes in April. State of Origin representation (Under 16) year-round development programme within NSW. Large squad of approximately 45 athletes, holistic programme. One game against Queensland in June.

(continued)

Table 30.1 (continued)

Age	UK	NSW/Australia
17–20	Academy Under 19 competition. 22 game league programme. England Academy (U-18) programme – year-round development programme for up to 40 players, annual two-test match series versus France and two-test series versus Australia every two years.	Club Under 18 Junior representative competition (nine games + finals + national final). State of Origin representation (Under 18) – year-round development program within NSW. Approximately 40 athletes, holistic programme. One game against Queensland in June. Under 18 test series versus England every two years. State-based competition (Under 20) 20-game regular season, four week development break. No work/study no play rule. Defined training times and limits on amount of training. State of Origin representation (Under 20) – single game against Queensland in July. Short term preparation, all players are NRL contracted, access is an issue. Junior Kangaroos – single game against New Zealand every year. Traditional performance-based selection and short-term preparation.
Adult (elite club)	Super League (30 game regular season). Challenge Cup. Reserve team/dual registration.	State Based 2nd tier competitions. NSW – IntrustSuper Premiership. 12-team competition, includes NZ. QLD – IntrustSuper Championship. 14-team competition, includes PNG. NRL (24-game regular season). Dual registration with state league clubs.
Adult (representative)	England Knights. This is a development programme for those players considered to be two to four years away from full international representation. There are up to four playing opportunities that coincide with the Senior international programme each Autumn.	State of Origin (three-game series, NSW V QLD). Prime Ministers XIII (emerging international programme versus Papua New Guinea).
Adult (international)	2018 – Autumn three-test series versus New Zealand. 2019 – Autumn Great Britian Lions tour for three-testtest series versus Australia. 2020 – Autumn three-test home series versus Australia. 2021 Autumn World Cup (in England).	2018 – single test versus New Zealand. 2019 – home three-test series versus Great Britain. 2020 – three-test series versus England (away). 2021 – RLWC in England.

what Australia *is* doing since there are a number of different development models depending on which State Governing body is controlling and delivering the process and an athlete's geographical location.

Checking for differences – method

Building from this template, and to investigate the Australian TDEs more closely, we have gathered information from those with the responsibility of setting strategy and delivering the programmes.

Participants

In the context of an up-to-date comparison of the two countries, it was important to be able to solicit the views from key decision-makers in the process as well as those at the 'coal face' of player development; namely, club leaders and coaches. The participants were selected due to their positions as expert strategic leads for performance and TD with Governing Bodies, together with their full-time responsibility within clubs for overseeing the development of players aged 16–20.

The key individuals interviewed consisted of:

- National Rugby League (NRL) Elite Programmes Manager
- Heads of Academy from two NRL clubs
- Under 20 Head Coaches from two NRL clubs (same as Heads of Academy)
- Group interview of four U-20 players from each club.

The main thrust of the interview was questions on perceptions of the purpose underlying TD programmes and what elements participants' considered needed to be present for the creation of an optimal TDE that met overall aims and objectives for the sport in Australia.

Results

Overall, the markers of success differed according to the role of the participant. At NGB level, the success of senior teams in major competition were key drivers. The Australian senior team has enjoyed a period of domination and are current World Cup holders and Four Nations Champions. At face value, one would assume that this had been achieved through a systematically planned programme. However, at international level, countries have little time with their squads owing to club commitments and the demands made by broadcasters which does lead to very limited preparation time for a test match. "We prepared the Kangaroos for a test match on 2 training sessions. From a football point of view this is not ideal" (EPM, NRL).

That said, the State of Origin series is big business. In 2015, the three live televised games "were ranked among the top six highest rating TV events" (Bodey 2015). Consequently, there is a "perception that playing State of Origin would be the pinnacle of playing rugby league". (EPM, NRL). The image of the Kangaroos is not where it should be (in the eyes of the NRL) because of the status of State of Origin. In terms of a 'performance environmen', State of Origin is afforded over 30 days dedicated preparation time in a two-month period (May to July) "where they can build a lot more on what they are trying to achieve" (EPM, NRL). This provision will be examined in more detail later in the chapter.

It is clear that the international programme would not be so successful had it not been for the perceived healthy state of the NRL competition and State of Origin. As far as the NRL is concerned, they are pleased that both NSW and QLD have development programmes that feed this in terms of Under 16, Under 18 and Under 20 representative teams.

However, in terms of optimum TDEs, there does appear to be a gap between theory and practical application. At state level, there has been little attention focussed on a systematic process. Whilst NSW has won 16 of the last 18 junior SOO games, this has not translated to success for the senior team that has only won one series out of the last 11. Therefore, moving forward, the stated aim of the NSWRL Origin development programmes are "to get a larger talent pool available and exposed to high quality coaching in a good environment" – a philosophy that is not always reflected across all Junior Representative participant clubs.

How does this compare to the aims of the RFL's system? This philosophical stance does match that of the UK. In the knowledge that RL is a 'late maturation' sport, steps are being taken to educate key stakeholders (coaches, local administrators) that the development of talent is a long-term process and should not be clouded by craving short-term successes (e.g. winning trophies with Under 13 club teams) and that identifying and developing talent should not be done solely on current performances.

However, in both NSW and the UK this is still being hampered by a lack of understanding of what player development actually is. Historically, State level age banded activity has been about short-term representative teams preparing to play either domestic competition or the annual State of Origin fixture. This view is supported by an Under 20 player, who noticed that throughout Under 16 and Under 18's representative programmes coaches were mostly pre-occupied with technical and tactical aspects in order to win games. Coaches and significant others were "confusing winning with development" and, consequently, had a tendency to identify current performance rather than develop talent. This approach was, in part, put down to the large numbers of participants where it is very easy just to find the next best to step in, as illustrated by the participation figures in Table 30.2.

The NSWRL Junior Rep programmes are seen as some of the best within Australia at producing talent for the NRL, with over 900 athletes taking part each year. However, the graduation rate of athletes who take part in the programmes who then go on to make at least one appearance in the NRL competition is around 4% for the Under 16 competition and 12% for the Under 18s.

Consequently, from the point of view held at State level, NRL clubs are selecting players based merely upon current performance and physical and technical ability. As the data quoted above suggests, ability *may* be being confused with maturity (Barnsley & Thompson, 1988)). This can be linked to the requirement to 'win now' for an NRL coach, an approach that is mirrored in the coaches at Under 16 and Under 18 level, rather than

Table 30.2 Participation figures (2017)

Age Group	National Total Participants	
	Australia	United Kingdom
3–9 years old	42,315	7098
10–12 years old	35,294	6307
13–18 years old	50,957	10670
	128,566	**24075**

taking a longer-term view to player development, perhaps understandable given the job security of most NRL coaches.

Interestingly, players reported that they had learned that psychosocial qualities were pre-determinants of success, with commitment and mental toughness highlighted as two key features. Players pointed to the fact that "you've got to be willing to cut out a lot of your social life for it" and "If you can't push through the sessions they don't want you here". Reflecting on these comments, this is a 'survival of the fittest' approach and a reflection of greater playing resources/easier replacements, rather than a conscious effort to develop resilience and mental toughness.

Whilst this plan at state level is still emerging, Club A (domiciled in NSW) has made the strategic decision to actually broaden its approach. Club A made their talent identification programme a lot broader, involved more players at a younger age rather than being too selective at younger age groups (Under 14). Four hundred players aged 12–17 have been involved in Club A's programme. This has resulted in 87% of players selected to Club A's three age-banded programmes having come through their development pathways. This has been achieved by having "the support of the General Manager and NRL Head Coach" (HOYP, Club A). This view was supported by the Under 20 coach who noticed that a "change of NRL head coach saw more resource allocated to juniors". One driver for this approach was that "In the past we spent a lot of money on the re-location of kids. We felt that we could use that money wiser and the results we have had in the last two years are the best we've had" (HOYP, club A).

Conversely, Club B has been required to take a different approach. Club B is domiciled in the state of Victoria where RL is considered a 'developing' sport. According to the HOYP, the aim of their system is to get a "born and bred Victorian NRL player". The origins of Club B's development model emerged out of a necessity to fit in with the rest of Australia so that they could access competition, primarily at Under 16 and Under 18. However, selective environments are evident at Under 12 with a state team. "The first real intense programmes are the Under 12 state programmes. We try and get the better athletes into a system that they are starting to be educated to the (Club B) way". Similar to Club A, Club B believes that in order to be more successful they must generate a larger playing pool from which to select. However, owing to the fledgling nature of the sport in Victoria, the availability of adequate facilities (e.g. rectangular fields) and "the growth of numbers of players has out grown the supply of coaches" (HOYP, Club B).

Interestingly in Club B, there appears to be a lack of 'philosophical congruence' evident throughout the club. Where this club is concerned, there is a perceived negative impact upon talent development created by the political and financial climate of the club. From discussions with both the Head Coach of the Under 20's and the HOYP, it is clear that the private owners of the club are solely concerned with first grade success and "they don't see putting half a million dollars into development and running 16s and 18s teams as their brief" (HOYP, Club B).

Discussion

Whilst at face value the Australian system appears to be bearing fruit (especially where results are concerned), it does lack some validity against empirically researched characteristics of what an optimal TDE should look like. Indeed, due to phases of early selection, this does magnify the relative age effect. There is a similar trend with club teams.

The data presented are consistent with the trends found in English RL. However, these trends *may* be present due to differing reasons.

Theory versus practice

In England, there is a well-documented scarcity of player supply to satisfy the needs of all the Super League Club Academies. Therefore, a need to recruit the perceived 'better players' at 14 magnifies this. This often manifests itself in recruiting players on current performance rather than potential and, therefore, due to the nature of the sport, the relatively older players are initially selected for development programmes. This is also compounded by a new ruling (from 2016 onwards) that movement by players between clubs at ages 15 and 16 is now subject to compensation payment. (RFL Operational Rules Tiers 1–3).

In Australia, in contrast, it is the competitive nature of youth programmes through 'junior reps' that drives the relative age bias. In the absence of long-term development programmes, competition is seen as the predictor of developing talent and largely ignores a holistic model. From interviews with key stakeholders, this development model is clearly based upon the competition structure rather than recognised models of talent development.

Coaching versus competition

One of the main limitations of the Australian system is the learning disposition of the coach. "There is agreement in the literature that dispositions (e.g., values, interests, and attitudes) direct the cognitions of individuals" (Griffiths & Armour, 2013, p. 678). The historical reliance on competition means that administrators and coaches know no different and have yet to be challenged. Although NSW enjoys a huge playing population (almost 50% larger than Queensland), it *could* be accused of massively under-achieving since the senior team has such a poor run of results at SOO level. At age-banded level, NSW are enjoying success on the field but this appears to be at odds with sound TID principles where long-term aims and objectives are compromised by the demands for short-term success. Therefore, there is a need to carefully consider the role that competition plays throughout the pathway and the importance placed on it by coaches in the role of talent development.

Similarly, in England, a historical over-reliance on competition is prevalent in the community and schools' game. This has a potentially damaging impact on the size of the playing pool and, despite the RFL's best efforts to instil a long-term player development philosophy, this is compromised by the volume of competitive playing opportunities that drives a 'win at all costs' mentality in coaches. Again, this flies in the face of what the research tells us and will require a major shift in philosophy to bring about change.

RL in the UK has begun to educate coaches and system builders about developing athletes for the long term. Since 2013, there has been a concerted push to educate coaches at the base of the pathway to integrate sound TD principles into their coaching. This has come in the form of a 'talent development curriculum' and a series of CPD workshops. The content of the curriculum was derived through a literature review of TID research and applying this in a RL specific context within its current landscape via pilot projects. The philosophy of this programme is to help broaden the talent pool with more athletes aged 12–14 being able to access good talent coaching. The target coaches to deliver this on behalf of the sport are community club coaches and teachers (UKCC level 2 qualified). However, within their social milieu, there is still prevalent a sub-culture of short-term success being demanded at the expense of long term development.

Influence of UK academies

The vast majority of talent in UK RL is developed through Super League Academies. The relative scarcity of available players and the fact that the majority of Academies serve a very small geographical area means that the search for, and recruitment of, Academy players is of paramount importance. The whole tone of recruitment and development is impacted because the administrative and political backdrop forces clubs to make decisions on players at an early age (e.g. at 14). These players will remain in club systems and rarely exit due to a need to succession plan and the fact that compensation is payable should a player move between clubs at age 16. In the absence of a 'second tier' of competition within RL's TDE (see also Table 30.1) the playing population of the league is now becoming proportionately bigger towards those players identified at the age of 14. This could be setting a dangerous precedent for RL since irrefutable research and data analysis tells us that talent emerges at different rates, there are multiple entry and exit points to the pathway and that RL is a late specialisation sport!

Political interference and financial constraints

This political interference in the talent system therefore demands that the 'development' function of programmes is of exceptionally high quality. From an NGB point of view, it would rather see financial resource distributed to less Academies. This would mean that its limited funding is not spread so thinly and higher quality environments can be fostered. This would also be proportional to the numbers of players in the potential 'talent pool'.

To compound this, the transition from age banded to senior RL in the UK is problematic since there is no 'next step' between Under 19 and senior RL. Consequently, progress through the pathway could be limited according to the club policy that an individual join at age 16. However, the Australian system allows for more competitive playing options post the Under 20 age group (see Table 30.1). Accordingly, players can be afforded opportunities at various levels according to their stage of development. This approach is backed up by the work of Webb et al. (2016) where the "variability throughout the pathway should be tailored to the exact nature of the organisation, its' surrounding contexts and the challenge faced" (Webb et al., 2016, p. 6).

At the elite level, there is a marked difference in the competition and training environments afforded to the players in the two systems. As has already been mentioned, elite players in the UK can play up to 37 competitive club games per year. This leaves little room for preparation of the international team and raises issues of overplaying and burn out for players, sometimes leading to a post-season 'club versus country' debate and players needing to be rested and therefore not being available for international selection. Conversely in Australia, the domestic club season is shorter and elite level players in the SOO system are provided with 30 days' additional preparation in high performance environments. Whilst the NRL is an intense competition, burnout *may* not be as significant as in the UK. To highlight this point, the respective captains of England and Australia at the 2017 World Cup both made their club debuts in 2002 (they are both one-club men). During that time, the England captain's club has been involved in 541 competitive games compared to his Australian counterpart, 422. This represents over seven games per year more, or, the 16 seasons of NRL is worth 12.5 years in SL (2002–17)! Less volume of club matches coupled with the SOO concept crucially provides a step between club and international competition in a high-pressured environment.

Perhaps one solution for England to catch up on Australia is to have more England players playing in the NRL. There are now seven of the current England squad with NRL clubs. This would make sense with players in a more intense competitive environment with appropriate rest and recovery through the season. However, this would 'devalue' the Super League by losing its best talent. This could be detrimental to its commercial and broadcast aspirations as the quality of Super League would be diminished by losing its better athletes.

Conclusion

This chapter has set out to compare the characteristics of TID of the world's two leading RL systems. It has examined both UK and Australian systems against current research and practice, and in the social milieu within which both systems operate. In any effective TID system, athlete progress is at its most effective when the transition between key points appears seamless. On the face of it, Australia appears to offer a seamless transition between levels of the pathway with progress to the international arena taking a staged approach. However, it is based upon flawed principles and is something that the system builders are seeking to address in a politically sensitive climate. We would suggest that the Australia system is reliant on its past history and not fully embracing change to maximise its enormous potential to the full.

In having a much smaller player pool, the UK system must seek to do things differently. The current system exposes flawed selection processes to the pathway at the key ages of 15 and 19. At 15, the system insists on a small number of athletes (200) being selected for further development via Academies. In a late maturing sport such as RL, a huge relative age bias is seen therefore many potential future elite players may remain undetected each year. At 19, player progression is somewhat of a postcode lottery dependent on which club you sign for and its attitude to the competition structure.

Both scenarios have been derived from a political and financial standpoint that are brought about the need to protect numbers participating in community RL (age 15–16) and the financial cost of development programmes post-19 years old. Therefore, to make further significant progress, the UK system must widen the base of the pathway and provide better development opportunities for more athletes by changing the culture and learning disposition of coaches that operate at community level and those within professional Academies with responsibility for TID. The UK must also have a coherent pathway with consistent messages for athletes post-19.

One important piece of learning from this chapter is that there are similar challenges being experienced on both sides of the world. However, because Australia is World Champion, the UK does not necessarily need to copy their system to close the gap. Instead, in the UK we must create better talent development environments that keep more players playing the sport and in recognised pathways for longer.

References

Bailey, R. & Collins, D. (2013). The Standard Model of Talent Development and Its Discontents. *Kinesiology Review*, **2**, 248–259

Barnsley, R., & Thompson, A. (1988). Birthdate and Success in Minor Hockey: the Key to the NHL. *Canadian Journal Of Behavioral Science*, **20**(2), 167–176

Bodey, M. (2015). State of Origin Scores Ratings Record. www.theaustralian.com.au

Collins, T. (2006). *Rugby League in Twentieth Century Britain. A Social and Cultural History*. Oxford: Routledge

Griffiths, M. A., & Armour, K. M. (2013). Volunteer Sport Coaches and Their Learning Dispositions in Coach Education. *International Journal Of Sports Science & Coaching*, **8**(4), 677–688

Martindale, R. J., Collins, D., Wang, J. K., McNeill, M., Kok Sonk, L., Sproule, J., & Westbury, T. (2010). Development of the Talent Development Environment Questionnaire for Sport. *Journal Of Sports Sciences*, **28**(11), 1209–1221

Ogden, J. & Edwards, J. (2016). Are Canadian Stakeholders Resting on Their Laurels? A Comparative Study of the Athlete Pathway Through the Swedish and Canadian Male Ice Hockey Systems. *Journal of Sport Management*, **30**, 312–328

Rugby Football League. (2017). Tier 1–3 Operational Rules

Webb, V., Collins, D. & Cruickshank, A. (2016). Aligning the Talent Pathway: Exploring the Role and Mechanisms of Coherence in Development. *Journal of Sports Sciences*, **34**(19), 1799–1807

Part VI
Living in the system
The performer perspective

As stressed in our introduction to the first section of this book, and then throughout, the most important individuals in any elite sport performance system are (or at least should be) the performers who take to the competitive arena. Indeed, the impact on the performer, squad, or team should be at the forefront of every decision and action taken by those involved in coaching, supporting, or leading in these systems. Of course, this is not to say that every performer will 'get what they want' as, inevitably, what is good for one individual might not necessarily be the best for another, or for the group as a whole. What performers want might also not match up with what they actually need if they are to improve or sustain their levels of performance. In this sense, living in elite sport systems is not always, or not even that often, a straightforward experience. As well as trying to make a system that is designed for 'most' work best for 'me' (or to understand how this system works best for me), a number of other pressures come into play when considering the stage on which their performance is ultimately delivered; whether that occurs in front of peers, fans, the media, and public week-to-week, a couple of times a year, or once every four years. In short, living in the elite sport system can be a hugely rewarding but also highly challenging process.

On this foundation, the purpose of this section is to present a variety of performers' experiences in different elite sport systems. Seeing our recurring themes through to the end, this set of performers represent different sports, different performing 'units' (i.e. those who have performed as individuals, in dyads, and in teams), and different domains (i.e. Olympic and professional). Importantly, they also come from those with different levels of experience as elite performers, with perspectives from those who are 'new on the scene' (i.e. Nico and Miguel Porteous), those who have been performing at the highest level for significant periods of time (i.e. Olaf Tufte and Sinéad Jennings), and one from a performer reflecting back on a long career after some years of retirement (i.e. Tore Andre Flo).

More specifically, our penultimate section opens with a contribution from 'Team Porteous' with Dave, based on the views of Nico, Miguel, their mother, Chris, and Tommy Pyatt, their personal coach. In this chapter, a perspective is provided on two athletes (Nico and Miguel) who have only just achieved elite status but with a fairly special twist: they are brothers who have made it in the same action sport of half pipe skiing. With reflections on their own experiences to date, combined with the thoughts of Tommy and Chris, this chapter offers a rounded view on the journey, support, key lessons, and next steps for both Nico and Miguel in their environment.

Moving to the other end of the spectrum, Chapter 32 then sees Olaf Tufte reflect on his long and successful career in elite rowing. Spanning the last six summer Olympic Games, Olaf identifies a range of factors that have helped him throughout his career, including perceptions and management of pain, sources of motivation, dealing with adversity, the ability to prioritise, planning for the four-year Olympic cycle, and the role of coaches and building your support team. Building on Olaf's account, we then continue with another Norwegian performer, but this time one looking back with some longer hindsight after a few years of retirement – and on a very different sport and challenge. More specifically, Tore Andre Flo presents a picture of performing for over 20 years in professional football, playing week-to-week, and at home and 'on the road', for various club sides across major leagues in Europe, as well as in major qualifying and finals competitions for his national team. As part of this perspective, the demands of men's professional football are outlined first, followed by a consideration of some important principles for 'surviving and thriving' in this domain, before Tore reflects on how these principles played out throughout his career.

Finally, this section concludes with a perspective that emphasises the challenge – and success factors – in balancing pursuits in elite sport with other professional and personal aspirations. To achieve this, Sinéad Jennings, with the support of Áine MacNamara, explores her journey in elite rowing and cycling while also training to firstly become a pharmacist then a medical doctor, whilst also raising a family. In this chapter, focus is placed on Sinéad's early experiences in sport and how this built a foundation for long-term involvement and success, the journey that Sinéad then went on across both of her focal sports, family decisions after missing out on the London 2012 Olympics, and then returning for the Rio 2016 Olympics. To conclude, Sinéad then reflects on what helped her to 'make things happen' both in sport, at work, and at home.

When considering the messages in this section, we hope that clear links can be made back to those in the sections that have preceded it. Most broadly, it is worth considering the role that coaches and sport science and medicine has played across these careers, as well as the impact of the policies, structures, and processes of the systems in which these performers operate or operated (positive and negative). More specifically, it is also worth considering the ways in which each individual has again worked to design approaches that work for *their* bespoke goals and context. Indeed, the ability to develop 'custom-built' solutions is not just a key characteristic for coaches, practitioners, or leaders to excel at 'delivering the system', but also for performers to excel at 'living the system'.

31

The new kids on the block

'Team Porteous' with Dave Collins

Introduction

This section aims to cover the performer's perspective of the elite sporting process and, to that end, we have secured input from a wide range of experiences. In this chapter, we examine the perspective of athletes who have only just achieved elite status but with a fairly special twist.

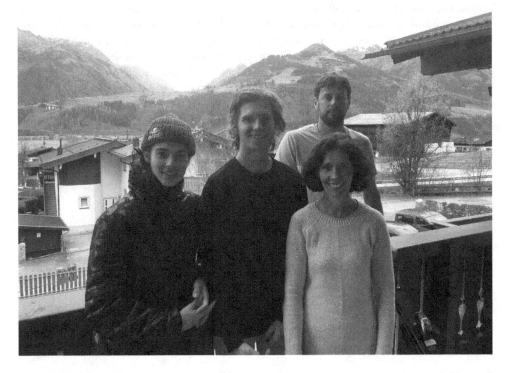

Figure 31.1   Team Porteous

First of all, we have two brothers who have made it in the same sport; the action sport of half pipe skiing. Secondly, we have the coach who, having started work with the athletes as eight and ten year olds, has worked with them all the way to the top. Finally, their mum offers a perspective on their journey and how she and her husband have seen and shaped the process over the last nine years.

'Team Porteous' are shown in the photo (Figure 31.1) above. The next four sections present each member's perspective in their own words. First we hear from Nico, now 17 and standing on the left of the picture. Nico is already an Olympic medallist and current Junior World champion. The second section is from Miguel, 19 years old and standing in the centre of the picture. Miguel has already medalled at the X Games, a commercial event which still retains its status as the unofficial World Championship. The third section is from Tommy Pyatt, standing at the rear of the group, who has coached the brothers for over nine years. Tommy now works for Snowsports New Zealand as a professional coach in freeskiing. The fourth section is from Chris Porteous who presents the parents' view. The chapter concludes with an overview of issues that have emerged, offering a unique insight into one family's experience of the pathway to the top. To facilitate discussion, I applied a timeline approach which we have used throughout our research. Each athlete's hand-drawn graphic is included and referred (for Nico, see Figure 31.2; for Miguel, see Figure 31.3) to help the reader with the timeline of events.

Nico's story

Up to the age of six to seven, I just went skiing. I loved it, had fun, and just tried everything that I could. You look at a lot of people and they're skiing every day of the week, best coaches they could possibly find and they're like six or seven. And I'm like nah. . . don't have a special programme, just let them actually fall in love with the sport rather than trying to make them into an elite athlete when they're so young. Because then they're just going to burn out when they do get to that 12–13 stage. I was never pushed then. I wasn't pushed but I pushed myself!

So I started freestyle skiing at about six. Tommy (the coach) came on the scene at my first junior nationals. I think I was six and Miguel was eight. He came in taught me how to slide my first box sideways. It was kind of like the base thing you learn in free skiing.

I had my first trip overseas when I was ten. For six weeks we went to Breckenridge, Mum and me and Miguel all went over, and that was kinda cool. I didn't really look at it as a full training. I looked at it as "oh cool we get to go overseas skiing". Nowadays, we never leave

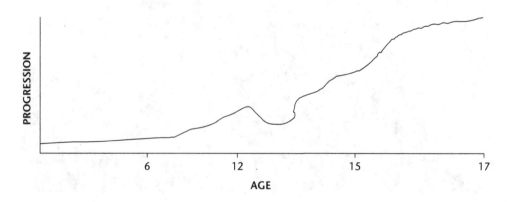

Figure 31.2 Athlete's perceived progress diagram – Nico

home to go skiing without "I'm going to train towards a goal". But back then it was just fun . . . "I'm going skiing!!"

It was also about then that I started taking terms off from school and stuff like that. We were living in Perth and I used to always take term three and term one off: term one off if we were in Colorado and term three off because we'd be in New Zealand.

Progress was good. At age 12, I did my first 12 (high rotation trick – short for three and a half full rotations – 1260 degrees). Also, I did my first training camp away without Mum. I went away with Tommy, Miguel, and an American kid and that was my first ever summer training performance progression camp. I had a whole bunch of goals which Tommy had set out so pretty much we went to a comp, I skied rubbish, I won, Tommy wasn't happy that I won because I skied rubbish! And so he made this list of tricks which I had to do and each time I ticked off these levels I would get a certain, you know, treat, so say I'd go to get a bag of lollies. Or I'd get to go do some activity and so the last one was to grab all four nines in four directions. That 'game' was a big turning point in my skiing – like a massive turning point.

I was still 12 and learnt my third direction of double, but then it was the end of the season. I came back to New Zealand. Then the next year, things started to go downhill really quick. I would have mad phobias over all my tricks and I would have full-on panic attacks and that's when I started to work with a sport psychologist.

This was very frustrating. My feeling was that "I am really wanting to do this. . . I really am wanting to go and risk my neck, travel around the world and away from home. Not be a normal kid you know not have normal friends". But the panic attacks just meant I couldn't do it! I discussed that a lot with Mum and Dad. They always said, and indeed, will always still say to me, "look, at any point if I don't want to do it, you don't have to". They were very clear that no-one was going to judge me for it.

But I stuck with it; both because I wanted to but also because I felt that other people around me did also. I think the other people having the pressure around me kind of helped a bit because I knew deep down inside that I wanted to stop. But I also knew that overcoming it would make me a better person. I showed myself that I could progress that fast in that short amount of time but then all of a sudden I had this kind of mental block. However, I knew I could be the best in the world. It was kind of like the driving force for me to keep skiing. I really enjoy it, but I was really scared of these tricks, but I really enjoy it and I want to be the best. It was a bit of a whole mumble jumble.

Fortunately, I had largely overcome this issue by 13 to 14. Transitioning from a young child to a teenager helped, plus the work with the psychologist. The way we were working was also good. . . focussing on training real hard in that period and taking it back to really true fun skiing. It was great that Tommy gave me the space. I was happy to be back. I progressed the fastest I've ever progressed. I would still get panic attacks and I would still feel really nervous but I continued to progress.

More recently, I have experienced little bumps rather than a major depression. One big cause is injury; almost inevitable in our sport. Even there though my feelings are mixed. Of course, I can't say that I like injuries: they're really bad but sometimes they can be really good. Because they give you a chance to reset, stop and think. Just mentally reset your hungriness and get back to what some would call a progression mindset. I can get off the treadmill, reflect, have a think then get back on. It just makes you fall in love with the sport again, because you realise just how much you miss it

Support

Across my whole career, Mum and Dad have always been there for me. They've been the biggest help I could ever ask for: from the way they help me, fund me, and don't ever put any pressure on me. Just 110% support. Never at a competition or anything have I ever felt pressure or Mum stepping in; just that they support me 110%.

It has also been massive to have Tommy as my coach throughout. That's down to one word – trust. Our sport's massive in trust because it's so high risk and a high injury rate where anything could go wrong at any second. You know you could die every time you go out. So, having trust in your coach and someone to push you at the right times and to not push you at the right times is perfect. Building a close relationship with a coach is the most important thing I think.

Having my brother with me is also fantastic. A training partner 24/7. Moral support, mental support always; never a nuisance on the hill (sometimes off!) but great. Keeps me in check.

Looking back – looking forwards

It's been a fantastic journey so far! I'm pretty proud of what happened in February this year, when I got a medal at the Olympics. But I also think probably one of the proudest moments I've had as well is watching Miguel get a silver at X Games.

Looking forwards, I want to try a few things differently before I really focus on the Games in 2022. I look at all these older guys and they're going off on film trips. Of course, sometimes I then remember and I'm like "heck you know I'm only 17"! But that's still a step I want to take. I feel like I've got to a point in training where I feel comfortable learning new tricks and comfortable learning new skills. So yeah, I think going back and just skiing powder and all. . . getting back to the roots of skiing.

Miguel's story

So, before ten, things were pretty normal. I was going to school and skiing every weekend: discipline-wise, I was doing pretty much everything. Importantly, however, always with the dream of being a professional skier in freestyle. When I was three my Grandma gave me a VCR tape that came in the front of a magazine she had bought. It was a big air thing and, at the time, it had a 14-year-old Aussie called Chris Booth who had won this big air event. I watched that

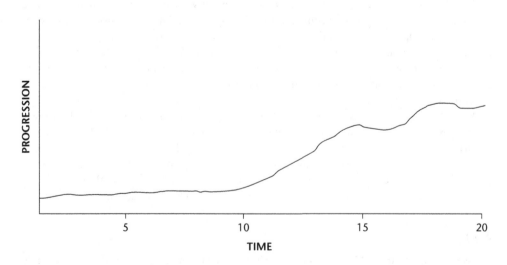

Figure 31.3 Athlete's perceived progress diagram – Miguel

hundreds of times from when I was three and that's how it all started! All that basic work was enjoyable but also absolutely essential. I would say without that I wouldn't be anywhere where I am now. You know the technical stuff starts right from ground zero.

So things started to move faster when I was ten. I guess Mum and Dad saw it was an OK time to let me start chasing what I wanted to do. I had been pushing the idea for a while. It was at that point where I started going overseas and things. Before that, I was skiing every weekend through the whole season and then on the school holidays. There were two weeks' school holidays and I'd ski 14 days from Saturday/Sunday to the next week.

At 12, I went to the states with Tommy and that's kind of when I started getting really serious. I had been doing ski racing but was still keen to do freestyle. So one of the race coaches told us that maybe we should go down to junior nationals for freestyle junior nationals, and I thought that was the best idea ever! I begged Mum for it and then we went down and hired Tommy. Mum came across Tommy's profile in the one of the Cardrona (big ski resort in NZ) ticket lifts and thought "oh he'll be alright" and it was Tommy's first year coaching. Tommy would've been 21; perhaps even 19, my age now. So, we worked with Tommy for like two weeks before nationals and did well. Then the next season was a bit more skiing and eventually that led to at 12 going overseas with Tommy. From then on, I was taking terms off from school; either northern hemisphere for their winter or to get more time in NZ during ours.

From a distance, my progress from then to 15 was pretty smooth. In detail, however, there were quite a few bumps. . . many from injury or from mini challenges like tricks I found particularly hard to master. At around 16–17, I was on a development squad. I'd done my first couple of world cups or big events, and I'd had a run in tricks that were great for me when I'd learn them, but then all of a sudden became quite irrelevant in the sport. So it was like I had to go back to all my basics and start again. Then, soon after, I didn't get selected for Youth Olympics and they picked someone else. Obviously I was bummed about it because I was aiming for that and so I went and skied for two weeks without a coach or anything. Just for fun and I really focussed on the fundamentals of my skiing. And, to be honest, that kind of fixed up everything that was wrong with what I was doing before – just in two weeks skiing for fun. So then the next competition was the Aspen Open (my planned alternative to the Youth Olympic Games). I went there and actually got third at that contest and because of that got invited to the Oslo X Games that same week. So, I flew straight to Oslo which was where coincidentally where the Youth Olympic Games was the week before. BUT. . . the way our sport is, the X Games was a much bigger deal than the Youth Olympics. So actually not getting selected was a huge backhanded help. It's funny how it's such a boys' club in our sport – the top competitions not the governing body competitions – they're such a hard club to get into but, once you're there, you seem to kind of maintain kind of invites and things. So that X Games was like I'd arrived.

Also around 17, from a technical perspective I went through what you might call a period of consolidation. The difficulty of my top tricks didn't change as quickly as before. However, the style with which I did them, or the way I put the run together, became more of a focus. Since then, however, I have taken another jump. There's not much evidence to go on so far but I feel there have been two main stages in my career, as you'd call it. So having made big gains last year I am now in a second period of consolidation.

Looking back and support on the pathway

Looking back, there have clearly been stages when progress seemed to stall, or at least be harder work than usual. Personally, I never have considered quitting, although people around me started thinking maybe I hadn't taken the best pathway. To be honest, I have enjoyed everything, even the challenges. Maybe they're not so great when you're having them but there are always little victories within the downs so I very rarely feel like there is no progress at all.

Mum and Dad have helped enormously. They have just been huge enablers of whatever I wanted to do as I'd always have their full support. That's what makes it so easy to be motivated or be making your own decisions for yourself. Because instead of someone making decisions for you or pushing you into anything or pulling you out of anything, it was totally "hey look if you want to do it it's up to you and you go do that and we'll help you as much as we can".

Of course, they have also definitely helped to ensure that skiing doesn't just absorb my whole life. Like I said, in those downs you've got to keep going but also get a break. You can't just be up the whole time and in our sport I think that is particularly important. Especially when you might be risking your neck daily!

My little brother has also been a huge help. Of course, I don't want to let him get too far ahead of me or beat me or anything! However, just having him there has been great. I think that, especially in the halfpipe where there's not a huge number of people travelling together, just having someone that's doing the same thing makes it a lot easier. You almost work off each other. He is more like a training partner than a little brother.

So going forwards, I am really confident that I am fully equipped. OK, perhaps I could've have stretched some more but I'm not sore so no problem!

The coach perspective

I've been coaching these guys since they were ten and eight; maybe even eight and six. This has been a wonderful but challenging job that has probably got harder as the boys have matured, developing their own opinions and drive, and so needing a different approach. Of course, that said I think it's probably easier to work with people for a long period of time. So long as you fit together well, the relationship gets so strong that you just don't have to talk a lot of the time; it's non-verbal.

In fact, I'd say it's a lot more challenging working with athletes for short periods of time. You have to work to get to know them and you don't know what techniques might work best. So, with long periods of time in contact, you come to know how they learn and how they operate. Furthermore, and once again so long as things are fitting well, the evolution of the relationship comes naturally. They just kind of change, aware of each time they get older and form more of their own opinions, and react differently to the feedback. I definitely wasn't driving the relationship changes. Of course, I would react different and work different at different ages and stages and definitely adapt, but it was more seeing "oh they're older and they're consciously thinking different". So now I'm going to react differently.

Family support

The parents have been great throughout. They've been the leaders for most of the growth pathway. I guess I just stuck to coaching. As I just carried on with my role, they've been the ones that have had to adapt to their kids getting older as any parent does. I think the parents have a particular style of pushiness. Unlike many sports parents, they're not forcing them to ski; the boys can always make the choice to stop. *But* they are very pushy in the way of do it or go. Things like when the boys don't want to go to the gym they'll be "no you're going" so there is pushiness. Perhaps that's because they have the power of "we're funding everything but we won't if you don't follow the high performance layout".

Importantly, that layout is kind of a group thing, with me and Chris deciding. The boys are taking more of a role as they get older. However, they keep coming up with new different ideas and then we have the challenge of adapting them to what we think's right because they have more crazy outlandish ideas the older they get! And you can't just shut them down anymore, you've got to be more clever about adapting them in the right way. As an example, their ideas will involve just wanting to buy a snowmobile and go powder skiing for the season; so I spend time reminding them that they're actually high performance athletes

Looking back, looking forwards

Looking back, I expected them to get to the top, I just didn't expect it to happen on such a sharp pathway. Within two years there was a lot of success that I thought would've taken a four to eight-year period. That said, it's been very useful to have the two. It wouldn't have worked I don't think with only one-on-one coaching. For example, it wouldn't have worked as a year-round role. Them having the support of each other, to be on the road with a friend or a companion, was the only way. I couldn't have travelled with one of them year-round, it just wouldn't have been a healthy environment. We would've had to bring in others to create a group. It's just simpler as brothers, I think. Especially when they get along as well as they do.

Of course, looking back there are things I could have done better. In the earlier years, I would've been coaching differently because I was learning with them. I was growing with them on a rapid pathway, from regional development athletes to national level and beyond. So I would've gone about the early stages differently. To be honest, I think every coach would say that because the whole sport is progressing so quickly. In hindsight, you wish you could've prepared them for where the sport is now. But that's not possible – you don't know what the future is holding.

Looking forwards, the biggest challenge right now is keeping them on track and not letting them sit back and feel comfortable. What I'm seeing right now is they're just resting on their laurels and trying to whip them back into shape for another four-year cycle is a big challenge. The biggest difference from the last quadrennial to the next is that they *were* chasing the game and having to play catch up. Now, they're so much closer to the level that the steps forward are going to be much smaller and incrementally smaller; the way we come to training is going be different. We need to periodise more; they're not going to be competing or training at their highest level all the time. In the last four years, there were so many times that they were.

The parent's perspective

I don't think I've ever actually had the conscious thought that I wanted the boys to be top class athletes. In fact, I don't actually think of them as athletes, to me they are just Miguel and Nico. As the whole thing started, I think Andrew and I decided that we have these two children and it's our job to get them to adulthood in the best way that we feel we can. And basically, that's supporting them in whatever they chose to pursue in their lives. So we have never seen success at skiing as a destination; rather, as part of the journey. It's certainly not the end point and it never has been. In fact, if you'd asked me ten years ago, there would be no way that skiing would be the enormous part of their lives that it is. We would've been thinking school, university, career. . . conventional, 'normal'.

Probably up until three years ago I saw skiing as a distraction to education, a full-on distraction. I often questioned what the heck were we doing letting them travel the world, not going to regular school! It was only within the last three years that I could see that some of the things that we were getting from skiing were valuable life lessons and that school would never have given them these opportunities.

So, up until around three years ago, it was trying to maintain a balance. However, an educator once said to me "let them go and do their sport". He said education will always be here for them but their sport isn't going to be. He was the headmaster of a private boy's school well regarded for its academic results. Once hearing this from him, I saw it as giving us permission to let them go and pursue their dreams. It made it OK for me to let them do it.

I suppose outside people would consider me pushy. To an extent I probably am; I do expect if we're doing something we are going to do it properly and try our best. Crucially, however, if they came and said to me I don't want to do it anymore, I'd say that's fine. . . let's go and do the next thing. We work hard as parents to keep skiing in perspective. I think it's important that they actually see there's life outside of skiing. And I think that's what scares me really. Ensuring that they know there is this life of going on outside skiing. That it is possible to have fun and fulfilling lives without skiing and there's other things in life to enjoy.

Another thing to keep in perspective is disappointment. I don't see this as a sport-specific thing however; I don't think it's any different to disappointment at school. Life's full of disappointment. It doesn't really matter where it comes from; it's just another part of life. We acknowledge the disappointment but we don't dwell on it. Just as, at the same time, we don't dwell on their success. We don't make a big thing like "oh my goodness you've got a medal at the Olympics, that's fantastic". There's not one photo in our house of the Olympics, of Nico wearing a medal, just the same as there's no photo of disappointment. It's just that sometimes, this happens, sometimes, that happens; just get on with it and get onto the next thing.

How it started – how it progressed

I think we were at our local ski field at Christchurch. One of the coaches said "oh you could go to the junior nationals" but we didn't even know anything about the event. I suppose that was then maybe our pushy parent instinct! We said, "well you can't go to junior nationals if you don't know what to do, we'd better get someone to help you so you know what to do". However, I think the *real* turning point for them was when we left New Zealand. We and the boys loved skiing and moving to Perth they knew that we wouldn't be able to ski as much.

We foolishly sold moving to Perth to the boys by saying, "you know, we'll come back to New Zealand and we will still ski". We would come back to New Zealand for a term and they'd ski and then we'd go back to school. I thought that would only last maybe a year and they would've settled into Perth life so well that they wouldn't want to leave. They would want to stay and go surf lifesaving, go surfing, hang out with their mates. But it didn't matter how good a time they were having in Perth, they still wanted to get back to New Zealand and still wanted to go skiing. Andrew and I knew that was really crunch time; that we actually had to start spending a little bit of time apart and our family wasn't a nuclear family anymore. But we made it work and I don't think it's detrimental to the boys' relationships with Andrew: it was a win–win in the end, but we did work at it to make it work.

Of course, as they progressed I was always thinking about school life. . . the need to be successful at exams. So Miguel hitting 16 was another one of my points in the timeline where I thought "we can pull, out this could be the time that we pull out". I thought up until then we could let him be a skier and then we could say "no, you're going to come back to school now". But it didn't work. . . I don't think we even suggested it! So then we came to that turning point I mentioned. Tommy and I sat down and we made that four-year plan; we were ticking boxes, but you can't give up just as soon as you don't tick one box: you know you have to keep going.

BUT. . . if they ever decided "oh no we don't want to do this, we want to go back to school, we want to just go and hang out with friends", it would be fine. We would've made it work for them and we always will.

Fortunately, they both wanted the same pathway. It would've been a lot more difficult if we'd only had one of them but that possibility was never an issue. For example, there was a time there when Nico was 12 or 13 and he wasn't enjoying skiing, we gave him every opportunity to back out and do other things.

The role of the coach

Tommy has been with the boys since the real start of their pathway. One big advantage has been the continuity. He's part of the family really; he knows those boys well, he knows what they've got as goals. Of course, there might have been disadvantages. Performance-wise, for example, I think they get very reliant on just one person. They haven't had the input from a lot of other people. So maybe that has stifled progress. Importantly, however, I don't think it has.

Our trust in Tommy is important. There's a high chance of them being injured and we actually had to trust that the coach had their best interest. That, rather than his best interest, or a team's best interest, or a programme's best interest, he was just looking after them. I don't think many parents would let their 12 and ten-year-old travel to performance camps and do the tricks that they were doing with this young 24 or 25-year-old male looking after their kids.

Advice to other parents

You asked me to say what messages I would send to other parents. Well, it's just my opinion but you did ask! My biggest point is don't put pressure on them. I don't monitor their success by podium finishes. I don't think dwelling on success and over-celebrating success are often positive.

I think what we have done is make use of skiing as a tool to develop the boys. Of course, I definitely think that education is important. But, coming from thinking that they could only be educated through the traditional pathways of a classroom, I have actually had to change my thinking and see that doing things a little bit differently isn't always that bad. There are positives there, even if some other parents may be critical of your decisions; either covertly or even to your face. Others always have their opinions on how you should be doing things or what you shouldn't be doing but don't let them blur your thoughts.

Some summary thoughts

I think it is interesting to read the boys' thoughts about their early career, especially in light of the current noise around early specialisation. From an age and activity perspective, both were early specialisers. Importantly, however, perhaps the combination of circumstances around them gave this a different feel; making them early participators rather than specialisers per se. This idea notwithstanding, both were committed to the sport early and clearly focused on what most would acknowledge as an early specialisation route. Of course, both may burn out or get fed up. Here again, however, the combination of parental support rather than pressure, careful coaching and the willing ness to make adjustments to meet individual circumstances may be the crucial factors.

There are also several examples of autonomy and luck, together with assistance from others. Both Tommy and Chris emphasise their role in giving the boys choices but also, crucially, ensuring that those choices carry personal responsibility. These ideas echo much of our work in talent development (e.g. Collins et al., 2016) and it is great to see the conscious focus on delegation and increased self-determination.

For me personally, however, as a parent, psychologist, and talent developer, I am completely impressed by Chris's open and honest stance on the boys' involvement. Readers are encouraged to consider her perspective against other relevant chapters, including those by personal and talent-development focused coaches.

Reference

Collins, D., MacNamara, Á., & McCarthy, N. (2016). Super Champions, Champions, and Almosts: Important Differences and Commonalities on the Rocky Road. *Frontiers in Psychology*, **6**, 2009. doi: 10.3389/fpsyg.2015.02009

32

Staying at the top in Olympic rowing for 25 years

Olaf Tufte with Geir Jordet

Introduction

25 years. How have I kept going for so long? That is a big question. I am driven by the possibility of becoming a little bit better tomorrow, no matter what. That is perhaps the most important thing for me; "Is it possible to do something better?". Even after winning the World Championships I trained in the afternoon because I've not felt that my performances were good enough and because, ultimately, it's the Olympics I intend to win. I want to be better. I hate to lose, but what I hate even more is to fail at something that I have practised. What this means is that I accept being beaten because someone else has performed better, but I do not accept failing at something I should have been better at practising. By the same token, it is certainly true that if one is to keep going in a sport for a long time enjoyment is extremely important. For me this is about passion; an inner drive making you want to take things just a bit further, and then a bit further still. Without passion I would never have continued for so long.

So it is this passion – combined with madness or idiocy – and the culture of which you are a part and in which you have grown up, that shapes you as an athlete. I have grown up in a culture where everything can always be a little bit better. It is an ethos I have carried with me from early on, and then I've since been thrown into a professional environment that has been very achievement-oriented. I believe that we become products of the environments in which we find ourselves. Suppose that someone plays football, eats pizza, and drinks beer; that then becomes their culture and people believe that this is how it should be. It is not people there is something wrong with, it is the culture. But who should change the culture? For me, this drive for improvement has been so important that I have always been driven to perform a little better tomorrow. In doing so, I have met a whole series of people who inspire me; everything from opera singers, to wrestlers and skiers. It makes no difference what they are doing, so long as the foundation of their drive is excellence in performance and they show a passionate interest in the process of getting to the top.

To keep at anything for as long as 25 years, it's essential that it should be fun. Spending time with like-minded, driven people is certainly a big part of this. One of the most fun things each year is the first World Cup regatta, where you meet all of the boys again, all the rowers, and you have to make some time to chat, especially because we are a big, happy family in the rowing world.

We are all individuals – some are screwed up in the head like me and find it fun to be in pain many times a day! This support from those around you comes not only from your friends and peers, but also from family.

For me, the reason that I can keep going comes from all of these many things put together. In what follows I will address some of them in more detail.

Pain

Pain comes in many different forms, one of which could be called 'external pain'. This is the pain you inflict upon yourself, which hurts and can go so far as to cause injury. Something else is training pain, an inner type of pain that you can actually control. You can let the pain have control over you, or you can take control over the pain and let it instead become a part of your plan. As an athlete, when you take part in tough training sessions or competitions you know that it is going to hurt. When I am preparing myself to race I go through every single movement in my mind, and I know with incredible clarity not only how painful it is going to be, but also how I will tackle it without it negatively impacting my performance. It is sometimes said about me by commentators on television that "he is good at lactic acid"; which I find a funny saying, because no one can be 'good' at lactic acid. Lactic acid is something you experience. The key is being so well trained that the lactic acid comes a little later for you than it does for others. If you can train at having some lactate in the body; you manage to wrap your mind around the pain, and instead focus on performing the patterns of movements that you must repeat again and again. If you aren't smart enough, the lactic acid will win in the end; the trick is being good enough to hold onto that which you have the ability to influence – the inner pain. It is usually lactic acid that is the inner pain. The need to have control in rowing is about managing extreme lactic acid and extreme ventilation at the same time.

One of the things I find most interesting about all sport – and even life itself – is that it is totally reliant on breath. If someone breathes correctly, they can manage much more. And if you manage to combine your breathing with keeping your shoulders low or being relaxed, you can achieve the most unbelievable things. A sprinter who runs 100 metres doesn't win if he has shoulders up to his ears. Messi doesn't manage to dribble well if he begins to think and tries to take control over his muscles without just letting it flow. He has to relax and play around with what he is doing in order to achieve perfection in the patterns of movement. It's about breathing. And by focussing on breathing, you take away the focus from the pain; and if you breathe properly then you have a much bigger chance of separating the waste materials that lead to increased lactic acid, which is the cause of experienced pain. In that moment you lose control over your breath, you begin to hyperventilate or feel that you have to have more air, but in doing so you actually get less oxygen, higher shoulders, more acid and it is then that your performance begins to stop and it hurts a lot. In rowing, for example, when we race 2000 metres we reach the finish line with over 20 mmol/l in lactate, which is pretty high. But the worst pain very often comes as soon as we stop rowing. That is because when we stop rowing everything in the body is freed and the inner pain is allowed to surface. Up until that point the primary focus was on breathing, keeping the dynamics of the movements going and ignoring the fact that it was painful. As long as we are smart enough during execution, we know exactly how hard we can push. The key is to find that trigger during training. If you have never practised dealing with pain in training how in the world can you expect to handle it during a race? You simply would not know what was happening. I believe that learning to deal with inner pain comes down to practice and observing how the body responds; each time you practise, you can go a step further. However, it is important to note that this practice is all about correct and good thinking, rather than being crazy. If you are crazy in the wrong way (i.e. overambitious, over aggressive, ignoring important limitations), then you destroy your body in the process while you push harder than your body can tolerate. This is all a matter of preparation.

Motivation

Personally, what drives me is seeing if it is possible to be better tomorrow. That is my primary motivation. But it hasn't always been that way, everyone goes through eras in life. For me in my teenage years, everyone in Norwegian sport was dumb, everyone else was wrong. In your 20s you are maybe pretty good and then you become "World Champion". Then you get past 30 and realise that perhaps Mum and Dad weren't so stupid when they were being strict; they gave me a pretty good toolkit to use in life, and there are also a lot of great people around who have looked out for me. You appreciate this and begin to realise that there are actually other people who may know something about what they're doing or telling you to do. When you get to your 40s, where I unfortunately find myself now, then you think even more. I feel that I am learning. I have a better understanding of the things that I can't do and have become even more curious. That, so far, is the lifecycle of me as a person.

When it came to athletic development in my teenage years and early 20s, it was all about winning as much as possible, all the time. Many are driven by winning the next interval, beating your best friend – you will beat him at any cost, no matter what you are doing. Then you become a bit more mature and begin to aim at the bigger races. You plan a little more in order to be in slightly better shape for the events that really matter; such as the World Championships and the Olympics. I would also by this time have enough sense about me to want to be in good enough shape when the Norwegian championship came, even though those events do not mean as much as the major international ones, I at least wanted something to show for my effort. It is then that you realise that you can do quite a lot, but you also understand that there are still many things to learn. So begins an interesting journey where the *path* to the goal is what is important. You must be smart enough to make the path as good as possible so that you may succeed at the end, by hitting those three to four days at the right moment when you reach the peak of your physical shape. All this comes from the fact that you have worked well not only in the preceding 11 months, but really the last 20 years. In order to accomplish this sort of long-term progress, you have to know something about a lot of different topics, but also a whole lot about yourself. You must be able to listen to your body, and to the coaches that pay enough attention to have a reasonable opinion about what is going on with your performance. It is about moving from the position where winning in the next five minutes is the most important thing in the world, to the most important thing in the world being building foundations so solid that you have the possibility of succeeding 11 months from now.

Adversity

Even to this day, I have always returned from injury in a better state than I was in before. The reason for this is that I haven't just sat on my ass when I have been injured. I find that while injured, I have time to do things that I don't usually have time for when I am 100%, such as better basic mobility training. Sometimes I have even moved into the elite sport centre and lived there for a while. Instead of sitting and watching *Home and Away* I have done all of the exercises I possibly could, such as when I had a prolapsed disc in my back and was only able to sit and cycle, I would do that for two to three hours at a time. I have also been known to do suspension training and flexibility training five times a day. Generally, I train much more when

I am injured than when I am healthy. When I become injured I seek out possibilities. The worst thing someone can say to me is what I can't do. I have no use for that type of advice. I only need to know what I can do and how much.

Sacrifice and lifestyle

I have never sacrificed anything in order to have my career. The day that I sacrifice is the day that I quit. I have prioritised incredibly hard, but that is because I want to win the Olympics more than I want to sit and make out in the back row of the cinema on a Saturday night. If you are structured enough you can manage everything, and train well enough at the same time. But you must be structured and disciplined. Some say I have sacrificed my youth and given up hanging out with the guys. No, I have not. I have simply prioritised hard. A part of that is focusing on my best friends, the ones who accept what I am doing. I believe that you cannot have more than ten really good friends, as you don't have time to take care of more than that. There are loads of wannabes and entourage friends, but you must find out who your real friends are. And your real friends are there no matter what, whether things are going well or going badly, and whether you are away for a day or a month doesn't matter. They are proper friends. By being structured I can hang with the guys, eat dinner, have a beer, drink a little wine and enjoy myself. But when they go out to bars or clubs, I head home. Because what happens when you go out? You split up, spend a bunch of money, end up going to the kebab place, eat junk food, and you don't get to bed before 5am and you feel terrible the next day. I would rather get home by midnight, smiling, having been with good friends, eaten good food, had a couple of beers and my body smiles back at me. Right after the guys get home I am already up and heading to training, and I am nearly finished with two training sessions before they get out of bed. Who is the winner of that evening then? But sometimes you take it a little bit further. On occasion, you have to act out and do things that aren't the best thing for you because the body needs to derail and disconnect and get a feel for what it really isn't missing. After you have stuffed yourself at McDonalds, you don't go to McDonalds for a good few months.

Through a long athletic life I have learned that it is the average that counts; how you perform on average over time. You cannot take back training, take back sleep, or take back eating. The average has to be good enough. That is perhaps the most important thing to teach younger athletes. I have learnt that enjoying life is not so dangerous, but over-usage comes with consequences. When you are young and you are hanging out with the guys, you end up over-using alcohol if you don't manage to stop, and end up drinking the whole six-pack before 7pm. When you are a bit older you open a bottle of wine, enjoy two glasses, have fun and that does not matter so much. But to chase down a six-pack of beer because you were thirsty is not healthy. You need to be really serious and at the same time you also need to allow yourself to enjoy life. Maybe that is going for a long walk in the woods, sleeping a little longer one day, or having a glass of wine with good food. If it is good for you and your mental health so that you can perform better tomorrow then that's great. But it is the average that counts. If it becomes a glass of wine every single day then that will have an impact.

Cycles

In rowing we work in Olympic cycles (i.e. four-year periods). We try to make a plan for the next four years because success in the Olympics is the most important thing for us. The four-year plan is also divided up into years in order to also succeed at each World Championship. We also divide the year up into training periods, which set out when we will focus on quantity, when we will focus on strength, but nevertheless keep up fitness levels. All these things are included in a normal cycle. I came to a point in 2012 where I had bombed at the Olympics for the first time. Between 2008 and 2012 things went really badly. I later found out that I had rowed with mononucleosis for four years, and subsequently took a year out to rest my body and think through what I really wanted to do. I came to the conclusion that I wasn't done with rowing. I believed that it would be possible to succeed again and become better. To achieve this I had to change my whole technical rowing pattern, which was a pretty long process, but I succeeded. I should have maybe stopped after Rio in 2016, but I got pissed off because we reached the goal, though not the dream. We reached the goal by being the fastest double in the world, but we messed up the dream of winning Olympic gold because we stumbled out of the starting blocks. So I got a bit angry and thought that I couldn't let this go, because we didn't get out of it what we should have. I tried again in 2017 to see if we could do it, but we fumbled a bit in the boat and it didn't work out again. By then I had already started a new Olympic cycle and I said that, "Whatever happens, to row Tokyo in 2020 as a 44-year old and succeed, that would be something!" I only know of one man who has taken a medal so late and he was 43 years old. I am 44. Ole Einar Bjørndalen failed at his seventh Olympics. Everyone says it is impossible. So I want to make the impossible possible.

I also know that I cannot do a whole Olympic cycle with everything I have around me now – family, three companies that take a lot of work, training, and being a farmer. I simply can't ignore all of that for another period so I have to take a year out of competing and work a little more and get a bit more control of my work and family life in order to then go back for two years at 100% and give it everything. That has been my plan. It has never been a lack of motivation to compete, but I had to make a plan in order to be able to get to Tokyo, so I had to work a little more on some of the other things in order to make time to be an athlete. I cannot just be an athlete because that would bore me. You also become stupid. When other athletes say to me that they don't have time to do anything other than train and rest either I turn around and leave or I laugh, because that is just nonsense. As athletes you have so much time that you can choose what to do with it; you can play video games, watch movies or series, read a little, work a little and take in many other types of stimuli. Very few of us can live off of sport alone and you arguably need a leg to stand on outside of sports. This is also a good opportunity to learn lots of new things and shift your focus, something which has been of utmost importance for me in my career to shift focus and not think of rowing strokes 24/7, because then you get sick of the sport. And then when I do come to think about rowing strokes, I will think 102% about rowing and that is what makes me much more effective. It is about being present. There are many athletes who are not, because they begin to bring other things into sport, or put sport into other things. Then you lose focus and do only half a job. Mentally, finding this balance and segregation is extremely difficult.

Now, at over 40 years of age, the biggest difference I notice from before is in recovery. It takes me a little longer to recover after hard training sessions. However, what has had the biggest impact on my ability to recover in my career hasn't been ageing, it was the mononucleosis. That led to me become significantly more sensitive. Before that, I was unstoppable in a way; I got up in the morning and ran intervals, a little food and rest later and then it was out to "die again" on the second session. I was everywhere the whole time, and there was nothing that broke me. Little sleep, lots of training, and all the training was hard. I got a couple of hours rest, ate a little food and then I was fine again. That's how I carried on the whole time. I believed that I was immortal, and as long as I got a little rest, things would work out. I ran my body into the ground after the Beijing Olympics. I did far too many things and my average amount of sleep between then and the 2009 World Championship was 6.5 hours a night. That is obviously not enough when you are a top athlete, father, and businessman. So things came to a halt for me, it's a bitter feeling I can still taste now many years on. I have had to strike out a completely new path and build myself up from the ground again. Very frustrating.

Coaches

All of the significant coaches I have had have been so close with me that they have almost been my back-up fathers. I have shared so much with them and they know me so well that when I have been in doubt, I have asked them what they have thought is best for me. I think that is critical. As an athlete you are always getting into situations where you experience doubt. It can be situations where you doubt whether you should train because you are scared that you aren't in shape, or doubt whether you should practice something because it is hard. It is then that a coach has to come in and say "this is what you need to do Olaf, in order to make it". Then you can rest your head on his shoulder and trust that he is right.

I have often said that I have trained extremely hard at certain times and people have shaken their heads and said that I am crazy, but I won nevertheless. After becoming older I have said that the most important thing is not to do everything right all of the time. Instead, for me it is more important to believe that what I am doing is the toughest and the best route for me, because when I am at the starting line I need to know that what I have done is the best I possibly could do. I have been the toughest and there is no one around here who has done a better job than me. That is what I need to be able to believe in order to succeed. Of course you will make mistakes along the way, but you don't see that until afterwards. What is most important is making as few mistakes as possible, and if you do make mistakes, hoping that they destroy as little as possible. Because if you don't make mistakes, then you don't learn either. You must dare to fail in order to succeed. Success is my job, and so I find this an important sentence to live by. When Tore Øvrebø was my boss (we won a couple of Olympic golds together), I would say (and I actually still say it): "I had the world's best rowing coach, but it took a damn long time to get him there". I have as good coaches as I want to have. In a way, I create my own coach. If I want a mean, bad coach then that is easy. If I want a good coach, then I have to allow him to become good. It is the same as being a father. If you want to have an unpleasant father then it is easy to get that. If you want to have a gentle father then you have to do a lot of things that make him happy and then he becomes nice and understanding.

In order for a coach to get to know Olaf Tufte the coach must know how things are for me. He needs to know what I am doing and why I think what I think. Tore Øvrebø and I are an example of this. We had a huge dispute early in my career because I was a farmer and when you are a farmer you can't wait until tomorrow to harvest grain or spray crops, you have to do it at the exact time it needs to be done. So we ended up having a disagreement when I had to rush off to catch the ferry home and Tore scolded me and said that I didn't understand what it takes to be a winner. I stopped rowing and answered back: "you don't know shit about being a farmer, you don't get it at all". Then it was Rolf Sæterdal who got hold of us and sat us both down and said "Olaf, now you have to explain to Tore what it is like to be a farmer. And Tore, you must explain to Olaf what is required to become the best". When I then told Tore how you have to think as a farmer and what the job is like he suddenly understood why I needed to take the ferry home. And Tore talked about the path to win a medal so I got an understanding of how important it was to plan everything so that I could manage to do the job. With this new mutual understanding, it then became possible to make a plan together. You must be able to get to know each other and you can accomplish this by being open and honest. Honesty is perhaps most important. When a coach asks how you're doing, don't complain – that's nonsense.

Rather, tell your coach exactly how you're doing and how things are going for you. Because different emotions you have can influence your feelings during training and sometimes you don't manage to separate the two. If you take a recently divorced person and compare him to a newly in love person then the person who is in love will win 99% of the time, because that person has so much energy and nothing bad can touch him.

I also think it is really exciting to build the team around me: physiotherapists, osteopaths, acupuncturists, gymnastic coaches, mobility trainers, and strength trainers. Finding new people is exactly the same as finding new training partners, I am really curious to learn ways we might work well together. I have mental coaches I work extremely closely with, and I have movement and mobility gymnastic coaches I work very well with. I use lots of information and facts from other gurus. I talk a lot with Johan Kaggestad, I continue to go back to Tore Øvrebø, even though Johan Flodin is my head coach who I really listen to. I can have discussions with others, especially other established athletes, about this and that. I also like to listen to the younger athletes in order to know what they know and how they think. And at the same time, I have to take time to sit and sort things out by myself. In a way, I have an inner circle of people who I choose to listen to a bit more and who I can go and spar with. If eight out of ten people are saying the same thing then you can usually accept that it's relevant. In this way, other people are to me extremely important in that I am always working to be as humble as possible in my approach to everything so as to be able to make choices based on the information and facts on the table. I combine this with my own experiences and feelings and so that I am able to have ownership of the choice that is made. If all the facts go completely against everything I believe then it impacts my motivation. In these cases, I either need to find motivation or talk with the people closest to me to figure out how to solve the issue.

Athletes from other sports mean a lot to me, because I get so much inspiration from training with others and getting their input. But most important here is friendship. Friendship with all of the fantastic people one meets along the way. To train with someone from another sport and get inspiration and tips you can take away with you is extremely important. If you train solely within the environment you are a part of then you become a product of that culture. I am perhaps sometimes perceived as a bit of a grumpy old man because I think that the youth of today are a little too relaxed and get too much handed to them on a silver platter. I sigh too much sometimes, but I rely on the fact that I have good enough people around me who push me regardless of age and who I can spar with. The better they are, the better you become. If you are training with a 6th division football team then you look like a jerk, if you're training with Rosenborg (one of the best football teams in Norway) then maybe you look pretty good, even if you're bad.

When I was a bit younger I was very concerned with being better than others. As I have become older I feel that when I watch others it is easier for me to feel joy around their great performances. At the same time, however, it is also extremely easy to feel irritated about good performances based on a bad work ethic. People who have done a bad job of building the foundations, but have succeeded anyway, irritate me. When I was younger I was extremely concerned with how I could beat people, how I could be better than them. Whereas now when I meet interesting people, I am much more focused on asking what I can learn from them. It's something I find really fun and interesting to do. It's now normal for me that when I see other athletes, I often look at what they are doing. If I know anything about what they are doing then I always think about how I would have done it if I think that they are doing it wrong. If I think that they are doing something interesting then I will ask questions. What do you do? How do you do it? Why do you do it? Curiosity. The best athletes and best leaders I meet are the most humble and curious people. The second best are, as a rule, the most arrogant.

Conclusion

For me, the path to success is essentially about one thing and that is hard work over time. Sitting within this there are many other factors. I tend to say that we often have shooting stars, both in sport and in business – suddenly they become good, but then just as suddenly they are gone because they don't have the foundation necessary to stay at the top. If you are suddenly successful in sports, but those around you have never been there and do not know how to take it further; how to handle all the attention and continue the success, then you are quickly done. Lottery millionaires are a brilliant example of this. Suddenly you win millions. You have never been used to handling lots of money. Three years later you are bankrupt. When you take the boring road you take it step by step. Replacing people around you with people who have been there longer than you and know more about the road ahead; you are making a strong foundation in order to stand where you are. So it is also that "slow and steady wins the race". It is a boring saying but the older you become the more you realise that it is this saying which truly makes the difference.

33

Playing home and away – and away and away

Tore Andre Flo with Andrew Cruickshank

Introduction

As highlighted at the start of this section, the best systems in elite sport will be firmly focused on the development and performance of those who take to the competitive arena. Of course, this is not to say that 'the system' is entirely responsible for competitive performance; clearly, responsibility is shared with the performers themselves. But what is it like to deliver on this responsibility as a performer and within the systems we have described so far in this book? To start to address this question, the purpose of this chapter is to offer a perspective on 'how to make things work' from the world of professional football. To do so, we draw on Tore's career as a footballer in the men's professional game; one which saw him play for ten clubs in four countries over 20 years, as well as international football in major qualifying and finals tournaments for Norway. As a forward, Tore played almost 500 games and scored 180 goals at club level and helped his sides to win six major trophies. On the international stage, Tore also played 76 times for Norway between 1995 and 2004 and scored 23 goals in the process; a total which places him as the joint-fourth highest goal-scorer in Norway's history. With the national side, Tore also played at the 1998 World Cup Finals in France as well as the 2000 European Championships in Belgium and the Netherlands.

More specifically, this chapter is made up of two parts. Firstly, we provide a general overview of men's professional football,[1] including a description of some key demands in a sport where top-level players usually represent multiple clubs (often in different countries and competitions) and, in some cases, their national team at the same time. We will also consider some particularly important principles for 'surviving and thriving' in this domain. From this base, our second section then moves to explore Tore's own career and how the 'surviving and thriving' principles played out in his specific journey. By our conclusion, we hope to have shed some light on living in professional football (and similar other systems), as well as what performers (and their systems) might need to make the most of their potential.

Living in the professional football system: some stand-out demands

For those less familiar with professional football, the first point that we should stress (and reflecting prior chapters) is that the game, especially at the top level, is BIG business! This is both in the sense of the volume of people with a stake in each team and the finances involved. As one example of the money involved at the top level, the current world transfer record at the time of writing is €222 million, spent by Paris St Germain to sign Brazilian forward Neymar from Barcelona in 2017. As another, the *average* wage for a current player in the English Premier League per year is now a multi-million-pound figure. Of course, these top-end examples are not characteristic of the professional game as a whole. However, and keeping the focus of this book in mind, it is fair to say that anyone playing in the highest ranking or highest resourced leagues around the world will receive a significant salary plus extra fees (e.g. via sponsorships and image rights). It is also fair to say that the vast majority of players will have an agent or representative who negotiates the best contract possible from any club – for the benefit of both the players and, to varying and sometimes problematic degrees, the agents themselves. In sum, money, to a large extent, can drive the game at the top end. It plays a major role in who's successful and who's not and can provide an extra lure for those hoping to reach the professional level; or even those with hopes for a family member, friend, or client to reach this level (a common challenge for those working in a club's academy).

As well as a driver of action, money can also be a driver of perception for the many individuals involved in the game: from players comparing their 'worth' in relation to others, to managers who hang their reputation on 'big money signings', to the directors, fans, media, and pundits who engage in a constant evaluation of whether each club is getting a return on its investment. Certainly, while finances drive many aspects of football, one element that it perhaps drives most significantly, for players, is expectation. For some, this expectation may be more internal in nature (i.e. "I need to perform because of the money the club has spent on me"); for others, this expectation may be a more external factor (i.e. "the media are giving me a tough time because of the money the club spent on me"). Either way, high expectations are rife in professional football.

Of course, this expectation isn't necessarily *caused* by money. For many with a stake in the game, expectations are largely derived from an emotional investment to the sport or a specific team; whether they are players, managers, coaches, support staff, a club or national team's wider staff, fans, or the media. In short, clubs and international teams typically mean a LOT to a LOT of people! Regardless of where exactly money comes into the equation, our point is that professional football is a highly pressurised environment where expectations are constantly generated, sometimes met or exceeded, and, at least as reported in the media, often fallen short of.

Arguably one of the clearest symptoms of this pressure is the managerial 'merry-go-round' that characterises many leagues in many countries (i.e. the regular hiring and firing of team managers). For example, the average tenure of managers around the globe is now often under two years, comfortably so in many cases. Paired with the tendency for players to move around a number of clubs during a career, another demand on players is the need to therefore perform under different managers with inevitably (and sometimes significantly) different approaches. This challenge is also extended for those representing their country, where the style of club play may differ markedly from national play (under management who will also come and go). The 'on-field' challenge of playing for club and country can also be complicated by the 'off-field' demands; including significant further travel, time away from home, and living in the company of less familiar team-mates (players spend much more time with their club than their national team over a season).

As well as the general features described above, professional football also presents a host of other, more specific demands on players over their careers. For example, the norm of moving clubs also means that there is a norm of moving home; sometimes to a new country with a new culture and new language. There are also a number of 'occupational hazards' to contend with, such as various levels of injury (from daily niggles to long-term curtailment), dips in form, and disagreements with and between managers, coaches, and team-mates to name a few! In sum, players who deliver on their full potential can experience a plethora of psychological, social, and financial rewards; however, achieving these outcomes – especially when combining club with international play – is clearly a demanding process. In this sense, and reflecting the regularity of matches and importance of winning, the pace of life can often feel accelerated in this world. So, what can help a player to survive and thrive?

Surviving and thriving in professional football: what can help?

Having outlined some particular demands of living in the football system, we now move to consider some broad principles of how players can survive and thrive in the game. Of course, a plethora of factors play a part in this process from across the bio-psycho-social spectrum. Therefore, the broad principles that we have chosen to explore are definitely not exhaustive. However, they are, we feel, crucial for a long and successful career in football or other elite team sports – and certainly played a part in Tore's achievements. Specifically, we focus on how challenges are *set, perceived*, and *managed*; or even more precisely, the role of:

- creating and shaping internal challenge;
- embracing and adapting to external challenge;
- managing challenge with a reliable and consistent support network.

Importantly, the rationale for this focus is grounded in the world of professional football (as described in the last section) plus recent research. Indeed, and as we hope to have stressed in this book so far, a career in elite sport is *filled* with challenge: some small, some major; some persistent, some fleeting; some 'on-the-pitch', some 'off-the-pitch'; some of personal doing, some of others' doing. Academic work has also consistently highlighted that perceptions of, preparation for, and responses to challenges are fundamental to performance; in fact, they have been shown to differentiate between those who achieve a little, a lot, or the most at the top levels of elite sport (e.g. Collins et al., 2016).

Taking the first of these principles, *creating and shaping internal challenge* relates to the challenge that is set and designed by performers themselves. In this respect, research has also highlighted many benefits of this principle and the linked concept of self-control, namely around its role in building and sustaining motivation, as well as enabling perspective and continuous personal growth (e.g. Toering & Jordet, 2015). Given the high pressure and continual 'bar-raising' objective in elite sport, such outcomes are clearly useful! For *embracing and adapting to external challenge*, this principle refers to the ability to accept and adjust to the openings, sticking points, and setbacks that elite sport constantly presents in a way that also supports growth and development. In a fast-paced, high pressure environment where players have to perform with an evolving set of team-mates and managers, being comfy with variation seems crucial. Our final principle of *managing challenge with a reliable and consistent support network* relates to the social support that performers can draw upon to 'release, reset, and refine'. More specifically, this principle reflects the idea that cognitive and emotional recovery requires a level of cognitive and emotional detachment from whatever is placing the demands on an individual (Balk et al., 2017); or, in other words, mental rest is needed to recover mental energy. Importantly, however, this principle also covers the 'bigger picture' or 'slowed down' style of thinking that is often difficult to engage with in the face-paced training and performance environment where focus tends to centre on what is happening today (especially in sports like football where matches are week-to-week).

While we now move to consider these principles in the context of Tore's career, it is important to note that all three are relevant for most, if not all, performers in football. We also feel that there is much crossover to other elite team sports around the world given similarities in the nature and level of challenge experienced by their performers; especially sports which are characterised by high levels of variation (e.g. those with a regular turnover in staff and players; different competition formats). To demonstrate the value of our three principles, and in line with the overall aims of this book, we now consider *how* they played a part in Tore's career. Firstly, however, it is important to set the context for this by providing an overview of Tore's specific journey in the game.

Setting the context: Tore's journey in football

In Figure 33.1, we have presented a timeline of Tore's career in professional football, as based on Tore's perceptions.

In this timeline, Tore has split his career into four major phases. Tore has termed the first of these "seeking a pro contract", which spans his first three clubs in Norway, up to signing for Chelsea FC in 1997. As noted, one particularly memorable event that was truly formative to Tore's growing skills and levels of performance was his debut for his national team. Turning to the second period, this has been described by Tore as his "peak phase" and covers his time with Chelsea FC, where he won the FA Cup, Charity Shield, Football League Cup, UEFA Cup Winners' Cup, and UEFA Super Cup, as well as a highly successful period with the Norwegian national side. As marked on the timeline, key events included: a hat-trick (three goals in the same game) against one of Chelsea's London rivals, Tottenham Hotspur FC, in his debut season for the club; plus his appearances for Norway at the 1998 World Cup, where Tore scored in a famous victory against Brazil that helped them to reach the second round of the tournament. After this period, Tore felt that the third phase of his career occurred between 2001 and 2006, which he has termed "up and down, without reaching my previous highs". During this third

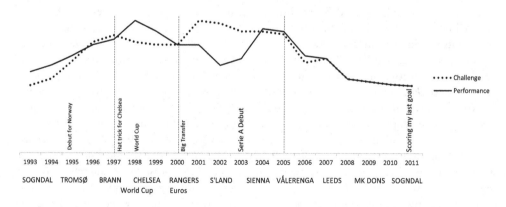

Figure 33.1   Tore's career timeline in professional football

phase, two particularly memorable events were a £12 million transfer from Chelsea FC to Rangers FC in Scotland and, four years later, his debut in Italy's Seria A for Sienna. Finally, "the end phase" ran from Tore's move from Sienna up to his final games for Sogndal, the club where he had started his career in Norway. In this phase, Tore recognised the particular significance of scoring his last goals in his final season in football.

Perceived performance level

As well as these phases and key events, Tore has also presented his perceptions on his levels of performance throughout his career, as marked by the solid line in Figure 33.1. As shown, Tore felt that his level of performance increased incrementally during the first two phases of his career – reaching his peak around 1998–99 – before sustaining a high level up to the start of the third phase of his career. In this third phase, Tore then reports a notable drop, up to his time with Sunderland, before returning with Sienna to the level he had sustained during his final year with Chelsea. Understandably in his "end phase", Tore felt that his performance level gradually dropped; however, it is notable that his performances during his final season, after first 'retiring', still matched the level of those a couple of years earlier.

Perceived level of challenge

Finally, the timeline also includes an indication of the degrees of challenge that Tore perceived throughout his career; in other words, how hard or tricky things were (see the dotted line in Figure 33.1). As shown, Tore experienced an increasing level of challenge throughout the first phase of his career; partly due to the increasing standard that he expected of himself and partly due to the expectations of others. In particular, Tore felt the pressure build up from the media, especially on moving to Brann and starting to play for the national side. Additionally, the supporters at Brann had, to a degree, turned against Tore when it was announced that he had signed for Chelsea; not for leaving the club per se, but instead for leaving under the 'Bosman ruling' which meant that Brann received a much smaller fee than the fans expected. Interestingly, Tore seemed well equipped to manage this increasing level of challenge given the corresponding increase in performance. Additionally, it is also telling that when stretched on his arrival at Chelsea FC, both on the pitch and off the pitch (given the move to a big city in a new country), his performance took another notable upturn while the level of challenge gradually settled. This level of challenge was still of a very high level of course, reflecting the standard of the competitions Tore was playing in for club and country, as well as a significant injury (when the medical staff were uncertain if Tore could recover and return to prior levels of performance).

Also interesting to note is the significant increase in perceived challenge when Tore transferred to Rangers FC for a substantial fee at the time – one that remains a Scottish record almost two decades later. More specifically, this increase in perceived challenge reflected the implications of a £12 million transfer; especially the increased expectation that Tore and the media placed on his performances. After two years at Rangers, Tore then joined Sunderland FC for a season that ended with the club being relegated from the Premier League; a period when Tore felt that his performance level had particularly dropped (relative to his peak). However, Tore then rose again to the test of playing with Sienna, before the level of challenge gradually dropped during the final phase of his career. Notably, and like the first phase of his career, Tore felt that his performance still matched this level of challenge.

Using the 'surviving and thriving principles': how Tore managed his journey

As suggested by the timeline and accompanying description, Tore experienced and achieved much across a long career. Against this backdrop, we now move to consider the role that the 'challenge principles' introduced earlier played in Tore's efforts to survive and thrive in the game. As before, we take each of these principles one by one.

Creating and shaping internal challenge

As noted earlier in the chapter, the ability to create and shape personally-meaningful challenge is a cornerstone of development and progression in elite performers. This idea of stretching oneself was also clear in Tore's reflections on the initial part of his career:

> I wasn't that big a planner, not as organised as young players are now, or proactive in managing relationships. But I had a dream to turn professional and play at the top of Norwegian football and I was going to work really hard to reach it.

In this sense, Tore benefited from having broad goals that were exciting and difficult but not impossible to achieve. Notably, part of this challenge – and Tore's commitment to achieving it – was grounded in his awareness of what others had achieved; especially his older brother:

> When I started playing my older brother got into the national team and that was another thing that opened it up for me and made me realise it was possible. It made me think, yeah, this *is* possible – if he can do it! I was also aware of other players who had got into the national team and felt that if they could reach it, I could reach it.

As indicated by this reflection and others, Tore seemed to benefit from setting himself both general (i.e. national representation) and specific targets (e.g. "I'm a striker and counted the goals a little bit"). These targets were often lofty: "I put a lot of pressure in the early period of my career." It is important to recognise, however, these targets were still *relative* to Tore's perceived ability and what he felt were his most likely routes for success. For example, Tore was clear on the type of challenge that he would require on leaving Norway; as well as when he would feel most ready to take this on:

> My initial clubs took me up the ladder in Norway, which is what I was hoping for, and made me realise what I could maybe achieve. My progress came gradually though – I never played for any of the national age group teams until the Under 21s – and I was glad I took it step by step and was patient. I wasn't the type of guy who could go abroad at 16 years old. So I said 'no' to many big, foreign clubs during the early phases of my career – they were very tempting but it was very scary at that time. I was enjoying the ways things were going and even when I reached my 20s, I didn't feel quite ready to move abroad and it ended up being a clever decision for me.

Supporting the importance of creating shaping positive and exciting challenges, Tore felt that his 'surviving and thriving' in the early part of his third career phase was hampered by a different type of focus. Namely, Tore felt that his own and others' expectations when playing for Rangers led to him force and chase good performances; in short, trying to "make it happen" much more than "let it happen" (which was a different balance to the one he had enjoyed in Norway and at Chelsea):

> I always felt 'I need more', 'I need more', 'I need more' at Rangers. I tried to push myself too much. Instead I needed to feel free and light when I played, like I had for most of my time with Chelsea, with no worries.

Indeed, it was telling that when the Tore was able to focus on a more personally exciting and meaningful challenge, greater satisfaction and performance also returned:

> Sunderland was the toughest season on the pitch. It was difficult to play up-front for a struggling team that eventually got relegated and I needed to do something new and start afresh; that's why I went to Sienna. I had a dream to play in Italy when I was young; it was something I wanted to try and it was the perfect time to go to a club with no real expectations, happy with every point they could get, who could surprise everyone outside of the club that were certain that we would be relegated.

Similarly, finding and designing his own challenge was still apparent as Tore moved through the final phase of career:

> This final period after Sienna happened because I loved playing football. I didn't have to play for a big European team, I was just happy playing and there was still a challenge – the clubs were still trying to achieve something. And when I finished by missing a penalty for MK Dons in the playoffs [in what was meant to be Tore's last professional game in 2008], it was in me for a few years after – a terrible, terrible feeling to retire with. So it drove me to build myself up again and return. I thought: 'I can't finish my nice career with that, I need to do something else' to help me to get over the MK Dons experience.

Overall, Tore's experiences highlighted the role that personally-generated and shaped challenge can play throughout a career:

> You need a lot of motivation – you will hit a time where you won't be as motivated and you need to find a way to get back into it. To go out and train every day you have to have something to inspire you – a clip of Maradona could give me enough for a week.

To be clear, it wasn't simply the case that *any* challenge supported surviving and thriving, but more the 'right' type of challenge that was shaped and approached in the 'right' type of way.

Embracing and adapting to external challenge

As well as creating and shaping internal challenge, Tore's experiences also point to the benefits of embracing and adapting to external challenge; both on and off the pitch. In this sense, 'carving out' your career certainly seems to be valuable, but elite sport will always throw up speedbumps, traffic jams, and roadblocks! In this sense, Tore had to find ways to adapt and approach new and often unpredictable challenges across his career. For example, Tore didn't try to fight or become distracted by the increased level of attention that was being paid to him by foreign clubs or Norwegian media during the first phase of his career:

I felt the pressure build up from the media – especially when I moved to Brann and started playing for the national teams; the media interest flew up in the sky. It was a challenge to tackle as I didn't like to read anything from the media. I picked up anything that was negative, even a little thing in amongst lots of positive things. So, I tried to avoid the media as much as I could and when I was on the pitch playing, or around the football environment, I didn't feel the pressure or expectations that I was more aware of outside. I was just enjoying playing and how well it was going.

Indeed, the commitment to his game, including proactive work on his 'mentality', seemed to serve Tore well for adapting to changes in his environment throughout his career; including when Tore moved to Chelsea:

I was *very* nervous around all of these superstars who pushed each other and I knew I needed to play really well; but when the training started it was a bit of a relief. The nerves I had came out in positive energy and I just went out at played – I focused on the football and ended up surprising myself. I also didn't try to be anyone I wasn't and the superstars helped me to go under the radar a little.

Tore's tendency to "see the positive in things" also helped with a host of other challenges that he faced, including his return from a serious injury at Chelsea, learning to speak Italian, as well as his transfer from club to international play:

Sometimes it was lovely to get a new environment by playing for the national team. I loved coming back to Norway to meet Norwegian players and speak Norwegian, to have a different type of atmosphere and a different type of pressure. It was a bit more relaxed than normal club life – and you came back fresh for your club.

As well as these effects, the value of embracing and adapting to external challenge was also reinforced by Tore's lessons from his time with Rangers. More specifically, Tore highlighted the difficulties that can be faced when a major challenge isn't quite anticipated, engaged with, or adjusted to:

The transfer fee was a crazy amount of money that made everyone around me crazy. One day you were a cheap player and then the next you were a really, really expensive player and the expectations became so high it was impossible to meet them. The media pressure in particular was ten times more at Rangers than Chelsea – it was something much, much bigger than I had ever experienced before. Celtic [Ranger's biggest rivals] were doing well at the time so the media would be having a particular go at Rangers anyway. So I could score two goals but get pulled up on the chance I missed – and it was impossible not to notice. Even if you tried to avoid the media reports people would come and say 'don't take notice of what they're saying in the paper'!

I really tried but I always struggled to get to my top level at Rangers. I do think the price tag was a weight on my shoulder: it held me back as I never felt that people were satisfied, they always wanted more. I felt that everything I did was not good enough. The manager bought me for a lot of money and I felt that he needed me to do really, really well because of the money too. And so I never got that feeling of relief [after playing well]; that weight off my shoulders – even though it didn't go that bad! Overall, I should have handled the Rangers experience much better; I should have embraced the price tag rather than force myself to justify it.

In short, the level of challenge perceived by Tore only seemed to increase when he attempted to fight or vindicate the transfer fee. Significantly, Tore's lesson in this case (to embrace the situation) also matched the approach that he found effective in dealing with other external challenge; such as playing for different managers with different styles and different methods:

> You have to have an open mind and accept that things change: you can't think 'it needs to be like this, or if I can't play with him then it won't work'. You have to adapt and be professional no matter what happens; work around things when players that you connect with better move on. Of course, every player has a style they prefer or a way of playing that they like but that also didn't always match the manager and every club is so different. So you have to adjust and be the player that was needed for the team. It didn't always work but I tried.

Managing challenge: a reliable and consistent support network

Considering the final of our three key principles, it was also clear that Tore's ability to create and shape his own challenges, plus embrace and adapt to those imposed on him, was helped by a reliable and consistent support network. More specifically, good relationships were built with team-mates and members of the coaching/support staff at each club; however, the 'come and go' nature of top-level football makes it difficult to rely on those within a club for long-term support. Instead, or at least in addition, a network that operated beyond each club was particularly useful.

More specifically, Tore's network, which had evolved naturally, was made up of a 'support and sounding board team' within the game itself. For example, Tore forged strong bonds with two influential coaches, whom he stayed in contact with throughout his career. One of these was a coach who had worked with Tore's older brother and later became the assistant coach for the Norwegian national team:

> Harald Aabrekk was someone who I had trained one-on-one with and who I could talk to and discuss things with. He knew how football functioned and had played himself at the top level in Norway. He was *the* factor in my decision to go to Tromso and we always kept in touch, even when we weren't involved with the same team.

The other key coach was Egil Olsen, who managed the Norwegian national team for part of the time that Tore played for his country:

> Egil Olsen was a big believer in me and helped me to wait for the right club to move away from Norway to. I took on board everything he said to me and it gave me unbelievable inspiration; he could say something little and to me it meant a lot. He was very supportive, alongside Harald Aabrekk; and he really believed in me.

As well as personal 'support and sounding boards' within football, Tore also noted the huge influence of his 'support and switch off team' outside of football. In this respect, Tore valued the empathy and normality that his family could offer in particular:

I didn't have much pressure from my family early on in my career – they were very easy going and my mother was relaxed and made football not so important. My girlfriend, who is now my wife, was also very supportive and it was very important for me to have her with me at Chelsea; somebody to help me outside of football and to think about something else – sometimes it's really good to speak a language that nobody else understands too! The main person across my career for this type of support was my wife. You need people around you can to talk, calm you down, inspire you, but not push you.

In short, this type of support was invaluable in allowing Tore to get a mental break from the game and, by virtue, to be mentally fresher and ready for when it was time to turn back on to 'football mode'. In fact, this stability seemed essential in a professional environment which was quite the opposite.

Concluding thoughts

In this chapter we hope to have highlighted the nature and level of demands typically faced by performers in professional football. As described in our Introduction, many of these demands stem from: (a) the nature and level of expectations; (b) the nature and level of change in those with whom you work with (i.e. the "managerial merry-go-round"); and (c) the level of difference across goals, resources, and context in each different playing environment (i.e. club-to-club and club-to-country). To survive and thrive in this domain, we have therefore pointed to the value of players creating and shaping their challenges, embracing and adapting to external challenges, and managing challenges through a reliable and consistent support network. Of course, much more than this is needed, as previous books and research has indicated. However, we hope to have demonstrated that they are nonetheless significant for those presently or soon-to-be living in the world of elite team sport. In the context of this book, we also hope to have pulled a number of ideas together from prior chapters and offered a useful view on what it's like to live in this highly demanding, yet highly rewarding world.

Note

1 Please note that reference to terms such as "football" or "the game" throughout this chapter are made in relation to the men's professional game (reflecting Tore's experience in this specific environment).

References

Balk, Y. A., de Jonge, J., Oerlemans, W. G. M., & Geurts, S. A. E. (2017). Testing the Triple Match Principle among Dutch Elite Athletes: A Day-level Study on Sport Demands, Detachment and Recovery. *Psychology of Sport & Exercise*, **33**, 7–17

Collins, D., MacNamara, Á., & McCarthy, N. (2016). Super Champions, Champions, and Almosts: Important Differences and Commonalities on the Rocky Road. *Frontiers in Psychology*, 6, 2009. doi: 10.3389/fpsyg.2015.02009

Toering, T., & Jordet, G. (2015). Self-control in Professional Soccer Players. *Journal of Applied Sport Psychology*, **27**(3), 335–350. doi:10.1080/10413200.2015.1010047

34

Life AND sport

Making it happen AND progressing while you play

Sinéad Jennings with Áine MacNamara

Editors' introduction

Sinéad Jennings became a first-time Olympian at the age of 39 at the Rio 2016 Games. Sinéad and her lightweight doubles partner Claire Lambe went onto to make history at the Games becoming the first ever Irish female crew to make an Olympic final. A former junior international triathlete and international level cyclist, Sinéad is also a three-time World medallist having the full set of medals, gold, silver, and bronze. Sinéad is a qualified pharmacist and medical doctor. She is currently finishing her training in GP and has a special interest in women's health and sports medicine. Originally from Donegal in the North West of Ireland, she is now living in Limerick with her husband Sam and three young girls, Clodagh, Molly, and Hannah.

Introduction

As I crossed the finish line in Rio 2016, I reached my goal of becoming the Olympian that I had always dreamed about. In the years preceding Rio I had read many newspaper articles talking about Sinéad Jennings 'The Olympian' and it made me cringe a little; although I had been close to qualifying for the Games (in two sports), I had never got there. Competing at the Olympic Games in 2016, and then performing in the final to get a sixth place finish with Claire Lambe, felt really satisfying – the culmination of a career in sport. In reality though, the pathway to get there had been anything but smooth.

My early involvement in sport as a foundation for later

Growing up in Donegal in the northwest of Ireland my sisters and I played everything from basketball to volleyball and camogie but swimming was my main sport. My parents were keen for us to play all sports from a young age and encouraged us in everything we did. In their minds, sport stopped us doing other, perhaps less desirable, activities and they were happy that they always knew where we were! The encouragement I got from my parents was really important and transcended sport into every aspect of my life – indeed, school was a priority in our house.

Table 34.1 Key sporting achievements

Key sporting achievements
• Olympic Finalist, 2016, Lightweight Doubles with Claire Lambe
• World Silver Medal 2008 Lightweight Singles
• World Rowing Champion 2001 Lightweight Singles
• World Bronze Medal, 2000 Lightweight Singles
• 2017 IRONMAN Dublin 70.3 Third Place
• Former International Track Cyclist
• Former Junior International Triathlete

Sport was a family affair and my parents and sisters all played a huge role in both my introduction into, and subsequent involvement in sport (Côté, 1999; Kay, 2000). Dad was into cycling and when we were young I would have spent many afternoons out for spins trying to hang on to the back of his bike. I was encouraged to cycle competitively and I won an All-Ireland title when I was 13 or 14 years of age. Unfortunately, there wasn't a pathway in cycling for women at that time so I didn't really progress after that. However, lots of the guys who were involved in cycling competed in triathlons and they encouraged me to give that a go. My swimming and cycling background helped me make a relatively smooth transition and soon I was competing nationally and internationally. I went to the triathlon Europeans Championships as a junior and finished 15th.

'There or thereabouts'

Upon reflection, the early opportunities I had in sport were a great learning experience and gave me a solid grounding for what was to come later in my career. I learned the value and importance of hard work (though I don't think it ever really felt like hard work back then!) and sticking with something (Gould et al., 2010). Interestingly, I never felt pressure or expectation from others to succeed. Despite some success as a junior, I was never earmarked as the next 'superstar' but I was always 'there or thereabouts' in the talent pool (Collins et al., 2016). This status, or perhaps lack of status, allowed me develop in a positive and appropriate way without excessive pressure or expectation. In fact, I was usually terrible when I tried something new but I always persisted and worked hard until I was able to perform well. Looking back, I can see how this attitude was different from some of my peers. Lots of other girls, some of whom I would have thought of as way more talented than me, dropped out of sport or didn't commit to the training and sacrifices required to reach the next level (MacNamara et al., 2010). I think the key to fulfilling my potential was that I enjoyed the process as well as the outcomes of sport. I enjoyed training and pushing myself to be the best I could be. I found lots of satisfaction in making improvements and progress; in fact, that was what I really thrived on (Côté et al., 2009). My internal motivation – really wanting it - made a huge difference and drove me to the next level (Mallett & Hanrahan, 2004).

Identity formation

Although sport played a significant role in my life it wasn't the only thing that was important to me. This gave me a bit more freedom in terms of my investment in sport and the choices I made around engagement. Most importantly, my self-worth and identity wasn't fully tied up in being an athlete (Miller & Kerr, 2002) and because I didn't solely have an athletic identity (Brewer et al., 2000) I was able to balance my involvement and invest energy in other academic and social pursuits. Of course, I dreamt of becoming an Olympic champion, but this never felt overbearing. I think it also helped that my parents valued and emphasised other aspects of our lives – school work and university ambitions – and while they supported us in sport, it was never the be-all and end-all (Brewer & Petitpas, 2017). I always knew that their approval wasn't tied up in me being an athlete (Petitpas & France, 2010) and this gave me the freedom to explore different activities, as well as educational opportunities without pressure. I think that this lack of identity foreclosure was crucial to my sporting, educational, and family choices throughout my career.

The start of my rowing career

After I left school, I moved to England for university. A pharmacy degree in Sunderland took up a lot of my time and I really enjoyed my university days. Although I remained active during university, I didn't invest in elite sport, or compete consistently or competitively at a high level during my undergraduate years. Looking back, this might seem like a lost opportunity but, on reflection, this 'break' allowed me time to explore different aspects of my life rather than being tied up in being 'the athlete' (Petitpas & France, 2010). This relatively slow and delayed introduction into elite sport may also have played a role in the longevity of my career. Up until this point, I had accumulated a reasonably high training volume as a junior athlete in sports other than rowing. Ironically, delaying my entry into a rowing specific training and development programme may have been the best foundation for my later success in rowing (Gullich & Emrich, 2006).

At the end of university, I moved to Edinburgh to continue my pharmacy studies and that was a turning point in my sporting journey. I joined the rowing club and thought I would just do it socially but quickly realised that rowing isn't really like that! In a way I fell into rowing but I loved it from the start. There were great athletes and coaches in the club who took me under their wings. Although I was very much a novice, Hamish Burrell (my coach at the time) spotted something in me and invited me into his high-performance programme. I thrived under Hamish's coaching and made really quick progress physically, technically, and perhaps most importantly, in my belief that I could be good. I started rowing with some very modest ambitions – winning a Novice championships was probably the height of my goals – but under Hamish's regime soon had World Cup and Olympic finals in mind. By the end of the first year with him I got a bronze at the 2001 World Championships in the lightweight singles. The following year I was World Champion, again in the lightweight singles. It was a good start and I was hungry for more!

After winning the World Championships in 2001, my eyes were very much set on qualifying for the Olympics in 2004. I had been successful in the single but that was not an Olympic event. At the time, the women's rowing programme in Ireland was not very structured and even though we had some success there was always some factor that impeded our progress – funding, resources, availability, not making weight. There was also a lack of depth in the talent pool; I was quite a bit faster in the single scull than the other girls at the time and there was a big gap between me and the other rowers in the selection pool for the double lightweight boat. In the end, I struggled to find a suitable partner and didn't qualify for the 2004 Games – missing out by 1/100th of a second.

A cycling detour

Moving into the qualifying cycle for the 2008 Bejiing Olympics, two important changes happened in my life. I moved into the heavyweight singles (an Olympic category) as, I thought, that offered me the best opportunity of qualifying. I also decided to return to university to study medicine. It was always important for me to maintain a dual-career (Aquilina, 2013) and medicine was always something that I wanted to do. Unfortunately, I wasn't supported by the national association to compete at the Olympic qualifying regattas in the heavyweight single. However, I did win a silver medal at the 2008 World Championships in the lightweight singles. Although I was happy with that achievement, I was starting to question where my future in rowing was going to be. I was also aware that I needed to consider my medical career as well as my personal and family life. Sport was an important part of my life. However, I always knew that other things were important as well – my career, my family, my husband. Ultimately, I wanted to do sport to the highest level possible but I wanted to achieve in other aspects of my life in parallel. This fuelled my decision to study medicine and become a doctor.

While I was at the Rowing World Championships in 2008 I was approached to join the cycling programme that was attempting to qualify an Irish 3km team pursuit for the Olympics. That opportunity was really tempting; after all my dream was to compete at the Games and it didn't look like that was going to be attainable in rowing. At the time, I didn't think that qualifying for London in rowing was achievable, so I went to cycling because I really wanted to get that success. I was motivated by the idea of being able to get to the Olympics – it was a do it now or never type of decision! Although rowing and cycling have different technical demands, there was also a lot of crossover between the sports. I think that the psychological skills and characteristics that I was able to bring from rowing, as well as the experience, power, and endurance built up during my rowing career, made me an attractive cycling 'recruit' (MacNamara & Collins, 2015; Vaeyens et al., 2008).

Soon after transferring to cycling in 2011, I took some time out to have my first baby, Clodagh. Having a family was a very important decision for me and I wasn't willing to jeopardise that opportunity for sport (Palmer & Leberman, 2009). It seemed to be a logical stage in the cycle and I knew that I would be able to return in time to have an opportunity to qualify for the Olympics. I returned to the cycling team quickly after giving birth, motivated by the chance to qualify for London 2012. Interestingly, while the process of returning to elite sport brought added pressures to motherhood such as balancing the demands of training and competition and travelling to camps and events, I didn't consider it a difficult decision (Appleby & Fisher, 2009). In fact, motherhood allowed me to gain a new and multifaceted identity outside sport, while also including sport as an integral part of my identify (Palmer & Leberman, 2009).

In the run-up to London 2012, we had a strong team and we knew that a solid performance at the final World Cup in Kazakhstan would give us an Olympic ticket. Unfortunately, a puncture and a misunderstanding of the rules by the officials meant that we lost out on the chance to qualify for London. Unfortunately, I missed out (again!) on Olympic qualification by the smallest of margins and my Olympic dream was on hold (again!).

Family decisions

After the disappointment of missing out on the London Olympics, I took another break from sport and, effectively, retired from elite competition. Reflecting on this, I was fatigued from the ups and downs of the previous few years and needed time to focus on my career and family life. I used this time to complete my medical studies and began training as a General

Practitioner. My husband Sam and I also decided to have another baby and I gave birth to my second daughter Molly in 2012. Although I didn't have any concrete plans to return to rowing at this stage, I always remember Sam (himself an Irish Olympic rower) saying that we should have another baby now because if something happens in the next future (in rowing), I would still be able to go for Rio.

After Molly was born, I got back into training really quickly and was able to work that around my family life. I wasn't training for anything in particular but I got myself into decent shape running with double buggy and won a half marathon six months after giving birth in sub-79 minutes. At that stage, I wasn't necessarily planning a return to elite rowing but Rowing Ireland approached me about getting involved with the qualifying campaign for Rio 2016. Don McLachlan had been appointed as a new coach and there was a very good group of athletes involved. However, I was already pregnant with my third child at this stage so Olympic plans had to be put on ice!

Motherhood and elite sport

I was back training three days after Hannah was born. I was on six months' maternity leave and I decided that I would commit to a proper training programme during this time. I was really focused on the Olympics and motivated to come back with a bang! Interestingly, even though I now had three young children I found that I was able to commit more time and energy to training than I had in the last Olympic cycle. My parents, Sam, and my coaches were indispensable parts of this support network that allowed me to negotiate the logistical demands required to commit to training at this level (McGannon & Schinke, 2013). I think another key reason that allowed me to negotiate motherhood and sport was that I (and my support network) never viewed these as competing demands but we always saw them as complimentary (McGannon et al., 2015). Of course, one or the other had at times to take a backseat but I never felt that the demands of motherhood and sport were polarised; instead, I was able to resolve that tension and this helped me be successful (I hope!) at both (Appleby & Fisher, 2009).

There were a couple of factors underpinning my reasons to go back to rowing. I had tried to get to the Olympics for so long and there was so much heartbreak along the way. In the Rio cycle, there were talented athletes to train and compete with and with whom I could form a partnership. Don McLachlan, the coach, was also really committed to the programme. In the end, despite the juggle of family and work, I thought I would be a fool not to try and I would regret it for the rest of my life. Of course, I was hesitant – what if I make all these sacrifices in terms of career and family, and I still don't make it? One of my big mottos is 'give it a go and have no regrets'; I would have hated to have looked back on my career with regrets. It was this intrinsic motivation that drove my decision to return to rowing. Interestingly, I think that having an identity outside sport – as a mother and a doctor – also helped me return to elite sport and protected me against potential threats to my self-esteem; even if I wasn't successful in Rio, my self-worth wasn't completely bound in being a rower (Grove et al., 1997).

The path to Rio 2016

Claire Lambe and I really only formed a partnership one year out from Rio, which made qualification look like a long shot. I was injured for some of 2015, but returned in time for the World Championships. In France, at the World Championships, we earned our place at the Rio Games. It was such a great feeling after all the ups and downs that I had experienced in my career. It was a childhood dream of mine to compete at that level and I was so proud that I hadn't ever given up on that dream. All the focus had been on qualifying for the Games but following our qualifying performance, Claire and I quickly reassessed our goals and we went to Rio to fight for a medal. In the final we came close in finishing fourth. In some ways, the competitor in me wonders what we could have done to finish in the medals but I am so proud of what we achieved. I had made it the Olympics and we had performed on the biggest stage in the world.

Coming home from the Olympics, I knew that everything had been put on hold for Rio and now it was payback time. I had exams to do in medicine, the girls were in school and they needed a lot more of my time so priorities changed. I had given so much to my rowing career, and had been supported by my family and friends along the way, and now I knew it was time to flip my priorities around. I had always seen myself as a mother and an athlete so I didn't find this change of priority too difficult (Appleby & Fisher, 2009). I still try and train every day and that is important to me but now it is a case of fitting it around my job and family life. I feel happy enough with my decisions – I am still driven to get better and improve – but it just looks different now.

Finding a way to make it happen

I knew that I wanted to be the best in the world – even though, especially when I was younger, I might not have always said that out loud. Winning the World Championships so soon after getting serious in rowing really gave me the confidence to think that I could go all the way. I never lost confidence in my ability, despite all the setbacks, and I knew that if I really wanted to I could still make it happen. Although there were lots of ups and downs in my career, looking back now I can see how those setbacks helped me in the long run even though it didn't feel like it at the time (Collins et al., 2016). I used the disappointments to look inwards, assess what happened and seek out ways to improve – lifestyle changes or even technique changes – that ultimately made me better. The bumps and detours that I experienced throughout my career allowed me the opportunity to bulletproof the psychological skills, resilience, and mental toughness I needed to stay on the journey and ultimately achieve my goals.

A balancing act

Of course, sport was only part of my story. I was also a student, pharmacist, doctor, mother, and wife during my rowing career. I am proud of the way that I was able to balance everything and although priorities changed at different stages, I think that I always gave 100% to everything that I did. When I first started rowing Hamish, my coach at the time, said to me that "you can't be a world class rower, then switch off at work, and then switch on later but you need to world-class in everything that you do". I really took that advice on board and was conscious that I wanted to be the best I could be at everything I did. At the beginning I wanted to be a good pharmacist and be a world-class rower. Then when I chose to go back to university and do medicine I always kept that in the back of my mind and found a way to manage my dual-career (Burden et al., 2004). Of course, this meant that there were lots of plates to keep spinning – even more once the girls came along later in my career – but I think that each part of my life contributed to the other. Although many athletes talk about how their athletic success comes at the expense of other aspects of their lives (Cosh & Tully, 2014), I think that a combination of my personal motivation, support network, and a performance environment that valued commitment, hard work, and determination allowed me maintain this dual-career status.

As I said earlier, I think that I viewed each facet of my life as complimentary rather than competing (Appleby & Fisher, 2009). At various times, I made the decision to back off training when I had exams but then I would try and compensate for it after the exams. It was important to be clever in finding the individual balance that worked for me rather than following a blueprint that might not be the right fit. My sporting career has certainly been non-linear but the ability to negotiate the transitions within, as well as in and out, of this wave-like pathway has been a key feature of my success (Wylleman & Lavallee, 2004). I am proud that I was able to keep things progressing in all facets in my life. Indeed, this is a really important part of my transition out of elite sport – even if I am no longer an elite rower I am still a mother, wife, and doctor.

I made my own luck!

Looking back on my career, it might seem that there were a lot of lucky breaks that helped me reach my ultimate goal – meeting Hamish Burrell in Edinburgh in the early years and then partnering with Claire Lambe in the run up to Rio, for example. On reflection though, I think that I made the most of the opportunities I got by being ready and willing to jump in and work hard (MacNamara et al., 2010). Even from a young age, I always worked hard to make the most of my potential and this was encouraged by my family as well (Côté, 1999). When I retired from cycling in 2011, Sam encouraged me to keep training in case the opportunity to get back into the rowing programme came along. The training, commitment, and sacrifices (Gould et al., 2002) that I had made prepared me for these opportunities by being in the best shape possible. Above anything else, I felt that I was in control of most of my career decisions and outcomes. Of course, there were times when things happened that were outside of my control but I was still in control of my reaction to these events and what happened as a result of them. This internal locus of control gave me the belief that my world was controllable, manageable and meaningful.

Coaches, teammates, and family

I have been really lucky to have worked with some great coaches during my career. Hamish Burrell was my first rowing coach and his influence on me as an athlete and person cannot be overstated. Although I always had an inner belief in my ability, Hamish helped bring this out in me so that I could commit to world-class goals. Above all else, Hamish instilled the confidence and attitude in me to make the most of my potential. This wasn't limited to just sport but also impacted on my career decisions. Up until this point, I probably thought I wasn't clever enough to do medicine. But the confidence I gained from my early success in rowing – I had just won the world championships – and from the people around me at the time changed me as a person. I've always held on to the training and competition principles that Hamish taught me – the mentality that he gave me was so incredible and the belief he instilled in me helped me achieve my goals. I was also extremely lucky to have worked with the coaching guru Thor Neilson who empowered me to be self-sufficient and to make things happen myself. Finally, Don McLachlan was the coach who eventually got me across that line to Olympic competition.

Supportive coaches also really helped the transition back to rowing in 2014 and was a crucial part of our ultimate success. A key aspect of this was the recognition of individual differences amongst athletes. The coaches recognised and acknowledged my personal situation, what I could bring to the high-performance environment and together we were able to figure out a way to make it work (Wylleman & Reints, 2010). For example, Don McLachlan, the national coach, allowed me the flexibility to adapt the training programme to my logistical needs and training history. I was 39 years of age at the time so, reflecting this and my background in the sport, the quantity of training was adapted to meet my needs (MacNamara & Collins, 2015). Importantly, I was also allowed to stay at home in Limerick with my family to train rather than relocate to the national training centre in Cork. These concessions were really important to me – I wouldn't have been able to join the programme if it meant relocating my family. Dom, as coach, respected this and understood what I could contribute to the team. This flexible approach was a really positive and important factor in our success – we found a solution that helped us rather than working on a blueprint that was successful elsewhere.

Throughout my life, the people around me have inspired me to be the best I can be. Earlier I described the role my parents played in setting foundation and fostering the positive attitude needed in sport. My sisters were also really important motivational figures for me (Hopwood et al., 2015). In 2012 I travelled to London to watch my sister Caitriona compete for Ireland in the Olympic marathon. At that stage, I probably thought that my Olympic dreams were over and was trying to convince myself I was happy with that decision. I was really inspired watching Caitriona run and I left London knowing that there was a box left to be ticked in my career.

My husband Sam is also a huge influence on me. From a sporting perspective, he has competed at two Olympics which meant he understood the sporting, training, and competition pressures of striving to reach that level. More importantly was the support and backing he gave me as I came in and out of my rowing journey. I think anyone other than Sam would have thought I was crazy making some of the decisions that I did! In fact, when the opportunities arose Sam was the first to tell me to jump straight in – I would be the one saying the reasons why I couldn't, or shouldn't, and he would be the one giving all the reasons about why it could happen. I think that he always thought I was an even better athlete than I was; he had such confidence in me without which I don't think I would have succeeded like I did.

Having children was always something that was important for me and although I really wanted to have children I also didn't want it to be the end of my sporting ambitions. Without doubt it was harder to compete and train with a young family. When I was a student, given that I had a pretty hectic schedule, it was much easier to prioritise training and, to an extent, myself. I found that much more difficult with children and once Clodagh was born, they certainly became the priority; if I couldn't get to a training session, then I couldn't. My outlook certainly changed – I was still fully committed to training and competing at the elite level but my family became my priority. This meant that training was probably compromised a little bit but I was very organised and determined that no aspect of my life suffered too much. The ability to compartmentalise was crucial; when I was training, I was 100% committed to that; when I was with the girls, I was 100% focused on them. It was really beneficial that I was surrounded by family that understood this type of lifestyle and the commitment it involved.

I think the support I got and needed from my network changed over the years. When I was young, I was really motivated to please others and make them proud of me. In the middle years, this was still important though the financial support that I got from my parents was also crucial in helping me through university as well as in sport. Once Clodagh, Molly and Hannah were born, logistical support was the crucial factor (Holt & Dunn, 2004). I was really lucky that both my parents and Sam's parents helped us with childminding; who was going to look after the kids while I was training or away at competition was really important to me in ensuring that I was fulfilling my role as mother and athlete (Appleby & Fisher, 2009). That support was a massive help in creating the environment that allowed me 'keep all the balls in the air'.

Conclusion

The pathway to the top is rarely smooth and neat; mine certainly wasn't. However, the ups and downs that I experienced along the way made me the athlete and person I became. Indeed, the different worlds that I occupied during my career, whether as a rower, cyclist, doctor, or mother, helped me developed a broad suite of skills that I could use to cope with the challenges and opportunities that I encountered along the way. What would I like to be remembered as? Perhaps as someone who made the most of every opportunity that came my way.

References

Appleby, K. M. & Fisher, L. A. (2009). "Running In and Out of Pregnancy": Elite Distance Runners' Experiences of Returning to Competition After Pregnancy. *Women in Sport and Physical Activity Journal*, **18**(1), 3–17

Aquilina, D. (2013). A Study of the Relationship Between Elite Athletes' Educational Development and Sporting Performance. *The International Journal of the History of Sport*, **30**(4), 374–392

Brewer, B. W., & Petitpas, A. J. (2017). Athletic Identity Foreclosure. *Current Opinion in Psychology*, **16**, 118–122

Brewer, B. W., van Raalte, J. L., & Petitpas, A. J. (2000). Self-identity Issues in Sport Career Transitions. In D. Lavallee & P. Wylleman (Eds.), *Career Transitions in Sport: International Perspectives* (pp. 29–43). Morgantown, WV: Fitness Information Technology

Burden, S. A., Tremayne, P., & Marsh, H. W. (2004). Impact of an Elite Sport Lifestyle on Educational Choices and Career Outcomes. Self-Concept, Motivation and Identity, Where To From Here? *Proceedings of the Third International Biennial SELF Research Conference*

Collins, D., MacNamara, Á., & McCarthy, N. (2016). Super Champions, Champions and Almosts: Important Differences and Commonalities on the Rocky Road. *Frontiers in Movement Science and Sport Psychology*, **6**. 2009. ISSN 1664–1078

Cosh, S. & Tully, P. (2014). "All I Have to Do is Pass": A Discursive Analysis of Student Athletes' Talk About Prioritising Sport to the Detriment of Education to Overcome Stressors Encountered in Combining Elite Sport and Tertiary Education. *Psychology of Sport and Exercise*, **15**(2), 180–189

Côté, J. (1999). The Influence of the Family in the Development of Talent in Sport. *The Sport Psychologist*, **13**, 395–417

Côté, I., Lidor, R., Hackfort, D. (2009). To Sample or to Specialize? Seven Postulates About Youth Sport Activities that Lead to Continued Participation and Elite Performance *International Journal of Sport and Exercise Psychology*, **7**(1), 7–17

Gould D., Dieffenbach K., & Moffett, A. (2002). Psychological Characteristics and their Development in Olympic Champions. *Journal of Applied Sport Psychology*, **14**, 172–204

Grove, R., Lavallee, D., & Gordon, S. (1997). Coping with Retirement from Sport: The Influence of Athletic Identity. *Journal of Applied Sport Psychology*, **9**, 191–203

Gullich, A. & Emrich, E. (2006). Evaluation of the Support of Young Athletes in the Elite Sport System. *European Journal for Sport and Society*, **3**(2), 85–108

Holt, N., & Dunn, J. (2004). Toward a Grounded Theory of the Psychosocial Competencies and Environmental Conditions Associated with Soccer Success. *Journal of Applied Sport Psychology*, **16**, 199–219

Hopwood, M. J., Farrow, D., MacMahon, C., Baker, J. J. (2015). Sibling Dynamics and Sport Expertise. *Scandinavian Journal of Medicine and Science in Sports*, **25**(5), 724–733

Kay, T. (2000). Sporting Excellence: A Family Affair? *European Physical Education Review*, **6**, 151–169

McGannon, K. R. & Schinke, R. J. (2013). "My First Choice is to Work Out at Work; Then I Don't Feel Bad About my Kids": A Discursive Psychological Analysis of Motherhood and Physical Activity Participation. *Psychology of Sport and Exercise*, **14**,179–188

McGannon, K. R., Gonsalves, C. A., Schinke, R. J. & Busanich, R. (2015). Negotiating Motherhood and Athletic Identity: A Qualitative Analysis of Olympic Athlete Mother Representations in Media Narratives. *Psychology of Sport and Exercise*, **20**, 51–59

MacNamara, Á. & Collins, D. (2015). Second Chances: Investigating Athletes' Experiences of Talent Transfer. *PLoS ONE*, **10**(11). e0143592. ISSN 1932-6203

MacNamara, Á., Button, A. & Collins, D. (2010). The Role of Psychological Characteristics in Facilitating the Pathway to Elite Performance. Part 2: Examining Environmental and Stage Related Differences in Skills and Behaviours. *The Sport Psychologist*, **24**, 73–81

Mallett, C. J. & Hanrahan, S. J. (2004) Elite Athletes Why Does the "Fire" Burn So Brightly. *Psychology of Sport and Exercise*, **5**, 183–200

Miller, P. S., & Kerr, G. (2002). Conceptualizing Excellence: Past, Present and Future. *Journal of Applied Sport Psychology*, **14**, 140–153

Palmer, F. R. & Leberman, S. R. (2009). Elite Athletes as Mothers: Managing Multiple Identities. *Sport Management Review*, **12**, 241–254

Petitpas, A. J. & France, T. (2010). Identity Foreclosure in Sport. In S. J. Hanrahan & M. B. Andersen (Eds). *Routledge Handbook of Applied Sport Psychology* (pp. 282–290). New York, NY: Routledge

Vaeyens, R., Lenoir, M., Williams, A. M. & Philippaerts, R. (2008). Talent Identification and Development Programmes in Sport: Current Models and Future Directions. *Sports Medicine (New Zealand)*, **38**, 703–714

Wylleman, P. & Lavallee, D. (2004). A Developmental Perspective on Transitions Faced by Athletes. In M. Weiss (Ed.), *Developmental Sport Psychology* (pp. 503–524). Morgantown, WV: Fitness Information Technology

Wylleman, P. & Reints, A. (2010). A Lifespan Perspective on the Career of Talented and Elite Athletes: Perspectives on High-intensity Sports. *Scandinavian Journal of Medicine and Science in Sport*, **20**, 88–94

Part VII

Integration

Making it all work

So, there we have it! A view on modern elite sport performance systems: what makes them great, what makes them difficult, what makes them work, and what makes them fail. Of course, this view is a partial one. As emphasised in the first chapter, our aspiration for this book was not to try and cover every single element, or discipline, or factor in elite sporting performance; or *what* those who work and live in this environment do. Instead, our aim was to provide an insightful and informative view of this world through a breadth of perspectives, plus a range of presentational styles. In this sense, these perspectives have been much more focused on *how* and *why* elite systems – and all of those involved in them – develop, perform, and learn the way that they do in relation to *their* specific sport and context.

In this respect, we hope that a number of implications for working and performing in elite sport have become apparent, or emphasised, as the sections have progressed. Firstly, for long-term survival and success, it is clear that coaches, practitioners, leaders, and performers all need to have skills in adapting to their environments. Indeed, we feel that our contributors have done an excellent job in pointing to the complex and dynamic nature of their environments; as well as highlighting how these complexities and dynamics are rarely played out in exactly the same way in different settings (even within the same sport). In line with this, our contributors have also emphasised a message that there isn't *one way* or a *definitive set* of principles on how to do things in elite sport. Instead, it has been highlighted that such an approach is much more likely to result in the coach, practitioner, leader, and performer falling behind or, at the very best, standing still. Problematically, or in fact positively as we see it, elite sport provides little reward to those who stand still. In short, the need to understand, work to, and take advantage of your context is essential.

Secondly, the interpersonal side of elite sport systems is also critical to how this world operates. Indeed, any system in which passionate, committed, and driven people work closely with other passionate, committed, and driven people will throw up problems over power and politics; especially when these people have different levels of responsibility and influence. In this respect, many coaches, practitioners, leaders, and performers in elite sport are, one way or another, fascinated or obsessed by the world in which they operate and are driven to achieve personal success within that of the collective. Naturally, this can bring significant challenges for co-ordinated action; but it is also one of the primary reasons why teams, departments, and organisations in elite sport continue to push the boundaries and standards of performance: the rewards of finding, developing, and executing the 'next edge' – individually and collectively – are highly magnetic and addictive! In sum, therefore, the balance of personal and collective interests lies at the heart of optimal functioning, performance, and success.

As the third and final implication to draw out at this stage, and somewhat linked to the last point, optimal systems in elite performance sport cater for individuals but, first and foremost, are driven by a collective effort. So, although there needs to be 'foundation of balanced interests' – or, in other words, a shared goal – there also needs to be an established *way of working* that continually drives everyone to achieve this. In this respect, and based on the range of people, disciplines, and resources involved – including elements not considered in this book – an elite sports team, department, or organisation will only deliver on their full potential if they gather, interpret, and act on information as efficiently, consistently, and coherently as possible. More specifically, and resonating with the ideas on interdisciplinary work described in previous sections; this 'way of working' includes a shared understanding of the challenges in achieving the goal, a shared understanding of who is responsible for working on what part of the solution, a shared set of standards on interrogating this plan and solution, a shared set of processes for implementing this plan and solution, and a shared approach for evaluating the overall process and outcomes. Based on these implications and those listed above, the final section of this book now moves to consider some broader factors – and raise some broader questions – on 'making it all work'. In doing so, our last contributions look at the role and needs of future research, a perspective on practitioner development, and the development of high performing teams in a more general sense.

More specifically, Dave and Andrew open this final section with a chapter on the role of research in driving the performance system and how this might be enhanced in the future. As part of their discussion, Dave and Andrew consider some of the embedded challenges and possible solutions for such research, the interaction of researchers' goals and epistemologies, the benefits of 'pragmatism' as a guiding philosophy, and thoughts on some immediate next steps. Subsequently, in Chapter 36, Dave then returns to collaborate with Helen Alfano and Geir to present a perspective on the development and performance of elite sport practitioners. Overall, their position covers the need for environmental appreciation, role appreciation or clarity, interpersonal skills, the ability to function in a team, skills in PJDM, and expertise-based learning and development. Finally, to wrap things up, the last word goes to Stuart Lancaster, who, with the support of Veronica Burke, offers a view on the development of high performing teams. More specifically, Stuart identifies some essential components in building a long-term, high performing team based on a 'performance pyramid', plus the skills required by leaders to deliver this.

We hope you enjoy the final flurry!

35

Driving the performance system

DOES research help?

Dave Collins and Andrew Cruickshank

Introduction

This book has predominantly taken a 'hands off' approach to research, focusing rather on the challenges, interpersonal features, and ways of working across the breadth of elite performance roles, responsibilities, and contexts. Importantly however, the very nature of elite performance, the inherent and constant need to be cutting edge, makes the concept of research central to how things *should* work. We say should since, as several examples in this book have shown, researchers (especially academic ones) and practitioners often 'enjoy' a strained or strange relationship. Accordingly, in this chapter we explore how research can make itself more palatable and useful to elite performance. We firstly explore the inherent challenges of research in this hyper dynamic sphere, offering some methods which can help to counter them. We then consider what the researcher is trying to do, and how this viewpoint can help or hinder the application process. We then present pragmatism, a scientific approach with a rich history, as a potential 'best fit' method before concluding with some next step suggestions.

Research in elite performance – embedded challenges and possible solutions

As we said earlier, researchers and practitioners are often 'strange bedfellows'; apparently competing agendas (as one example, simplicity versus comprehensiveness), outcome aspirations, and career paths add to other more esoteric divides to lead to a silo mentality. When we move into the elite performance sphere, the additional levels of challenge and push to succeed merely exacerbate the problem. One element of the divide was described by one of our colleagues, a former scientist in a national institute, who reported the coaches' view of the scientists as "answering questions that didn't need to be asked"! In short, the relationship, even though increasingly accepted as an important feature of elites support systems, can be an unhappy marriage.

Of course, it is important to understand the challenges from both perspectives. For the practitioner in elite sport, there is the necessity to be always seeking the next edge; to seek out new methods which will confer the illusive competitive advantage. For the scientist, where reputations are built largely on peer reviewed publications, the need for speed and secrecy are a double challenge – "we need the answer quick, even as a rough approximation and, once we have it, you can't tell anyone!" Unfortunately, we would have to suggest that this position is sometimes less than productive. Secret Research and Development (R&D) projects are probably fine when there are commercial products and objective data involved. In simple terms, when clear advantage can be demonstrated against quantitative data which accurately operationalise the target variable. As an example, X runs an average of 2.5 seconds when using this supplement in double blind trials (cf. Andy Jones' work on nitrates reported in Chapter 9). When a more complex mix of variables are involved however, as is often the case in elite settings where coaching approaches involving interpersonal issues are being applied, then the lack of external checks provided by peer review can be very limiting. Indeed, Dave would advance the view that "maintaining competitive advantage" is often a good excuse used by administrators to increase the scienciness of interventions (cf. Collins & Bailey, 2012). The problem is that, whilst peer review is a far from perfect system (e.g. Smith, 2006) it is probably the least bad approach that we have. In the present context, it offers some crucial quality control to test ideas before they are applied. This is a perhaps neglected but crucial angle as, in elite sport, we are playing with people's livelihoods, life aspirations and, most crucially, identities and consequent mental wellbeing. Furthermore, as a common weakness in performance sport research, work rarely if ever considers the failures from the system (see Taylor & Collins, in press, for one exception). Without this, the assumptions of an approach may never be challenged and the idea perpetuates as 'obvious and face valid' because champion X or medal winning programme Y have used it, so. . .!

Of course, we readily acknowledge that, in the fast-moving world of elite sport, there probably isn't a chance to set up tightly controlled double-blind experiments. Furthermore, that is even if the clunky and personal-interest ridden peer review process would accept the paper, or even perhaps see the application. As such, we would suggest that innovation in elite sport should be less evidence-based and more evidence-grounded; in other words, the logic for applying an approach would draw on evidence from other work together with a theoretical justification for why the data can apply to this new context (once again, cf. Jones in Chapter 9). Our experience tells us that hard pressed coaches will often balk at this even slight delay, claiming (justifiably) that time in a quadrennial/season is of the essence. A fair point but, if we are to maintain our ethical stance as scientists and avoid some of the damage to individuals inferred in the previous paragraph, then some quality assurance process surely has to be applied to R&D potentials? Indeed, in our experience, such checks are often conducted by the developers themselves, doing this as part of their responsibility to provide a genuine product.

One other word about the secrecy issue. The idea of critique and experimentation is central to the approaches suggested by several relevant authors in this area, most notably Schön (1987), and as highlighted already by Dave in Chapter 1. As such, one should expect both scientists and practitioners in elite performance to employ this approach. So, looking forward to the next section, responsible researchers in elite environments might be encouraged to specifically explore, consider, and comment on the weaknesses and limitations of their work and its implications, as well as selling the strengths. We have seen several situations where scientists have presented ideas based on lab studies and encouraged coaches to "give them a try" in a field setting. It seems the height of irresponsibility to offer research to elite environments without fully considering and commenting on the drawbacks as well. The 'competitive advantage' card needs to be played carefully and appropriately!

Researcher goals and epistemology – important considerations

So, given that the urgent needs of elite performance for rapid *and* effective innovations are to be met, it is worth considering the approaches which may be most useful for researchers to take. The first is what outcome deliverables the researcher is chasing.

Other authors (e.g. Collins & Collins, 2018) have already written on the influence which promotion systems in academe may have on the focus and practical orientation of university or institute-based researchers. National assessment systems such as, in the UK, the Research Excellence Framework or REF, have driven a focus on publishing papers which score highly against external criteria. We would suggest that applicability to elite performance environments might not be one of these, even though real-world impact is. Coincidentally, this is also clearly an issue against the confidentiality challenges highlighted in the previous section. The main point here is, whether from a social constructivist "this is what my community rate", or a personal "this will get me promoted" stance, that applied research may not be as valued and hence, become a rarity.

Science through, of, and for sport

In any case, and wherever the motivations have come from, other work has already highlighted the different foci or purposes that research in sport can take. Described by Collins and Kamin (2012), there appear to be three stages of progression, or perhaps more accurately levels, which researchers can take. At a fundamental level, researchers may just exploit or employ sport as a potential laboratory or topic for study. Termed science *through* sport, the focus here is the scientific results; outcomes which could perhaps be obtained by investigation with other participant groups but which, often for pragmatic (with a 'small p' – so different to the next section) reasons, has used athletes. The second stage identified by Collins and Kamin saw researchers developing a bespoke new science focused on the sporting environment itself. Termed science *of* sport, this may generate a completely new sub-discipline (e.g. sport psychology) or, perhaps more traditionally, describe the subset of the parent discipline itself; for example, exercise physiology. In the last category, science is used for a sport-focused purpose; in the present context, elite performance. Science *for* sport places the application as the primary focus and would appear to be the logical goal for those working in elite performance environments.

As highlighted by Collins and Kamin (2012), researchers can be effective in all three domains, although they suggest that this might be less common than many believe. More pertinently, however, they suggest that researchers need to be very clear on their goals within any project. Without this clarity, risky assumptions may be made by both author and consumer, with consequent errors of expectancy leading to less than optimum application. As an example, consider the issues highlighted by Collins, Carson and Toner (2016) who challenged the universality of advice on attentional focus offered by some researchers. Collins et al. observed that several such studies seemed to infer uncritical extrapolation from simpler but experimentally tight laboratory studies to wider applied environments. In this particular letter, they suggested that high-level gymnast participants performing a standing single rotation might lack direct inferences for those same performers doing something closer to their limit; and, of course, the tasks they were training for. The fact that the author's response presented their external focus as a *"conditio sine qua non"* (Wulf, 2016) suggested that the distinction may not have been acknowledged! This is one of many examples where researchers quite legitimately pursuing one goal from the through/of/for set may need to be, at least, cautious in how their results are used elsewhere.

Researcher epistemology

Running as a close parallel to the goals they set for their work, the researcher's epistemology may also play a role in how well data from their work may impact elite performance. We will consider just one distinction which is, we suggest, increasingly common in sport. This is the distinction between quantitative and qualitative investigation, and how findings from these approaches may be generalised and transferred to others. Most specifically, we would highlight issues of this as 'within' then 'between study' issues where, although one study or series of studies may be epistemologically consistent, these results are then extrapolated in potentially questionable ways to application-focused papers.

In this regard, Stelter, Sparkes, and Hunger (2003) highlight that "qualitative research can mean different things to different people". This breadth, at once a strength and a weakness, does make things hard to pin down. However, if we may, one guiding principle does seem to be that investigation is focused on a personal perspective. As such, and as highlighted by Collins, MacNamara and Cruickshank (2018), research which employs elite athlete autobiographies as a source of knowledge are excellent for portraying *that person's* perspective. Subsequent extrapolation to generate guidelines for work with other elites must, at the very least however, be treated with caution. Again as highlighted by Collins et al., this is a common problem for elite performance research as, by definition, participants are in short supply! This practicality notwithstanding, researchers need to be very clear on the epistemological stance they are taking, once again acknowledging strengths and weaknesses of what they have done in generating what they have found.

It might be useful to present a positive applied exemplar. The work of Hanin on the Individual Zone of Optimal Functioning has adopted a mixed-methods approach (descriptive and quantitative likert data) to examine the personal perspectives of an athlete's perceived ideal pre-performance state (e.g. Robazza et al., 2004). Clearly, the focus here can be seen as science *for* sport, but the use of the epistemology is consistent with both purpose and application of the knowledge gleaned.

Putting these two sub-sections together, we want to emphasise how important it is to see an implicit but also overtly expressed coherence between goals, epistemology, method, and outcome. This coherence, together with careful process, will help to ensure that research for the promotion of elite performance is optimally effective.

One particular approach – pragmatism

So, given that each individual's personal goals and epistemology play a significant part in determining the utility of research for elites, is there one method which might have more to offer? Or, at least, that might be emerging as a front runner in the 'potential contribution stakes'? In this next section, we consider pragmatism; an approach which is receiving an increasing amount of use and attention from those really committed to research *for* sport.

Pragmatic research: what is it?

As outlined above, and just like leaders, coaches, sport scientists, and other specialists can approach their practice from different philosophies, the same is true for those who research it. More specifically, these philosophies are made up of a researcher's beliefs on what the world of elite sport is like (e.g. whether the factors at play are more concrete and consistent across different environments, or more fluid and relative to each). These philosophies are also made up of beliefs on what type of knowledge is to be generated via research (e.g. precise, 'black and white' facts, or more general, 'shades of grey' principles). Finally, these philosophies are made up of a researcher's beliefs on how this knowledge is best acquired (e.g. by observing, measuring, and analysing things as objectively, or in the most 'error-free' way as possible; or by interpreting events and constructs with much a much more subjective and contextual lens).

When it comes to elite sport, just like most other performance environments, research is based on a range of philosophies. Very broadly speaking, disciplines with a history in the 'harder' sciences (e.g. physiology) have tended to take a more objective and experimental approach, while those with a history of being in the 'softer' sciences (e.g. psychology) have been more likely to adopt a more subjective and experiential approach. Overall, however, one factor which seems to tie much prior research together is the ultimate goal that is being worked towards. Specifically, much research in elite sport has explored different factors for the primary purpose of *understanding them*; in other words, to *KNOW* more things or to *KNOW* things better (cf. 'the science *of* sport' approach mentioned earlier). In contrast, and unfortunately for those working within elite sport, much less research has explored different factors for the primary purpose of *enhancing them*; in other words, to *DO* more things or to *DO* things better (cf. 'the science *for* sport' approach mentioned earlier). Thankfully, as far as we see it, this is where pragmatism comes in! Indeed, and as one example in the numerous disciplines which support elite performance, this lens can solve many of the issues that have plagued coaching practice ("it's not evidence-based enough") and coaching research ("it's not applied enough") to date.

Of course, there is much detail behind the pragmatic philosophy and we encourage those interested to consider a range of works on the topic in sport and elsewhere (e.g. Bryant, 2009; Collins et al., 2018; Corbin & Strauss, 2008; Giacobbi et al., 2005; Maxcy, 2003; Morgan, 2007), plus recent studies which have attempted to harness the principles, as we have sought to do so ourselves (e.g. Cruickshank & Collins, 2015; Savage et al., 2016; Davies et al., 2017). To emphasise some of the most important components here, however, the primary concern for the pragmatic researcher – or 'pracademic' – is in conducting research that will answer important *practical* questions for *specific people* in the *here and now*; not questions to understand something for the sake of understanding alone, or for the sole benefit of the researcher and their academic careers! In this manner, the pragmatic philosophy encourages researchers to deal with the world that we all face day-to-day; whether that world is actually 'real' in the strictest sense, or 'real in the same way for everyone'.

Continuing this theme, pragmatism is built on the idea that research should make a real difference to the people, groups, environments, and systems that it studies. In fact, for pragmatists, this is *the* reason why research is undertaken. Truly valuable research therefore starts with questions that are, first and foremost, *practically meaningful* for *specific* contexts. So, instead of asking questions like "what qualities do effective leaders in elite sport have?", a pragmatist would be more inclined to ask questions like "what qualities do effective leaders in elite sport have *when it comes to rebuilding a team for a new Olympic cycle in the current UK climate?*" All in all, pragmatic research is driven by a desire to *do* something to help people or groups with a *specific, real world* challenge, issue, or goal.

How does pragmatic research work?

In terms of how it drives an actual project, the pragmatic philosophy places a number of requirements on researchers. As described above, pragmatism starts by shaping the actual *purpose* of any research (i.e. to develop a specific solution, or progress our knowledge of a genuine performance challenge, issue, or goal to help those who engage with it). Second, it encourages researchers to focus their questions around specific processes and contexts rather than overly generalised factors and situations (i.e. how things actually *work* or are *played out* in a *particular* elite sport domain). Third, it encourages researchers to explore constructs or concepts with diverse people, groups, or events to tease out commonalities and contrasts; thus acting as an internal 'check and challenge' to provide the most accurate, practical findings.

Fourth, pragmatism encourages researchers to select methods for collecting and analysing their data that are relevant to their specific question, rather than the other way around (so no method is 'inherently' better than another; it depends on the nature and stage of the research). In this way, taking a quantitative *and* qualitative angle in the same study (i.e. 'mixed methods' or 'multi-methods' research) is promoted when this helps to generate meaningful and useful findings (e.g. a study that wants to explore the physiological, psychological, and social impact of a new pre-season training programme). Certainly, and as noted earlier, the multifaceted nature of many constructs in elite sport (e.g. periodisation) means that a combination of rich qualitative data and robust quantitative data often offers the best grounds for identifying useful solutions.

As a fifth requirement, pragmatism also encourages researchers to take advantage of what they already know about the challenge, issue, or goal that they are investigating. In this way, researchers can bring their own applied experience and expertise to the table when they are collecting and interpreting data; so, rather than trying to remove or hide them, experience and expertise on 'how things work' are recognised as paths for generating new insights and finding innovative answers. Moreover, the applied experience or expertise of the researcher can significantly lift their credibility with, and ability to relate to participants; and often lead to the collection of higher quality data than researchers who come to projects 'cold'.

Sixth, the pragmatic philosophy further requires researchers to recognise that the 'end point' of their work is not the write-up of their findings, or even publication in an academic journal. Instead, pragmatists need to consequently share and 'test' their findings with those working in the applied world to gauge the extent to which this knowledge: (a) 'makes sense'; and (b) can be used to drive new, better, and shared action. In other words, and emphasising an earlier message, do the findings help *us* to *do* more things or *do* things better?

Seventh, and finally, pracademics also carry a responsibility for regularly evaluating and updating the findings from their research. In this sense, pragmatism works against the principle that the world is always evolving – which elite sport tends to do a high speed – and so the findings from pragmatic work are therefore always provisional and fallible. As such, these findings need to be regularly evaluated and updated to ensure they remain as relevant as possible for those who will benefit from them *today*.

One other thing to emphasise at this stage is that the pragmatic philosophy is not only relevant to 'scientists' in the traditional sense; it is also highly relevant to those working in elite sport (including leaders, managers, and coaches), especially given growing exposure of the 'scientist-practitioner' model in professional training and education. Take, for example, an incoming leader who is looking to improve the ways in which sport science services are integrated after limited buy-in from coaches and athletes to date. Following pragmatic principles, the leader is focused on understanding a *process* (i.e., gaining buy-in) that will improve the system's performance in the future. To tease out the sticking points and why these have arisen, the leader also follows the principle of exploring different perceptions. More specifically, the leader considers opinions across the sport science and medicine team, coaches, performers, and 'outside observers'; some of whom have been in the system for a number of years, others who have more recently joined. As well as different perceptions, the leader also evaluates trends in relevant data to see if any other factors might be influencing things (e.g. the age and stage of the performer group; the goals that have been identified in their performance plans). Additionally, collecting and analysing this 'data' is progressive, so that emerging answers are checked and challenged against further data, with the leader also comparing these against their previous experiences. Subsequently, a solution is generated and shared for feedback from relevant groups, with the evaluation of this solution based, first and foremost, on the difference that it then makes to gaining future buy-in. This solution is then continually monitored and updated by the leader so that is remains relevant as the system evolves (e.g. as coaching and sport science staff come and go).

Can you believe it? Evaluating pragmatic research

When it comes to evaluating the quality of pragmatic research, it is clear that a lot depends on the aims and nature of the study. Indeed, rather than being able to apply the same set of criteria to every piece of research, the findings from different pragmatic studies need to be considered in context. For example, evaluating a study that explores hormonal responses to a new training programme clearly requires a different set of criteria compared to a study which explores how channels of communication can be improved across middle managers in elite sport organisations. In this sense, the quality of the *research process* (e.g. the methods that were used) and the *internal coherence* of the study (e.g. how well the methods matched up with the purpose) are informed by established standards and norms in scientific research. Of course, understanding these standards and norms can be a challenge for those less familiar with academic enquiry; in fact, it's often a challenge for those who are familiar! However, one marker that anyone working in elite sport can consider when it comes to pragmatic study is *external impact*; in other words, the *quality of the consequences*.

Indeed, central to the pragmatic philosophy is the call for 'consumers' of research to apply the "so what?" principle; i.e. what difference do these findings actually make to real world practice? Firstly, for the *specific* type of person, group, environment, or system on which the research focused. Secondly, for the *general* type of person, group, environment or system on which the research focused. If this difference is difficult to work out, difficult to see the value of, or difficult to agree with, then these should signal doubts over the quality of the work. In this sense, a piece of research might be expertly planned and executed against all relevant academic standards (in terms of how the data was collected and analysed), but if it doesn't offer any sufficiently meaningful results and implications on a *practical* level, then the quality of this work, from a pragmatic perspective, is poor. That said, a piece of research that does generate meaningful results and implications is not automatically 'good' when the research process and internal coherence is poor (i.e. the meaningful results might be an error borne from poor procedures). Therefore, the extent to which you can 'believe' a pragmatic study depends on both the quality of the research process *and* the quality of the implications. So, as with most things, confidence in a piece of pragmatic research runs on a continuum: a consumer can take greatest confidence from research that has a quality process and a quality set of implications; some confidence from research that has a poorer process but a quality set of implications; or little confidence from research that has a poor process and a poor set of implications. As a starting point for engaging with any piece of pragmatic research, however, the findings should, first and foremost, mean something to peoples' practical lives.

Next steps – the future for research in elite performance

We hope that the need for research in elite performance is clear, and also, the need for quality and personal commitment to pursuing the performance outcomes as coherently and effectively as possible. Indeed, we would suggest that there is a genuine need for those working in elite performance to carefully review their approaches and make sure that they are on the right track. In that respect, we hope that the ideas presented in this chapter offer food for thought, or maybe even a checklist, for research in the area.

There are also some wider questions, pertaining particularly to the Professional Judgement and Decision-Making (PJDM – see Chapter 1) around study design on elite performance questions. Consider as one example the relative status of pragmatism as an approach which is almost 'purpose built' for this topic. Despite being long established as a philosophy to guide scientific research (Bryant, 2009; Morgan, 2007; Giacobbi et al., 2005; Corbin & Strauss, 2008), the pragmatic approach has been largely overlooked or underplayed in elite sport to date. We would strongly support a more frequent usage, whilst also extant literature might use some of the critical points to re-examine the claims made.

In closing, readers might like to consider some of the points made in this chapter and how they might apply to the breadth of disciplines presented. There is clearly no 'one size fits all' solution, so PJDM would also appear to have a role to play in this element of elite performance support as well.

References

Bryant, A. (2009). Grounded Theory and Pragmatism: The Curious Case of Anselm Strauss. Forum: *Qualitative Social Research*, **10**(3): Art. 2

Collins, D. & Bailey, R. (2012). "Scienciness" and the Allure of Second-hand Strategy in Talent Development. *International Journal of Sport Policy and Politics*, **5**(2), 183–191. doi: 10.1080/19406940.2012.656682

Collins, D., Carson, H. J., & Toner, J. (2016). Letter to the Editor Concerning the Article "Performance of Gymnastics Skill Benefits from an External Focus of Attention" by Abdollahipour, Wulf, Psotta, & Nieto (2015). *Journal of Sports Sciences*, **34**(13), 1288–1292. doi: 10.1080/02640414.2015.1098782

Collins, L. & Collins, D. (2018) The Pracademic in Adventure Sport Professional Development and Education. *Journal of Adventure Education and Outdoor Learning*, **19**, 1–11. doi:10.1080/14729679.2018.1483253

Collins, D. & Kamin, S. (2012). The Performance Coach. In S. Murphy (Ed.), *Handbook of Sport and Performance Psychology*. (pp. 692–706). Oxford: Oxford University Press

Collins, D., MacNamara, Á. & Cruickshank, A. (2018). Research and Practice in Talent Identification and Development – Some Thoughts on the State of Play *Journal of Applied Sport Psychology* doi: 10.1080/10413200.2018.1475430

Corbin, J., & Strauss, A. (2008). *Basics of Qualitative Research: Techniques and Procedures for Developing Ground Theory* (3rd ed.). London: Sage

Cruickshank, A. & Collins, D. (2015). Illuminating and Applying "The Dark Side": Insights from Elite Team Leaders. *Journal of Applied Sport Psychology*, **27**(3), 249–267. doi: 10.1080/10413200.2014.982771

Davies, T., Collins, D., & Cruickshank, A. (2017). This Really IS What We Do With the Rest of the Day! Checking and Clarifying What High-level Golfers Do During the Meso-levels of Performance. *The Sport Psychologist*, **31**(4), 382–395

Giacobbi, P. R., Jr., Poczwardowski, A., & Hager, P. (2005). A Pragmatic Research Philosophy for Applied Sport Psychology. *The Sport Psychologist*, **19**, 18–3

Maxcy, S. J. (2003). Pragmatic Threads in Mixed Methods Research in the Social Sciences: The Search for Multiple Modes of Inquiry and the End of the Philosophy of Formalism. In A. Tashakkori & C. Teddlie (Eds.), *Handbook of Mixed Methods in Social and Behavioral Research*. Thousand Oaks, CA: Sage

Morgan, D. L. (2007). Paradigms Lost and Pragmatism Regained: Methodological Implications of Combining Qualitative and Quantitative Methods. *Journal of Mixed Methods Research*, **1**, 48–76

Robazza, C., Pellizzari, M. & Hanin, Y. (2004). Emotion Self-regulation and Athletic Performance: An Application of the IZOF Model. *Psychology of Sport and Exercise*, **5**, 379–404. doi: 10.1016/S1469-0292(03)00034-7

Savage, J., Collins, D., & Cruickshank, A. (2016). Exploring Traumas in the Development of Talent: What Are They, What Do They Do, and What Do They Require? *Journal of Applied Sport Psychology*, **29**(1), 101–117. doi: 10.1080/10413200.2016.1194910

Schön, D. (1987). *Educating the Reflective Practitioner*. San Francisco, CA: Jossey-Bass

Smith, R. (2006). Peer Review: A Flawed Process at the Heart of Science and Journals. *Journal of the Royal Society of Medicine*, **99**(4), 178–182

Stelter, R., Sparkes, A. & Hunger, I. (2003). Qualitative Research in Sport Sciences—An Introduction. *Qualitative Social Research*, **4**(1), Art. 2, http://nbn-resolving.de/urn:nbn:de:0114-fqs030124

Taylor, J. & Collins, D. (in press). Should have, Could have, Didn't – Why don't high potential players make it. *The Sport Psychologist*

Wulf, G. (2016). An External Focus of Attention is a *Conditio Sine Qua Non* for Athletes: A Response to Carson, Collins, and Toner (2015). *Journal of Sports Sciences*, **34**(13), 1293–1295. doi.org/10.1080/02640414.2015.1136746

36

Working in the jungle

How should elite sport practitioners operate and be developed?

Helen Alfano, Dave Collins, and Geir Jordet

Introduction

Many strive to work in elite sport with high performing athletes but delivery in these environments presents a maze of complexity. With time tight, repeat performances essential, and environments highly pressured, selection of the most appropriate delivery models is essential for the sport practitioner. Sport clients, both organisations and individuals, will demand relevant and 'useful' input. If the model selected or the focus of delivery is deemed unnecessary or uncomfortable, the likelihood for 'buy in' (the desire to accept input and work with a delivery provider), impact, and even continued use of the provision or practitioner may be limited. This concept was supported by Martindale and Nash (2013) who investigated the perceptions of coaches to support provision.

Even when the approach and content are optimum, there are other practitioner-related issues that will affect the receipt, and therefore the impact, of the intervention. It seems fair to assume that the *quality* of service delivery is also key and that, if sufficiently high, this will directly impact on the level of success achieved. From our own experience, ongoing investigations, and the current literature (both academic and anecdotal), it would seem that technical expertise in a defined area that is essential for successful delivery *but* it is not perceived as the limiting factor by those who work in elite performance sport (Anderson et al., 2002; Ballie et al., 2015; Ingham, 2016; Kyndt & Rowell, 2012). Rather, it is the *application* and *presentation* of that expertise that appears critical. It is therefore important to understand what good application looks like.

This application/presentation of knowledge and delivery of good practice is linked to an ability to understand context, flex and align to that context and, ultimately, to meet the client's requirements, both as an individual and in a team. There is, therefore, a need to appreciate and apply relevant contextual support within the environment, the role, the people, and the team you are exposed to within each elite sport. Importantly, this 'how to do it' set of skills represent an important addition to the already 'what to do and why' which will come from the specialist's knowledge of his/her subject, together with an appreciation of the context which makes sure that the content is going to make a contribution. So, focusing on the 'how' knowledge is applied gives us the basis of four headline 'must haves' for delivering in elite performance environments: environmental appreciation, role appreciation, interpersonal skills, and team functioning.

Environmental appreciation

The ability to assess, adapt, and align to the environment of a sport is a critical area for high performance delivery. Where delivery or support is unsuccessful you will often hear statements such as "they weren't on board", "were not on the bus" or "just didn't fit" used by the primary consumer of support, as exemplified by a quote from a current Performance Director (PD): "They need to understand their subjects, but also the world they operate in and how that subject can be best used in that world". The suggestion is that an ability to embed and immerse oneself in the environment is often challenging, especially in the crucial early days' experience when impressions can be make or break.

It is important to note that this isn't necessarily a trait characteristic; you either have it or you don't! Many support providers have had a good 'fit' in one sport only to move to another and struggle for the same 'fit', limiting their impact and influence. Our research and experience would suggest that this alignment to the sport only seems possible if an accurate assessment of the environment has been made *and* the ability to adapt existed, *raising the question as to how this is best developed*. Reflecting our PD quote above, the sports practitioner also requires the ability to make an informed decision on *how* to deliver with this information. This idea offers support to the previously identified concept of Professional Judgement and Decision-Making (PJDM) and its link to performance delivery (Martindale & Collins, 2005 & 2013). We expand on this later in the chapter.

Returning to environment, the skills to make an accurate assessment are critical, and supported by a knowledge and appreciation of aspects such as the sports network, organisational hierarchy, performance determinants, vision, culture, and expected behaviours. The environment one might find in a weight-making combat sport could be very different to that of a classic endurance event for example. Aspects such as the demands of the sport, the type and profile of athlete, the background and role of the coaches, and the competition structure will differ greatly. The model of the sport you need to *fit* to, the dynamics and the place or person you need to influence may also differ. One may require an athlete-centred delivery model, whilst the other a coach-focussed approach. Identification of the appropriate model of delivery with an appreciation, indeed preferably a deep understanding, of the environment can be viewed as a first rung on the ladder towards good practice. Of course, mechanisms which support the development of environmental appreciation include familiarisation, which can be sought through deliberate immersion, exposure, and time on task. However, these are certainly things which would sensibly be developed as part of professional training.

With that said, practitioners may benefit greatly from already having a deep understanding of a particular sport, acquired through their own athletic career, coaching experience, and/or years of specialisation working in this sport. Highly context-specific knowledge may on some occasions give a fuller and more functional understanding of a specific practical challenge that is attempted solved, potentially helping the practitioner add even more value in the process.

Role appreciation or clarity

Do I really know why I'm here? Do I really know what I contribute to? Do I really know what the full intent and objective of the team is and where I fit in that jigsaw? These are all relevant and meaningful questions for the practitioner in an elite sport setting. Indeed, successful delivery may be defined by the appropriate use and impact of your technical expertise or role, therefore seeking clarity, understanding and delivering to that defined role and expectation is critical. We would ask how delivery can ever be effective if you are unsure what is expected of you and how? Those who are able to define their role, have clarity of role across situations and within the team, knowledge of what to deliver and an ability to be held accountable to that, seem more likely to deliver effectively. The most successful support providers will look to seek clarity from the sport or role consumer, with the most optimal outcomes and decisions on a delivery model often coming when the questions are asked "what would you like from me? And how?" In similar fashion, if the consumer isn't sure about what they want and/or vague in how they communicate this, they are quite literally limiting the service they are paying for!

Accordingly, an understanding of Role Clarity (RC) as a construct, often linked to role performance, may support delivery, with a lack of clarity previously identified as a major barrier to successful application of sport science (Martindale & Nash, 2013). Role clarity can be described as an objective presence of adequate, role-relevant information, where the individual subjectively feels that there is enough relevant information to perform. The links for this construct with positive individual performance, feelings of efficacy, and delivery to requirements are well noted (e.g. Bray et al., 2005; Eys et al., 2003). This clarity is also positively correlated to the functioning effectiveness of a team performance, extending the importance of this construct (Eys & Carron, 2001).

Of course, role appreciation does needs to be underpinned with technical expertise, an understanding of boundaries, and selection of the appropriate delivery model. There must be an ability to deliver within boundaries of competency and expertise. Obvious examples here include working within the confines of medical confidentiality for those to whom this applies. The negative consequences of stepping outside boundaries commonly pose a challenge to successful delivery. For example, a Strength & Conditioning (S&C) coach offering supplementation or nutritional advice has the possibility to limit both the 'buy in' and impact for S&C delivery as a whole, the coach themselves, and the nutritionist, especially if the advice does not work, is ill-informed, or poorly timed due to lack of understanding or knowledge of the area. Never mind the impact on the coach's working relationship with the nutritionist.

Such disciplinary concerns notwithstanding, the ability to deliver with an element of flexibility within a role is essential. For example, there may be a requirement to adapt to an athlete's response to an intervention, or to coach demand. The boundary-conscious practitioner might see it as his/her role to upskill or educate the coach but their readiness and requirements for input might not match his/her intentions. An intention to support outside of your role where required is also favourable. For example, when Helen worked in Paralympic sport there was an ongoing requirement for assistance with lifting bags when travelling to support the athlete or fellow team member, very much outside of her sport science role and delivery. It may also be the case that in smaller support teams a practitioner plays multiple role at times, an S&C coach who might report on daily wellbeing or a physio on 'game' day responsible for ensuring recovery drinks are provided and recovery complete. The intention to support in this way can be positive on the perceptions of others and support the feeling that there is a 'fit'.

In some sports, systems, or countries with less resources, the principle of multiple roles can be taken even further. Sometimes, it could be extremely beneficial if members of staff have combination skills and multiple areas of responsibility. Examples of such could be the sport psychologist running smaller exercises on the field during a training session, the physical therapist actively helping athletes regulating stress prior to competition, and a head coach doing the post-match video analysis him/herself. A key to such setup is that the person in question must indeed possess dual competencies, that there are clearly delineated roles, and that everyone involved communicate exceptionally well. While there are apparent risks with such a model, related to lack of time and/or not focused enough service delivery, benefits might be harvested from a tight and functional performance staff unit where everyone (compared to a setting with more specialised members of staff) sits even closer to the athletes and ultimate performance product.

Another desirable characteristic for the elite sport practitioner is that of an ability to be accountable for ones' actions and delivery. This is underpinned by an ability to be vulnerable, open to feedback and the capacity, willingness, and skills to reflect on personal delivery. However, this is only really possible when the role and outcome is clearly defined and the organisation or sport has a part to play in setting higher-order vision, strategy, and hierarchy, and supply effective management to support the process of defining the role and setting objectives for delivery.

Interpersonal skills (and understanding people)

"You can have all the technical knowledge in the world but if you can't get on with somebody you'll never get in and be a part of it in order to give that technical knowledge". This quote from a current British Performance Director demonstrates the importance of interpersonal skills for practitioners. These roles in supporting elite performance are front-facing service delivery roles, defined by human interactions with individuals and as part of a team, in order to access human performance. 'Buy in' and influence (an ability to cause change in client behaviour) are critical pieces in the jigsaw of support services and personal delivery. Interactions with others, the ability to collaborate effectively, and professional relationships are important elements supporting delivery. Positive interaction skills or interpersonal skills seem to be a non-negotiable.

Interpersonal skills encompass communication, social, engagement, and influencing skills. With all interactions, an ability to self-manage with a considered approach is essential. Appropriate selection of when to interact, with whom, and how is key, again linking to delivery model selection and PJDM. It is also essential to understand who you need to influence and when. As an example, is it the coach, the athlete, or both who decide on training sets and, if there is a need to influence decision-making on this, who is it that you need to engage. Just adding to the complexity, is this person ready to hear the message and take on the information or are they focussed elsewhere or too busy and/or stressed to care? If the timing of an interaction is poorly considered, it can result in a loss of traction and action from a conversation and ultimately stall impact.

In terms of the *how* of interaction engagement skills, a strong appreciation of people (self and others) and self-reflection underpin this. Self-awareness (an understanding of how you may be perceived) and an ability to reflect on the responses received and adapt your approach are critical. If a message isn't landing in a meeting, the ability to appreciate this and consider another way of sharing this is vital. A strong appreciation of others, including their approach, style, preferred communication methods, and influence will support in critical conversations. It may be that they are not the right person to land the message to that person and another team member is.

The ability to select and amend style including pitch, tone, and language to suit the audience, which may vary greatly from well-informed highly experienced head coaches to an under-11 newly identified talented athlete, will also support interactions. As an example, within one sport we worked with, two athletes required a very different style of interaction. One was happy for an open, chatty, regular, and lengthy interaction, whilst the other preferred a more serious, facts-based, short interaction.

Another example, from another sport, is when one of us was required to communicate the results of a fairly complex player analysis to people on staff at a major football club – first to a group of coaches, then to a group of analysts. The coaches were not very knowledgeable or comfortable with numbers and statistics and, for most of them, there also was a substantial language barrier. Thus, the message was delivered focusing exclusively on the impact of the analysis on the field for the players in question, relying on a combination of video images and animated body language (including gross movements, gestures, and facial expressions). Following this session, the exact same basic content was presented to a group of quantitative analysts. Here, the focus and discussion revolved around regression analyses, potential outliers, and levels of statistical significance; mostly relying on logic and rationality, linguistic precision, and lots of data and statistics.

Listening and questioning skills are another must for effective conversations. An ability to listen well and respond appropriately builds 'buy in' to a conversation and the ability to ask the right questions at the right time is especially crucial where the focus is often on solving performance problems. Effective questioning skills also support in assessment and appreciation of the environment and in defining role clarity. The traits often positively linked to effective interaction include: compassion, respect, honesty, empathy.

Understanding the *how* of building effective professional relationships with regular, positive interactions with clients and team members is essential. The development of trust, linked with actions such as credibility and reliability (i.e. delivering what you promise, to a high level and in a consistent manner) are regularly required to support this and can be the critical aspect for long term delivery success. Developing 'empathetic intelligence' through tactics such as taking time with identified people, immersion in the environment of others, and regular reflections can support the development of awareness, interpersonal skills, and relationships.

Functioning in a team (the team player)

The final piece in the jigsaw for optimal delivery in elite sport performance is an understanding of the importance of the team, and an ability to work as a team member. Best practice in sports delivery is often characterised by its multi or interdisciplinary nature (cf. Dijkstra et al., 2015), and this area links to all the other *must haves* of good practice. *Anecdotally* those working in isolation are thought to have limited ability to appreciate the depth of a performance problem, possibly leading to a focus on the wrong thing or ill-timed delivery reducing the impact of an intervention. Those unable to work within a team may be associated with unsuccessful delivery due to negative aspects, such as client confusion and lack of clarity. Some obvious examples of areas where a multi or interdisciplinary approach is required for clear and impactful support include; returning an athlete to performance after injury and supporting those athletes with mental health challenges.

In a team there is a need to combine and exchange knowledge, discover problems and generate solutions, and some practitioners may be required to operate in a number of different teams, with an ability to engage effectively with each, even when there may be inconsistent and limited exposure to them (e.g. for a multisport practitioner/medic). The desire, ability, and skills to function effectively as part of a team are critical for high performance support work; a concept demonstrated in many other performance domains (see Salas et al., 2003). Functioning teams are often characterised by all members having a shared and organised understanding of: roles, objectives, intent, boundaries, and of each other. Evidence has linked accurate expectations and common knowledge of the team and task with a co-ordinated response of actions and readiness to perform effectively (Fiore et al., 2012). The construct of Shared Mental Models, overlapping mental representations of knowledge by members of a team (Van den Bossche et al., 2006) could be useful here and these may give a commonality in view of the environment, resulting in similarity of response to a task across the team and generating a level of predictability in behaviour.

The sports practitioner will be required to navigate working with others and differences across a support team in terms of philosophy of delivery, working ethos, and codes of confidentiality may exist as obvious examples of challenges. In order to be effective a desire to broaden horizons of interest past personal domains, an understanding of the 'bigger picture' of the system and network, and *how* the team will operate are essential. Openness to collaborate, supply guidance, and sharing are therefore important and an awareness of other team members' skills, knowledge, abilities, preferences, and task-relevant attributes will be critical, supporting decision-making on who requires what information and how to adapt behaviour in response to team needs. For example, a decision on a training set for an injured athlete in the gym environment will have a wider impact on the athlete's targets around return to play; the physio's input that day and the coach's capacity to add sport-specific stimulus or training on top.

The interpersonal skills discussed earlier are just as critical here and underpin communication, collaboration, relationships, and engagement of others that is required; be they fellow practitioners, coaches, athletes or sports stakeholders. Additional skills for the effective *team player* include the ability to lead the team when required towards a goal or objective and the ability to challenge, and support others effectively. Modelling vulnerability and openness are supportive of this. Professional respect for others supports team delivery and it is often the demonstration of negative traits such as ego or self-interest that leads to a breakdown in team working.

Again there is a critical role for organisation and management of the sport to support team functioning; providing the right leadership, environment (with constructive challenge, feedback, and regular critical review) and opportunity for increased likelihood of successful delivery.

Professional Judgement and Decision-Making (PJDM): getting the content–style blend right

Of course, all these stylistic, communication concerns are essential components of practitioner effectiveness. Additionally, however, the practitioner needs to know her or his stuff, and make the right decisions on what particular blend of knowledge is required. Going into detail on each and every discipline is outside the scope of this chapter, and we would encourage readers to look at the other specialist-related chapters to get an 'across the disciplines' picture. Undoubtedly, however, all will require a strong set of skills in PJDM, meaning that the support content and blend is optimised for the particular context and client needs. This *what* focus combines with the *how* stuff covered above to make for an effective professional.

In summary, PJDM should underpin all aspects of the support professional's work. Obviously, different sports need different styles and procedures; weight lifters are different to figure skaters, physically, mentally, nutritionally, and mechanically! Crucially, however, this obvious difference needs to be extended to offer even more finely grained differentials. Clearly, different individuals will need bespoke interventions; then presentation may well change seasonally or with maturation. Finally, intrapersonal changes day to day will necessitate modification to both content and approach. Effective work will require you to vary at all these levels; using your knowledge, experience, and skills in ever more subtle combinations. In fact, our ongoing research into this topic suggests that developing your ability to personalise and contextualise appropriately is the main element of maturation and development as a support professional.

Preparing for the jungle

So how do we best develop the practitioner, or prepare them for the jungle with the skills and attributes to deliver good practice and meet client demands? All of the 'must haves' discussed above may be linked to the concept of expertise and expertise-based learning. Expertise has been associated to, and researched within, the sports coaching domain for a number of years now based on the understanding that coaching involves much decision-making with a key cognitive basis (Nash et al., 2012). This link to expertise has also been explored in the psychology arena (e.g. Martindale & Collins, 2013) but not across other sport science and medicine disciplines; yet, like the coach, *all* sports practitioners must utilise different types of knowledge to solve problems and make decisions, a key feature of expertise. Indeed experts are able to make "valued judgements to identify and deploy optimal techniques in any situation" (e.g. Collins & Moody, 2016 – in strength and conditioning). Literature exploring expertise has captured its key features or nature, all of which it could be argued are important for, or offer support to, the developing practitioner striving for optimal delivery (e.g., Feltovich et al., 2006; Hoffman, 1998; Kahneman & Klein, 2009; Nash & Collins, 2006; Nash et al., 2012; Shanteau & Weiss, 2014). Key features of those with expertise include the following:

- Having deep domain-specific, organised knowledge developed over time.
- Having an awareness of personal strengths and limitations.
- Having an ability to recognise patterns faster than others, leading to an economy of effort.
- Having a sense of typicality that supports anomaly detection and so the need to adapt, resulting in being more flexible and adaptable to situations.
- The development of mental models and routines that gather, manage, and interpret essential information only to allow processing capacity to be focussed on the environment at hand.
- Having an understanding *why* a situation has arisen and *how* the relevant factors interact, rather than just *what* the situation is or factors are.
- Having an ability to form multiple representations and interpretations of a challenge, thus supporting the revision of old strategies and creation of new automaticity in decision-making.
- Demonstrating a strong use of reflection (both on- and in-practice).

Understanding the nature of expertise allows us to suggest that it is practitioners with *expertise* that we want to build, rather than just competency (see Collins et al., 2015 for a more detailed argument on this). Reflecting this, we make a case now for expertise-based training or learning, alongside an emphasis on development of PDJM skills, as a valued approach to developing the practitioner. This should support an ability to perceive, evaluate, judge, and plan in order to select the most appropriate model of delivery at the optimal time – a focus on the *application* not just the knowledge. This type of training is already established as best practice in many other fields (e.g., the military, avionics, and medicine: Ericsson, 2009). It focuses less on 'outputs' (although still critical) and what the practitioner understands or has competency in, and more on the thinking behind actions or on the *why* and *how* they did or do something. The target then is developing critical thinking or cognitive skills, as a wide range of cognitive skills from deliberate thinking to rapid cue-based thinking are necessary for optimal delivery. These critical thinking skills combined with good reflective skills should allow knowledge to be applied effectively in the varied environments a sports practitioner finds themselves in.

Literature on expertise-based training suggests methods to systematically train the cognitive subskills of expertise. Fadde (2009) offers a cognitive task analysis approach, focused on extracting the cognitive demands of a task alongside the skills needed to effectively negotiate it which could support the practitioner and those responsible for their development. The approach includes building an understanding of the task and its elements before assessing the areas of expertise required and finally simulation of the scenario to explore the cognitive processes required. Hutton et al. (2017) identified six principles for accelerating adaptive expertise or performance skill, shown by those who can consciously and effectively *vary* their performance *appropriately* across contexts. These included: provision of flexibility-focused feedback to support learning and adjustments, coupling of context and critical thinking across scenarios, presentation of tough scenarios, learning in relatively complex contexts, and active reflection to encourage critical thinking and analysis. These suggested approaches ultimately stress the need to practise problems and stretch your skill sets but also to extend or seek opportunities to practise relative to a client, context, or challenges. Scenario or problem-based training opportunities and an environment where it is safe to fail for practitioners should be sought. To prevent the development of practitioners who struggle when the 'model' doesn't work and can't think of others ways to approach something, atypical scenarios should be presented with limited direction given on what a practitioner *should* be doing, this will also encourage personal philosophical development. Supervision and support will be critical for this type of practitioner development, with regular contact, discussion, observation, and reflection on actual practice then allows for development of independent, flexible, and creative thinking (for example, was there *another* way to do this?).

In conclusion

Sport clients demand relevant and 'useful' input; therefore the selection of the most appropriate delivery models is essential for the sport practitioner. The *quality* of service delivery is also key, with technical expertise in a defined area an essential for successful delivery *but* not the limiting factor. There is a need to appreciate and apply relevant contextual support within the environment, the role, the people, and the team you are exposed to within each elite sport.

Solid appreciation of the environment, or sports context, can be viewed as a first rung on the ladder towards identification of the appropriate model of delivery. Alignment to the sport and its environment is critical and only seems possible if an accurate assessment of the environment has been made *and* the ability to adapt exists. Those with role appreciation; who are able to define their role, have clarity of role across situations and within the team, knowledge of what to deliver, and an ability to be held accountable to that, seem more likely to deliver effectively. If this role clarity is underpinned with technical expertise, an understanding of boundaries and a flexibility to work outside the role, where required and appropriate, the chance of successful delivery is increased again.

In these front-facing service delivery roles, interactions with others, the ability to collaborate effectively, and professional relationships are important elements supporting delivery. Interpersonal skills, therefore, are a must for the sports practitioner. Appropriate selection of when to interact, with whom, and how is key, as is a strong appreciation of people (self and others) and self-reflection which underpins the *how* of engagement. The generally accepted concept of multi and interdisciplinary team-working for positive impact on performance means the ability to extend this and work as a team member is essential. Functioning teams are often characterised by all members having a shared and organised understanding of: roles, objectives, intent, boundaries, and of each other. The construct of Shared Mental Models could be useful here, giving a commonality in view of the environment, resulting in similarity of response to a task across the team and generating a level of predictability in behaviour.

Finally, PJDM should underpin all aspects of the support professionals' work, utilising knowledge, experience, and skills to deliver successfully. The development of PJDM skills alongside the development of expertise could add value to the sport practitioner. Expertise-based training models which focus on critical thinking, cognitive skills, and the *why* and *how* support is delivered through exposure and reflection on supported, relevant practice opportunities could be the key to unlocking the best prepared practitioners.

References

Anderson, A. G., Miles, A., Mahoney, C., & Robinson, P. (2002). Evaluating the Effectiveness of Applied Sport Psychology Practice: Making the Case for a Case Study Approach. *The Sport Psychologist*, **16**, 432–453

Ballie, P., Davis, H., & Ogilvie, B. C. (2015). Working with Elite Athletes. In J. Van Raalte & B. Brewer (Eds.), *Exploring Sport and Exercise Psychology* (3rd Ed.) (pp. 401–425). Philadelphia, PA: Elsevier

Bray, S. R., Beauchamp, M. R., Eys, M. A., & Carron, A. V. (2005). Does the Need for Role Clarity Moderate the Relationship between Role Ambiguity and Athlete Satisfaction? *Journal of Applied Sport Psychology*, **17**, 306–318. doi: 10.1080/10413200500313594

Collins, D., Martindale, A., Burke, V., & Cruickshank, A. (2015). The Illusion of Competency versus the Desirability of Expertise: Seeking a Common Standard for Support Professions in Sport. *Sports Medicine*, **45**(1), 1–7

Collins, D., & Moody, J. (2016). Role and Competency for the S & C Coach. In I. Jeffreys and J. Moody (Eds.), *Strength and Conditioning for Sports Performance*. London UK: Routledge

Dijkstra, H. P., Pollock, N., Chakravety, R., & Alonso, J. M. (2015). Managing the Health of the Elite Athlete: A New Integrated Performance Health Management and Coaching Model. *Br J Sports Med*, **48**, 523–531. doi:10.1136/bjsports-2013-093222

Ericsson, K. A. (2009). *Development of Professional Expertise: Toward Measurement of Expert Performance and Design of Optimal Learning Environments*. New York, NY: Cambridge University Press

Eys, M. & Carron, A.V. (2001) Role Ambiguity, Task Cohesion, and Task Self-Efficacy. *Small Group Research*, **32**(3), 356–373

Eys, M. A., Carron, A. V., Beauchamp, M. R., & Bray, S. R. (2003). Role Ambiguity in Sport Teams. *Journal of Sport & Exercise Psychology*, **25**, 534–550.

Fadde, P. J. (2009). Expertise-based Training: Getting More Learners Over the Bar in Less Time. *Technology, Instruction, Cognition and Learning*, **7**, 171–197

Feltovich, P. J., Prietula, M. J., & Ericsson, K. A. (2006) Studies of Expertise from Psychological Perspectives. In K. A. Ericsson, N. Charness, P. J. Feltovitch, & R. R. Hoffman (Eds.), *The Cambridge Handbook of Expertise and Expert Performance* (pp. 41–67). New York, NY: Cambridge University Press

Fiore, S. M., Ross, K. G., & Jentsch, F. (2012). A Team Cognitive Readiness Framework for Small-Unit Training. *Journal of Cognitive Engineering and Decision Making*, **6** (3), 325–349. doi: 10.1177/1555343412449626

Hoffman, R. R. (1998). How Can Expertise Be Defined? Implications of Research from Cognitive Psychology. In R. Williams, W. Faulkner, & J. Fleck (Eds.), *Exploring Expertise* (pp. 81–100). New York, NY: Macmillan

Hutton, R., Ward, P., Gore, J., Turner, P., Hoffman, R., Leggatt, A., & Conway, G. (2017). Developing Adaptive Expertise: A Synthesis of Literature and Implications for Training. 13th International Conference on Naturalistic Decision Making, Bath, UK

Ingham, S. (2016). *How to Support a Champion: The Art of Applying Science to the Elite Athlete*. United Kingdom: Simply Said

Kahneman, D., & Klein, G. (2009). Conditions for Intuitive Expertise: A Failure to Disagree. *The American Psychologist*, **64**, 515–526. doi:10.1037/a0016755

Kyndt, T., & Rowell, S. (2012). *Achieving Excellence in High Performance Sport: The Experience and Skills Behind the Medals*. (1st ed.). London: Bloomsbury

Martindale, A., & Collins, D. (2005). Professional Judgment and Decision Making: The Role of Intention for Impact. *The Sport Psychologist*, **19**, 303–317

Martindale, A., & Collins, D. (2013). The Development of Professional Judgment and Decision Making Expertise in Applied Sport Psychology. *The Sport Psychologist*, **27**, 390–398.

Martindale, R., & Nash, C. (2013). Sport Science Relevance and Application: Perceptions of UK Coaches. *Journal of Sports Sciences*, **31**(8), 807–819. doi:10.1080/02640414.2012.754924

Nash, C., & Collins, D. (2006). Tacit Knowledge in Expert Coaching: Science or Art? *Quest*, **58**, 464–476

Nash, C., Martindale, R., Collins, D., & Martindale, A. (2012). Parameterising Expertise in Coaching: Past, Present and Future. *Journal of Sports Sciences*, **30**, 985–994

Salas, E., Shawn Burke, C., & Cannon-Bowers, J. (2003). Teamwork: Emerging Principles. *International Journal of Management Reviews*, **2**(4), 339–356

Shanteau, J., & Weiss, D. J. (2014). Individual Expertise Versus Domain Expertise. *American Psychologist*, **69**, 711–712. doi:10.1037/a0037874

Van den Bossche, P., Gijselaers, W., Segers, M., & Kirschner, P. A. (2006). Social and Cognitive Factors Driving Teamwork in Collaborative Learning Environments. Team Learning Beliefs and Behaviors. *Small Group Research*, **37**(5), 490–521

37

Creating long-term high performing teams

Stuart Lancaster with Veronica Burke

Introduction

In order to truly understand how to build long-term high performing teams it is important to change our mindset on how we 'view' a team. A strong team has a strong 'team spirit' and that spirit can grow or diminish in its size depending on many factors, a lot of which are in the leader's control. In this chapter I would like to try and describe what are the essential components in building a long-term high performing team that has a strong 'team spirit' and ultimately a chance of reaching its full potential.

Using the Performance Pyramid (see Figure 37.1) the starting point is for the leader to assess in each of the layers on the Pyramid (Culture, Identity, Higher Purpose, Behaviours and Standards, Ownership, and Player Led Leadership) and this will then guide their decision-making on where to focus their attention on building or enhancing the team that they are working in. Where you score your team's effectiveness will directly affect the proportion of time that will need to be spent on the different dimensions of the Performance Pyramid. The key here is always to start at the bottom and ensure the foundations are strong with a good culture.

Your judgement on where to focus your attention as the leader depends on your knowledge of the organisation and your entry point into it. For example, if you came through the organisation from within you may already have a good insight into the culture and environment, where the team sits in relation to its maturity or whether it needs renewing. Having coached England Saxons team from 2007–11, I was able to observe the England senior team's evolution during that period, so when I came in as head coach, I felt I had a good insight into what needed to be done, how it needed to be done, and at what level to start building a long-term high-level performing team. We focused on getting the culture right, selecting the right people, and making sure we were all aligned to a cause. From there we worked on building trust and building relationships, moving on to identity in the second year: what it means to play for England, the identity of England. Then we continued to work our way through the pyramid.

Conversely when I arrived at Leinster I had no real knowledge of the organisation, so I did my homework beforehand in order to find out as much historical information as possible about the team. My first month there was spent asking good questions about the

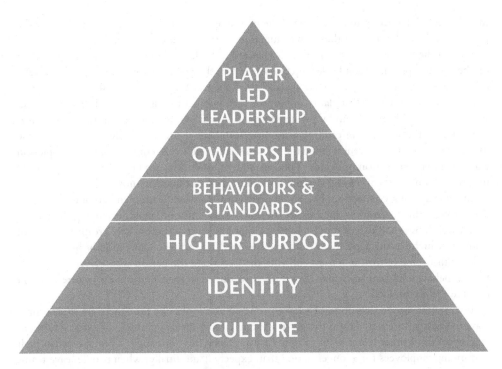

Figure 37.1 Creating long-term high performance teams

environment, while observing and learning about it, and making an assessment about where I saw strengths and where things needed to improve. Culturally I felt that Leinster was strong; there were some areas that needed adjustment, and the players needed a vision – in this case centring on the European Cup, which was achieved this year. Once I understood that Leinster's identity was very strong, I was able to move on to behaviours and standards, and then to continue working through the pyramid to the very top where the players ultimately drive the programme.

The pyramid is useful here because its layers can help you to formulate the right questions to ask. Find out as much as you can and how much the players are involved in driving all of this.

The Performance Pyramid

In this section, we will unpack the stages and features of the Performance Pyramid, elaborate on each and describe how they impact on one another.

Culture

A strong culture is the foundation of any long-term high performing team: it is the bedrock, best described as "the way we do things around here". Culture is hard to specify and certainly hard to measure. A useful way of understanding how to create a team with a strong culture is seen in Jim Collins' 2001 book, *Good to Great* (London: Random House). As Collins says, "Get the right people on the bus and then drive it somewhere great". Essentially Collins is saying that in order to build a strong team, you need the best people for the jobs who must fit in with the philosophy of how you want the team to function, both on and off the field.

One of the fundamental reasons why leaders fail in building teams is that they are not clear on their philosophy, i.e. their leadership purpose before they take on the leadership role, and as a consequence have no navigational compass to direct them during the ups and downs of building the team. Once you have that clarity of purpose then you get the right people in the right roles and motivate and inspire them by giving them the reason why you are going to create a great team. This is the first step in creating a strong culture and creating and selling a vision for the future. The next step is strengthening the relationships at all levels, connecting with people and extending that connection outwards. This capability is, of course, a skill that has to be practised in action and not just something that the leader knows about but does not deploy.

Imagine a strong connection, like an invisible cord, between team members and the leader. The stronger the connection, the thicker the cord. Time must be spent developing these critical relationships – working through problems, building trust and ultimately creating a sense of teamship which has the capacity to cascade downwards. It can take many months or even years to build that sense of trust in a team and you, the leader, are the person who everyone looks to for the behavioural standards that are required in this new high performing culture. So you become the role model!

If you want a good definition of what a strong culture looks like then there are three simple ways to assess your team. Teams that have a strong culture create an environment that talented employees from other teams want to join: "I want to be in your gang". They also retain high performing employees for a longer period than expected; and finally, when people leave teams that possess a strong positive culture they often say that was the best time in their career. To elaborate, when opportunities come up within your team – whether for players or management – the first question potential applicants will ask is "what is it like to work there?" They want to know if it is an environment where they can grow, feel respected, be given responsibility, accountability, and also autonomy to do their job. If the organisation's culture is strong and you have a great environment, then talented people will want to apply to work there. In fact, the organisation's reputation will often precede the job. In a competitive environment such as sport, where similar remuneration packages are offered by many teams, the point of difference can often be in the environment and the culture. Once talented people are on board, you want the workplace to be an enjoyable one. It is important for your people to achieve success, to be trusted, to feel as though their opinion is valued. The consequence is that even though they may want to move on to promotion elsewhere at some stage, they will find it harder to leave behind a great culture. You want people leaving with some reluctance and a heavy heart, with gratitude and mutual understanding between the employee and the organisation and on good terms, so if they are asked about the organisation they can say how much they loved working there.

Identity

Once you have established a strong culture it is important to invest time in understanding, developing, and growing the identity of the team. Great companies, sports teams, and long-term high performing organisations possess strong identities, and effective leadership is about growing this so everyone who works for the company or team has absolute clarity and pride in the organisation they work for. People want to feel part of something more than the numbers and the more they engage with the history of the team and connect to the wider community in which the team sits, the more they will commit.

Some teams already have this principle established, however, it is always useful to remind the people who drive the team forward what they stand for and why. Teams with a less well-established identity need a leader responsible for developing and growing the identity by delving into the organisation's history, understanding the anchors that define it, and building on these. I have been fortunate with England Rugby and Leinster Rugby to work in two teams that have strong identities that help build connections and foster the team's commitment. A leader who does not have an understanding of the existing identity needs first to ask questions, to ingest the responses, articulate their findings, and know what it means to the team members. For example, what does it mean to the players to play for their team?

Higher purpose

Higher purpose comes next in the Performance Pyramid and this dimension relates to the long-term goals that you are striving to achieve as a team. We will all have targets to hit and results to be achieved on a quarterly or yearly basis but the higher purpose is something beyond that, beyond winning the next match or tournament or piece of business – it is identifying a vision of where you want to go, and is fundamental to the creation of a long-term high performing team. Winning is, of course, very important, and with England the goal was to create a team that would succeed in multiple World Cup cycles, not just the next one. There needs to be longevity to the plan. England Rugby's higher purpose could be described as developing a strong culture and identity that permeates throughout the Rugby Football Union, all the way down to grassroots rugby. We also wanted to be respected in world sport so our organisation would be looked at in order to see how we were achieving our higher purpose. Serving the wider community is another example of a higher purpose that will inspire the people who work in your teams to go the extra mile for the organisation even if perceived success is achieved.

The art of leadership could be defined as the ability to identify the higher purpose, to articulate it in a passionate and inspirational way, and to drive people towards it. Being able to create and deliver such a message is the difference between a great coach and a great leader: the best leaders I have worked with have had the capability to create an inspirational image or style and to motivate others to want to achieve it. When interviewing candidates for a leadership position I would ask for an example of a higher purpose that they had created and defined for their organisation, a detailed description of how they identified and presented it.

When working on identifying this higher purpose it is important to carve out thinking time, away from the day-to-day running, managing, and coaching of teams, in order to allow creativity to flow – working on the business rather than in it. That element of perspective can help in developing a sense of direction. When troubled times occur you need to be able to return to your purpose, to the ideal of what you want to achieve, aligning values, behaviours, and standards towards the all-important goal. Without it, a team can struggle to find its way.

Inspiring team members towards the higher purpose is accomplished in a combination of ways. Initially this may mean addressing the group about what you are trying to achieve; but one of the most significant elements is in following the group contact within individual meetings to assess each team member's level of belief in the purpose or whether more time should be spent with them in order to explain how you see the vision and to engage them in it. These relationships, between the management team, the coach, and the players, are like a spider's web of interconnecting cords initiating from you, the leader, providing a strong connection within the group that will help drive the mission forward at all levels.

Another significant element of leadership is to build trust within the team. This means first showing you have integrity and are reliable: be consistent with your word and do what you say you are going to do. Once you have demonstrated that you are dependable the team members will know you can be trusted, both in good times and in bad. You are more likely to be forgiven for your own mistakes if you have developed a high level of mutual trust. Secondly you must give trust in order to get trust back: do not micro-manage or remonstrate with them if something goes wrong. The same goes for power – effective leaders give power away, entrusting their team members in the process and resulting in power being given back.

Behaviours and standards

It is important to create a set of values which will act as foundations for the behaviours and standards you want to see. For example when I arrived at Leinster the values of brotherhood, self-improvement, and humility were used as guiding posts for behaviours and standards. Brotherhood as a value would lead to behaviour such as supporting team mates during a game, looking after a player if he gets injured, not talking behind each other's backs, and so on. Self-improvement would lead players to continually practise to optimise their potential and make the most of set-backs as opportunities for learning. Humility in this context means maintaining a level of modesty, making sure you do not become arrogant or get carried away with a victory or too despondent over a loss. The aim would be for the leadership group and senior personnel to agree on what the behaviours and standards should be and to work together to drive them forward. In sport that would mean the head coach, the senior coaches and the senior players as a collective exemplifying the behaviours and standards for the rest of the team to follow.

Once you get these strong foundations in place you should be seeing behavioural changes that are visible from the top to the bottom of the organisation with a strong and deep-rooted commitment to high standards and behaviours that will drive the integrity of the team. Occasionally there will be issues in this area as people who work in teams are only human, however, the majority of the behaviours that you see should be positive, constructive, and deployed with a 'can do' attitude.

Ownership

Once you have the remainder of the stages in place it is absolutely critical for the senior team members to take ownership of the team's values. When the leadership group – including those at board and chairman level – owns the behaviours and standards, the vision, the identity, and the culture, those elements will trickle down throughout the organisation reaching even the youngest and most junior players as they are introduced. Making all members of the organisation feel like they are part of one big team, owned by everyone, is the ultimate aspiration. This sense of commitment to the team will in turn drive the culture, develop the identity, and enable team members to strive to achieve the higher purpose. As custodians of the behaviours and standards the leadership group will bring others along with them. Without doubt, this is the key to creating a long-term high performing team.

Player-led leadership

This is the final piece of the jigsaw and often the hardest to achieve. It is the culmination of all the layers of the pyramid combined with robust leadership from the people in the team, who ultimately 'own' the team and drive everything within it. This does not mean the leader at the top of the organisation abdicating responsibility. Rather, this describes a strong, resilient leader at the very top who, through their behaviour and values, empowers the people they lead to drive the team forward under their direction. When this can be achieved the dynamic of being inspired by the team members from within the team drives a deeper level of commitment from those who work alongside them, and is an extremely powerful force.

However, do not be under any illusion that you can turn around an organisation and create a high performing team in a short space of time. There is no quick fix and leaders need to be prepared for a long-term process that could take months or even years; it is very difficult to accomplish though achievable with great leadership. Small wins can be gained very quickly, but building the pyramid takes time and perseverance, and a strong desire to overcome the obstacles that will block your path.

External factors

In essence it is straightforward: follow the steps, build the layers of the pyramid, and success will follow. If only it was that simple! Building teams is never easy and you are constantly building the pyramid on shifting sands. The fluid nature of human relations, interaction, and behaviours consistently provides challenges for the leadership of any organisation. Additionally there are many external factors outside your control that can influence team performance and determine the health of even the strongest team as it goes through high pressure situations, for example play-off games or reaching cup finals; and in business, trying to hit an ambitious target on a tight timeline. Whatever the external factors may be, there are some that you can prepare for and anticipate and some that you cannot. Control the controllables! Looking at the Performance Pyramid and the long-term evolution of the team are good ways to assess and judge the leader's effectiveness or the organisation's current state.

In summary, there is no doubt that if you have established a strong pyramid based on the layers we have detailed above then you are far more likely to withstand the pressure and come out of the other side stronger rather than allowing cracks to become chasms in a poorly developed team.

Conclusion

In summary, the understanding and application of the Performance Pyramid is the key to building high performing teams. This requires a skilled approach from an outstanding leader – sound assessment, action, and evaluation which take account of the ever-shifting sand of external factors. This capability also requires the leader to have personal resilience – bouncing back from difficulties, keeping to the plan, and continuous reflection in action as the process of building the team continues.

Too often we position leaders at the top of organisations who might have the technical skillset in the role but do they really understand what it takes to build an outstanding team and do they have the skill set to 'move' the people they lead to achieve it? This surely has implications for leadership and coach development programmes for the future where we need to move beyond just the technical requirements of the role and develop the leadership skills of our emerging leaders so that in whatever organisation they work in they can really understand the process for building truly long-term high performing teams and have the skills to achieve it.

Index